HEALTH CARE FOR SOME

HEALTH CARE FOR SOME

Rights and Rationing in the United States since 1930

BEATRIX HOFFMAN

THE UNIVERSITY OF CHICAGO PRESS | CHICAGO + LONDON

BEATRIX HOFFMAN is professor in the Department of History at Northern Illinois University. She is the author of *The Wages of Sickness: The Politics of Health Insurance in Progressive America.*

The University of Chicago Press, Chicago 60637
The University of Chicago Press, Ltd., London
© 2012 by The University of Chicago
All rights reserved. Published 2012.
Printed in the United States of America

21 20 19 18 17 16 15 14 13 12   1 2 3 4 5

ISBN-13: 978-0-226-34803-2 (cloth)
ISBN-13: 978-0-226-34805-6 (e-book)
ISBN-10: 0-226-34803-2 (cloth)
ISBN-10: 0-226-34805-9 (e-book)

Library of Congress Cataloging-in-Publication Data
Hoffman, Beatrix Rebecca, author.
Health care for some : rights and rationing in the United States since 1930 / Beatrix Hoffman.
    pages cm
Includes bibliographical references and index.
ISBN-13: 978-0-226-34803-2 (cloth : alkaline paper)
ISBN-10: 0-226-34803-2 (cloth : alkaline paper)
ISBN-13: 978-0-226-34805-6 (e-book)
ISBN-10: 0-226-34805-9 (e-book)   1. Right to health—United States—History.   2. Health services accessibility—United States—History.   3. Health care rationing—United States—History.   I. Title.
RA395.A3H63 2012
362.1—dc23   2012000338

♾ This paper meets the requirements of ANSI / NISO Z39.48-1992 (Permanence of Paper).

FOR ANN BRIERLY + CAROL BRIERLY GOLIN

CONTENTS

INTRODUCTION

During the national debate over health care in September 2009, former US vice presidential candidate Sarah Palin claimed that reforms proposed by the Obama administration would bring "rationing" into the American medical system. Democratic proposals would "empower unelected bureaucrats to make decisions affecting life or death healthcare matters," Palin warned. Just a few days later, Harvard Medical School researchers released a study concluding that 45,000 Americans die every year because they lack health insurance and access to health care.[1]

Opponents of the 2010 Patient Protection and Affordable Care Act warn that the new health care law will lead to rationing, or limits on medical services. But many observers point out that health care is already rationed in the United States. "We've done it for years," said Dr. Arthur Kellermann, professor of emergency medicine and associate dean for health policy at Emory University School of Medicine. "In this country, we mainly ration on the ability to pay."[2] In fact, because the supply of doctors, hospitals, and treatments is never unlimited, medical care is rationed in every country, whether by the government, the private market, or some combination of the two.[3]

Why then does the idea of rationing seem so, well, un-American?

One reason is that health care rationing in the United States is almost never called by that name. The word "rationing" evokes the difficult days of World War II, when the government controlled the distribution of necessities such as food and gasoline. Wartime rationing was understood as a necessary and shared sacrifice as the country united behind the war effort. But the term has taken on more negative connotations in the decades since. Now, rationing makes Americans think of shortages, waiting lists, and long lines.

However, a classical economist would say that rationing also simply means the distribution of goods and services by price. Countries with universal health systems ration health care via controlled distribution, whether through national budgeting, government setting of prices and provider fees, restrictions on some services, or a combination of methods. The United States health care system rations primarily by price and insurance coverage—and, this book will argue, many other methods as well. Americans have learned to fear European or Canadian types of rationing, but don't see that the United States practices both price rationing and other types of rationing in health care.

Rationing in the United States is not a top-down, centralized policy imposed by the government. In the absence of a universal health program, rationing occurs in both the public and private health care sectors. It is practiced by government agencies, private health insurance companies, hospitals, and providers, in ways both official and unofficial, intended and unintended, visible and invisible. The American way of rationing is a complex, fragmented, and often contradictory blend of policies and practices, unique to the United States.

Rationing by price, or ability to pay, is familiar to most Americans. Often, this way of allocating health care means that poor and low-income people cannot get care at all, but it also means that they might get different kinds of care in a system that treats people differently on the basis of whether and how much they can pay. It also leads to many people going without insurance coverage simply because they can't afford it. But rationing by ability to pay is only one of many ways in which medical services have been distributed or restricted in the United States. Health care has been rationed by race, in the case of the Jim Crow health system and other types of racial discrimination; by region, in the case of the uneven distribution of health facilities and personnel throughout the country; by employment and occupation, in the case of the job-based health insurance system; by address, in the case of residency requirements for various kinds of health care; by type of insurance coverage, in the case of health insurance that limits benefits and choice of doctor and hospital; by parental status, in the case of Medicaid (childless individuals are often excluded); by age, in the case of Medicare and the State Children's Health Insurance Programs—and the list goes on. These types of health care organization (or disorganization), which allow access and coverage for some groups but deny it to others, or allow access to certain types of care but not others, have rarely been called rationing. But this book argues that they must be defined as such in order to more fully understand the workings of the American health system and productively debate ways to improve it.

The United States is unique because of the complex, sometimes hidden, and frequently unintended ways it rations care. The United States is also unique among affluent nations because it does not officially recognize a right to health care. Apart from the right to assistance in an emergency room (which has existed only since 1986, and even then only requires that patients be stabilized), Americans have no legal or constitutional right to medical care. Many other nations include a right to health care in their legal or constitutional documents, and virtually all affluent democracies other than the United States provide universal health coverage as a matter of right to their citizens. The scope and definitions of these rights to health care differ, and countries have created many different kinds of health care systems to help enforce them, but what they all have in common is that rights to access and/or coverage are universal, applying to all citizens of the country. The few rights in the US health care system—such as the right to emergency treatment and the rights of senior citizens and veterans to health coverage—apply only to particular groups of the population or to particular types of care. These selective, limited health care rights are another way that coverage and services are rationed in the United States, although we seldom talk about it this way.

Despite the lack of universal health care rights in the United States, the argument that health care *should* be a right is a powerful one in a country where "inalienable rights" are central to citizenship and national identity. Presidents from Franklin D. Roosevelt to Barack Obama have declared health care to be a right, not just a privilege. Opinion polls for several decades have shown broad public agreement with the statement that access to health care is or should be a right.[4]

This book tells the story of rights and rationing in the development of the American health care system since 1930. Since the United States recognizes few rights in the health care system, while refusing to recognize that rationing takes place at all, this is a challenging task. To uncover the history of rationing, the following chapters focus on the parallel themes of access to health care and the denial of health care. They tell the story of how Americans have sought access to medical services since the 1930s and how the system grew dramatically with the goal of bringing the benefits of modern medicine within reach of everyone. At the same time, the denial of access, and the refusal to make the benefits of health care available equally, have also defined the system. The history of access and denial is the history of the American way of rationing, and of a health care system whose impressive benefits are available to some, but not all.

The clash between the ideal of access for all and the reality of the denial of health care also helps uncover the history of health care rights in the United States. "The reason why there is a fuss over rights to health care is because so many are left out," writes the medical ethicist Larry Churchill.[5] *Health Care for Some* looks at the arguments Americans have made for treating health care as a right, and episodes in which health rights have been demanded by organized movements of workers, the elderly, African Americans, and others. It also looks at less explicit declarations of rights. When unemployed people crowded into free clinics, or senior citizens wrote to Congress complaining that they couldn't get health insurance, or parents sued a hospital after their dying child was turned away from the emergency room, they may not have carried signs saying "Access to health care is a right," but they were expressing something called "rights consciousness." Rights consciousness can be articulated, as when someone displays a bumper sticker reading "Health Care is a Right, Not a Privilege"; it can also be implicit, as in a feeling of outrage or dismay when hearing about someone being denied health insurance. This book looks at both types of rights consciousness and seeks to explain how they emerged from, and reshaped, the US health care system.

Rights consciousness conflicts with another pervasive notion: that health care is a product like any other, and that private competition and the profit motive should be important components of the US health system. Supporters of market-based health care argue that without financial incentives, medical innovation and quality would deteriorate. The idea that health care is a product to be bought and sold in the marketplace contradicts the notion that it is a public service to be provided on the basis of right. The tension between notions of health care as a right and health care as a commodity is a central theme of this book.

The large role of private, profit-making companies is unique to the US health system. Insurance and drug firms, medical device makers, hospitals, and others make a great deal of money from health care and have a vested interest in the status quo (although these interests shift and change over time, as this book will show). Companies and individuals that profit from treating medical care as a product, and many politicians who seek their support, have fought to ensure that health care does *not* become a recognized right.[6]

The acceptance of medicine as a commodity or product helps explain why the United States spends more on health care than any country in the world—17.4 percent of the gross national product in 2009, or $7,960 per person, and rising. All developed countries are experiencing burdensome and growing health costs due to technological advances and aging populations, but the gap between spending in the United States and elsewhere is striking. The same year the United States spent nearly $8,000 per person on health care, Canada spent $4,363, Britain $3,487, and Japan $2,878. France, whose health system was recently named the best in the world by the World Health Organization, spent less than $4,000 per person. Meanwhile, the United States in 2010 had 47 million people without health insurance, while these other countries left virtually no one uninsured.[7] It seems paradoxical that the United States spends far more money than Canada, Britain, Japan, France, and others, yet those nations enjoy higher life expectancies and better health outcomes, while covering everyone.[8]

This book argues that US-style rationing, along with the lack of universal health care rights for US citizens, has contributed to the comparatively high cost of health care in this country. Where other systems attempt to spread costs over the entire population, the United States spends vast amounts of money providing different types of coverage and different levels of care to different groups of people. Private insurance companies' administrative costs—time and money spent solely on paperwork and bureaucracy in order to determine eligibility and approve or deny claims—can be as high as *one-third* of their expenditures, depending on the type of plan.[9] Profits for health care companies and outsized incomes for many providers eat up a good portion of US health costs.

While decisions made privately by countless different entities add up to a lot of spending, centralized government decisions also contribute to the high cost of US-style rationing. The US Congress after World War II decided to fund high-tech hospital construction rather than develop a system emphasizing primary care or universal coverage. Starting in the 1940s, the government made employer health benefits tax exempt, which helped create the increasingly unaffordable and inefficient employment-based system of rationing medical coverage. And when private providers and health care companies wrested rights for themselves at the expense of the rights of Americans to health care, this too created massive costs. Government's desire to protect the rights of the private sector allows billions of taxpayer dollars to flow to private providers, hospitals, and pharmaceutical and insurance companies with little or no control over costs. Private power in the US health system has been built and maintained with the support of tax dollars, contributing to the limitation of universal rights, the persistence of unjust and inefficient rationing, and very high costs.

Health Care for Some is divided into four sections covering distinct eras in the history of US health care: the Great Depression, when widespread unemployment and poverty led to calls for government assistance in providing and paying for medical care; World War II and the postwar period, when medical miracles abounded, the hospital system grew enormously, and the private health insurance system was born; the fifteen years including and following the passage of Medicare and Medicaid, when new government programs and new activist movements transformed understandings of health care rights; and the three decades since 1980, which have seen a tremendous rise in the number of uninsured and a pitched battle between rights to access and market ideology. Finally, the epilogue considers the place of rights and rationing in twenty-first-century health reform. This book is a national study of the past eighty years, and uses evidence from all regions of the continental United States with an occasional focus on Chicago, where many rich historical sources on health care are concentrated and some of the most vigorous rights battles took place.

While *Health Care for Some* is primarily about the ground-level health system itself, more than national reform politics in Washington, the history told here is essential background to the health care debates and transformations of today. One reason that reform has continually faltered is because of our nation's failure to arrive at an honest understanding of rights and rationing in the health care system. Clearly defining how we already ration is an essential prerequisite for debating how reform proposals will ration similarly or differently. Understanding the history of rights and the denial of rights in health care is necessary for productively discussing how rights are included, excluded, or transformed in the 2010 health care law. History has the potential to cut through the overcharged political rhetoric and help put reform debates on firmer footing. At the very least, this story of Americans' struggles for access to health care should remind us what is centrally at stake: the health and economic security of all the people.

RATIONING AND RIGHTS

History and Definitions

Rationing

The term "rationing" describes the control and limitation of the consumption of a product or service. According to the distinguished health policy scholar David Mechanic, there are two major types of rationing in health care: explicit and implicit. In *explicit rationing*, medical care is distributed or denied according to official sets of rules. Explicit rationing occurs when, for example, Medicare or insurance companies create lists of drugs and procedures that will be covered or not covered, or when a national health system establishes waiting lists for particular kinds of services. *Implicit rationing* includes practices that are not seen as rationing but as "the nature of everyday life," such as the uneven distribution of health facilities and personnel, long waits for appointments, and different access to care for people with different kinds of insurance. Rationing by ability to pay is another kind of implicit rationing. Both explicit and implicit rationing can occur on the macro level of decisions and policies set by a health plan or health system. They can also both occur at the "point of service," where individual physicians or administrators make decisions to offer or restrict treatments and services to individual patients.[1]

Americans became familiar with explicit rationing in World War II, when the United States limited supplies of gasoline, fabrics, food, and other consumer items. World War II rationing tends to be romanticized: everyone was pulling together for the war effort and gladly shared in the sacrifices. This feeling of solidarity was widespread, but there was also plenty of complaining about rationing, and in some cases black markets allowed people who could afford it to buy extra supplies of rationed consumer goods.[2]

Official rationing took on an increasingly negative cast in the postwar years, when Britain continued to experience severe shortages and became known for grim austerity through the mid-1950s, in contrast to a US economy bursting with consumer goods. Yet economists would say that postwar America simply returned to classic rationing: the setting of prices by the market, or "rationing by the purse."[3] Also, not all countries establishing universal health systems practiced rationing in the same way. France, Germany, Japan, and other countries allocated resources via national global budgets for health care expenditures, and avoided the waiting lists that came to characterize parts of the British and Canadian systems.[4]

The concept of rationing medical care was not widely discussed in the United States until the 1970s. During the Nixon administration, Congress considered numerous plans for health reform, including ambitious proposals for national health insurance. Health care experts assumed that European-style official, explicit rationing by service (waiting lists or limitations on particular treatments) would become necessary under national health insurance, since the demand for care would increase much faster than the supply of doctors and facilities. Rationing was discussed in 1970s health policy journals in a generally positive light, as a way to efficiently and fairly distribute health care in the new system that many believed was inevitable. But in the mainstream media, references to rationing were overwhelmingly negative. The *New York Times* began printing horrific accounts of the National Health Service in Britain—including one about a woman who had been on a waiting list for a hip replacement for over fifteen years.[5] During later episodes of health care reform, the media and politicians repeated (and often exaggerated) stories of patients denied cancer treatment in Britain and Canadians flocking to the United States for MRI tests they couldn't get at home. As a result, the American public came to view "rationing" as a dirty word.

The few examples of official rationing in the US health system— "making difficult choices through explicit decisions"[6] —have received overwhelmingly negative publicity. When the state of Oregon in 1994 decided to expand Medicaid enrollments and said it would help pay for it by creating a priority list of covered and excluded services based on cost-effectiveness, outrage at the "dreaded rationing" erupted around the country.[7] Organ donation is another arena of explicit rationing; with the demand for organs far outstripping supply, hospital committees and an organization called the United Network for Organ Sharing determine who is eligible for transplants and who will receive them. The explicit choices made in organ donation, often on the basis of personal characteristics like age, ability to comply with medical orders, and history of drug or alcohol abuse, make many Americans deeply uncomfortable, raising the notion that physicians and committees are "playing God." Another kind of explicit rationing, by private insurance companies, became part of American health care with the rise of managed care in the 1980s, and also proved very unpopular as stories of HMOs denying treatments dominated the media (see chapter 9).

But far more common and pervasive methods of American rationing, including rationing by price, do not make headlines; it's just the way things are. The media does report "horror stories" about American patients who die, for example, after being turned away from an emergency room or having their insurance coverage canceled, but these are usually portrayed as isolated, shocking cases—not reflections of a pattern of health care allocation. In the case of the Oregon reform, for example, which rationed services within Medicaid, hardly anyone pointed out that Medicaid itself is a system of rationing by income. There was outrage at the former type of rationing, but silence in the face of the latter.

One purpose of official, explicit rationing is to save money. But as the variations in international health expenditures discussed earlier illustrate, American-style rationing has proven very expensive. One reason is that other goals have often come before cost savings. In the South, for example, it was undoubtedly more expensive for a community to build two separate hospitals, one for whites and one for blacks, instead of just a single hospital, but enforcing white supremacy carried a higher priority than efficiency in health expenditures. Also, rather than attempting to restrain costs, US rationing is often intended to help people or companies *make* money. Insurance companies denied treatments or excluded people with preexisting medical conditions partly to make their policies more affordable but primarily to improve their bottom line and provide value to shareholders. The proliferation of countless different health plans, each with different rules and types of coverage, has led to expensive paperwork, inefficiency, and high administrative costs. One study estimates that US physician practices nationwide spend between $23.3 and $30 billion per year just on interactions with insurance companies.[8]

In other countries, rationing is intended to apply equally to all citizens (however difficult this may be to carry out in practice). In the United States, rationing blatantly applies differently to different groups of people, medical conditions, regions, etc. Elsewhere, rationing controls the overall amount of health care a society provides. In the United States, rationing leads to too many services for some individuals, and too few or none for others.[9] Too many hospitals with empty beds, too many new procedures and devices, too many expensive tests and treatments, too many specialists—all of these drive the astronomically high costs of US health care. Alongside this overabundance are the 47 million uninsured, yet their far lower rates of using health services do not seem to reduce the costs to the system—on the contrary, hospitals charge more to make up for treating all those patients who can't pay, and emergency rooms become high-cost primary care centers for the uninsured. US-style rationing defeats the stated purpose of rationing to control expenditures.

Not everyone will accept the broad definition of rationing used in this book. Some health policy experts argue that the term should be used only to describe the allocation of medical care to individuals at the "point of service": the doctor's office or hospital.[10] However, because of the negative implications of the word "rationing" in the United States, this would imply that other forms of distribution or denial of care, such as by race, region, insurance coverage, or ability to pay, are more benign than official, government-sanctioned rationing at the point of service.[11] As this book will show, other forms of allocation often have not been more benign than official rationing. It is also unhelpful to define rationing only as policies made and enforced by central governments. In the complex and fragmented US system, actions taken by private companies, local governments, and other entities have mattered just as much, and often more, than top-down decisions in Washington when it comes to allocating or denying health care.

Rights

The right to health care, writes the influential political scientist Theodore Marmor, "in the most egalitarian expression, means equal access to equivalent medical services."[12] Although ideas about health care rights have been around for at least a century, the notion took on new meaning after the 1920s because of the dramatic rise of medicine's effectiveness. Previously, doctors and hospitals could not do much to help people. But with the spread of antisepsis and anesthesia, vaccines to prevent deadly diseases, lifesaving drugs to fight infection, and many other breakthroughs, medicine became a matter of life or death. As medical care became more effective, many began to argue that to withhold it was unethical, immoral, and unjust.[13] "The further medical care advances, the less can society contemplate its unavailability to people who may need it," as one labor representative put it.[14]

Alongside medicine's new power came new global understandings of human rights in reaction to the horrifying atrocities of World War II. International treaties following the war included health as a central component of social justice. The World Health Organization issued a statement in 1946 that "the enjoyment of the highest attainable standard of health is one of the fundamental rights of every human being," and the United Nations included a right to medical care in its 1948 Universal Declaration of Human Rights. Many countries in the second half of the twentieth century began incorporating health rights into their constitutions and / or implementing them in their medical systems.[15]

The idea of a universal human right to health care meshed with emerging notions of "social rights." Aspirations for social rights, or rights to protection from poverty, unemployment, sickness, and other social ills, dated as far back as the French Revolution, but spread rapidly after World War II as many countries began to adopt "cradle-to-grave" welfare systems. Government support—old age pensions, unemployment insurance, medical coverage—was to be given to all citizens not out of charity or largesse, but as a matter of right.[16] Social rights were earned on the basis of work and citizenship, and conferred self-respect and belonging, replacing the shame and stigma of charity or welfare. These rights included not just access to medical care, but also the right to *health security*—the knowledge that illness would not force an individual or family into poverty. "One run of sickness might wipe out the savings of a lifetime," as one writer put it. Health security required some coverage of wage loss during sickness, as well as medical bills.[17]

During this time, the United States embraced the increasing power of medicine but did not similarly embrace medical care as a social right. British sociologist T. H. Marshall argued that social rights were the final stage in a historical evolution that began with the adoption of civil rights (rights to property, free speech, assembly, and religion) and then political rights (the right to vote). However, in the United States individual rights have usually been seen as precluding or contradicting social rights. Individuals' right to be free from government interference and to choose freely in the marketplace would be threatened by welfare protections such as national health insurance. Even though some public goods, particularly Social Security and public education, have come to be treated as rights, broader, universal notions of social rights have been firmly rejected in the United States, with its strong tradition of "negative" rights (freedom *from* government interference), powerful anti-taxation movements, and the lingering Cold War tendency to define social rights as socialistic or communistic. Ideals of individual rather than social or collective responsibility for health have worked against the official acceptance of a right to health care in the United States.

Modern health and welfare systems outside the United States are built on notions of social rights, and this book argues that even in the United States rights and the denial of rights play a crucial role in the health care system. However, the acceptance of rights has been far from the only reason that societies have expanded access to health care. Arguments for greater access to the benefits of modern medicine have also relied on concepts such as charity, duty, military and national strength, and business efficiency.

These types of claims can actually contradict the notion of rights. The impulse and tradition of charity, for example, led to the creation of countless free hospitals and other institutions to assist the poor, but individuals accepted for care had to follow strict rules and sometimes endure conditions seemingly designed to erode dignity and self-respect. Since at least the time of Hippocrates, members of the medical profession have had a duty or obligation to put their patients' needs first. But physicians' obligations did not mean that patients had a right to care; doctors maintained the right to accept or reject patients except in emergencies. Some physicians have argued that doctors' professional rights, including the right to set their own fees, would be violated if people had a right to health care.[18]

Although rights imply obligations—someone has to enable fulfillment of the right—the same is not true the other way around. Like providers, governments have defined their obligations without simultaneously conferring rights on the public. In the late nineteenth century, many countries, including Norway, Sweden, Germany, and Mexico, included provisions in their constitutions about the state's duty to help protect citizens against poverty and sickness, using "the language of obligation rather than rights."[19] In many cases, governments increased their social responsibilities in the wake of popular upheavals, including revolutions, in which the people demanded a greater share of the nation's wealth.[20] The world's first health insurance system was created in Germany by Otto von Bismarck, the "Iron Chancellor," in the 1880s. Far from accepting the people's demands for rights, Bismarck believed that state-guaranteed insurance against sickness and unemployment would help his country avoid a revolution by quieting the masses.

Bismarck sought to strengthen the nation by providing citizens with greater security. In many other countries as well, the expansion of public health and calls for greater access to medical care were based not on the rights of the people but on the needs of the nation as defined by its leaders. Efforts by Western governments to reduce infant mortality at the turn of the twentieth century, for example, stemmed from concerns about "racial decline" and national weakness. War and the expansion of empires also called for greater attention to health, since diseased and poorly nourished citizens would weaken the nation's military capacity. Health provision could strengthen businesses as well as governments; in the United States, factory owners established health and safety programs, on-site medical clinics, and sickness insurance plans to ensure a healthy and loyal workforce. This type of health provision could work against rights, since employers, in common with Bismarck, hoped that workplace benefits would prevent workers from organizing labor unions and gaining more power.[21]

Imperatives of charity, duty, and efficiency continue to drive health care provision today. But since the 1930s, these notions have increasingly meshed with claims for rights. Many physicians, for example, came to believe that their professional obligations should include defending their patients' right to care. Some religious groups combine a tradition of charity with notions of rights. It is not always possible to separate rights claims from notions of duties, obligations, and needs, although this book tries to clarify the distinctions as much as possible.

Some argue that rights are not an appropriate foundation for a health care system. In 1983, the President's Commission for the Study of Ethical Problems in Medicine (appointed by Carter but completing its work under Reagan) concluded that health care was not a right but rather "a societal obligation balanced by individual obligation."[22] Conservatives insist that the right to health care is inherently un-American and would interfere with cherished individual rights, such as doctors' freedom of choice, or even the right of Americans to choose *not* to have health insurance. Another frequent argument against health care rights points to the number of people who engage in irresponsible behaviors like smoking, drinking, eating fatty foods, and reckless driving; why should their health costs be borne by those who live responsibly?[23]

The individualistic rights tradition in the United States leads some to believe that an American right to health care would worsen, rather than solve, the problems of the health care system. For many Americans, notes legal scholar Mary Ann Glendon, rights mean something you can sue over. Conferring social rights could lead to endless litigation in the courts.[24] Others argue that a right to health care would simply be too expensive for society to support. A common—and very American—interpretation of the right to health care is the idea that people are entitled to demand whatever medical services they wish, no matter how expensive or ineffective they may be. Haven't health costs soared because of the belief of well-insured Americans that they are entitled to all available services, treatments, and drugs?

Unchecked demand for high-tech, expensive, and cutting-edge medical care has indeed fueled the frenzy of United States health spending. But to equate a refusal to recognize limits with a right to health care is incorrect. Advocates for health care rights have always referred to reasonable limits on such rights. For example, organizations of the unemployed in the 1930s made demands for "*adequate* medical care," not unlimited medical care on demand (see chapter 2). Debates over the 1948 United Nations Declaration of Human Rights included lengthy discussions of how to reconcile the ideal of social rights with the reality of limited resources.[25] Health policy and ethics debates on the right to health care in the 1970s and '80s spilled a lot of ink debating how to define the terms "reasonable" and "adequate."[26] Although there may be individual Americans who hold to a "maximalist ethic"[27] and believe they have a right to every conceivable medical service and treatment—particularly if they can pay for them—no serious rights advocate has ever defined the right to health care in this expansive, impossible way.

The need to define limits helps explain why it has been so difficult to hold a national discussion of the right to health care in the United States. To talk of limits in health care brings up the dreaded specter of official rationing. Without a recognition that the United States already rations health care, the concept of reasonable limits on health rights sounds like an attempt to take something away, rather than another method of distributing the benefits of medical care that should be evaluated alongside what the nation currently does.

It may be that, even if such a discussion takes place, Americans still would prefer the US-style rationing described in this book to a top-down allocation of services, or imposition of global spending limits by the central government similar to practices in Europe and Canada. A rejection of official rationing makes sense in a country that so greatly values individualism and limited government. Yet Americans also will have to face the reality that the citizens of nations with universal health care enjoy many individual rights that most in the United States do not, such as the right to choose a doctor or hospital, the right to change jobs or residence without losing health coverage, and the right to freedom from fear of medical bills, also known as health security. How Americans lost these rights over the course of the twentieth century, or never had them, is one of the subjects of this book.

PROLOGUE

Rights and Rationing before 1930

Medical care in the United States was never an entirely public or private matter, but a constantly shifting amalgam of the two. Although many Americans think of a government role in health care as a recent phenomenon, notions of public responsibility for health have been around for centuries. Government officials since ancient times have had the authority to impose quarantine and other public health measures during disease epidemics. The care of the sick poor in the colonial United States fell under the responsibility of county or town authorities, a practice dating back to feudal England, when landlords assumed the support of peasants who lived on their land. Elizabethan-era poor laws transferred the landowners' obligation to local governments. In the North American colonies, the poor law tradition continued as towns were required to provide for their own.[1]

The local nature of poor relief meant that towns excluded non-residents from help. Some New England villages posted signs warning sick and impoverished individuals to keep away (this was the origin of "residency requirements" that still play a role in the US health care system). These policies sometimes led to harsh treatment. For example, Boston authorities early in the eighteenth century ordered a woman from Salem, who was on the verge of giving birth, to leave town immediately so they would not have to provide her with a doctor. Towns would also "warn out" new arrivals who might become public charges, which meant they could stay but could never receive public support.[2] Poor laws may have conferred obligations on town governments, but they gave no rights to the poor themselves.

Private medical practitioners abounded in early America, but public medicine was also part of the picture. Dutch settlers in the New World maintained midwives on their government payrolls. Local governments sometimes paid individual doctors for treating the poor; larger towns might appoint a single physician with this responsibility. New

England villages willingly funded caregivers and separate housing—
sometimes just a shack on the outskirts of town—for people infected
with smallpox and other contagious diseases. Municipal physicians
were less common in the Southwest, where tax revenues were insufficient and there was a stronger tradition of private rather than public
charity provision.[3] In the rapidly growing United States of the 1800s,
counties rather than towns became the unit of government that hired
physicians to care for the poor, and later in the century built the county
hospitals still central to the American "safety net" today.[4]

Before the late nineteenth century, poor people who got sick or
injured were usually placed in an almshouse or poorhouse and required
to work for their keep. Boston opened its public almshouse in 1662,
and other major Eastern cities followed suit in the early 1700s.[5] Although the medical care they offered was minimal, almshouses did
employ house physicians, and the almshouses in Boston, New York,
and Philadelphia eventually evolved into prominent hospitals. The earliest US hospitals devoted solely to the care of the sick were Pennsylvania Hospital in Philadelphia (founded 1752) and New York Hospital
(founded 1771). Early hospitals tried to distinguish themselves from the
stigma of the almshouse by insisting on admitting only the "worthy"
or "deserving" poor. Being a church member or industrious widow or
being known to a hospital board member denoted worthiness, while
prostitutes, beggars, unmarried pregnant women, and alcoholics were
unwelcome. Private hospitals also did not admit patients with chronic
or contagious illnesses or venereal diseases. Admission to private hospitals was by application, not by right.[6]

The 1776 Declaration of Independence named the inalienable rights
of "life, liberty, and the pursuit of happiness." Much later, in the twentieth century, some rights advocates would interpret this "right to life"
as including a right to health or health care, but there is no evidence
that Thomas Jefferson, in an age when medicine was not equated with
lifesaving powers, had such an idea in mind. "In those days," noted a
twentieth-century writer, "—pre-medical science—the right to life was
at the disposal of God, not man."[7]

The US Constitution (1787) made no mention of health, either. Care
for the poor, public health measures, and the regulation of medical
practice remained a state or local matter.[8] Following two major epidemics of yellow fever, in 1796 Congress considered whether quarantine should become a federal rather than a state responsibility. During
this debate (which was ultimately decided in favor of the states), Rep.

William Lyman of Massachusetts made what may have been the first recorded reference to health rights in US political debate: "The right to the preservation of health is inalienable."[9]

Early definitions of the right to health referred entirely to protection of the public health and not to actual medical services—a collective right rather than individual rights. However, in 1798 the federal government dipped its toes in the health care delivery waters with the "Act for the Relief of Sick and Disabled Seamen," a hospital insurance plan for merchant sailors and members of the US Navy. The program, based on a British model, put a tax on sailors' wages of 20 cents per month, which entitled them to medical care and hospital services in major port towns. This plan of taxation and government insurance aroused no controversy because it involved regulation of interstate commerce: merchant seamen had no permanent residence and continually crossed state boundaries. By being confined to seamen only, the program was a form of rationing by occupation. By the Civil War, the federal government had built two dozen hospitals with the funds, including merchant marine hospitals in fifteen cities along major American rivers, and more than 10,000 mariners were receiving benefits every year.[10] This extensive medical care program has been mostly forgotten, contributing to the misperception that there was little or no central government involvement in health coverage before Medicare.

Following World War I, federal hospitals serving veterans were absorbed into the new Veterans' Bureau (later renamed the Veterans' Administration), which greatly expanded the veterans' hospital system in the 1920s. In 1921 the federal government became further involved in medical care with the establishment of the Bureau of Indian Affairs Health Division (later Indian Health Service).[11]

Until the twentieth century, most Americans never went near a hospital. The vast majority of care took place in the home, at the hands of family members or neighbors. Local practitioners whose skill was based on experience rather than formal training, such as midwives, were common, and many patients engaged in self-care, using patent medicines and herbal treatments ordered through the mail or purchased from traveling doctor-salesmen. Physicians were called only when other measures failed. Even when summoned, doctors proved ineffectual at treating most diseases and conditions. Often the "cures" they attempted, including bleeding their patients or purging them with mercury-laced drugs, made even minor illnesses worse. Surgeons could perform many procedures successfully, but death rates from major surgeries remained high until improvements in anesthesia and antisepsis after the Civil War.

When patients sought professional medical care, did they have a "right" to it? Did practitioners have an obligation to provide it? Since earliest recorded history, doctors had expected payment for their services when the patient could afford to provide it. [12] In turn, the community expected doctors to devote some portion of their practice to caring for the poor, either without pay or with some form of reimbursement by government or private philanthropy. Physicians in the United States fashioned these longstanding notions of rights and duties into a Code of Ethics, formalized by the American Medical Association (AMA) in 1847. Physicians' obligation to their patients was clear: the first sentence of the Code asserts doctors' duty to "obey the calls of the sick."[13] Yet, "every duty or obligation," noted the 1847 Code, "implies . . . a corresponding right."[14] Doctors therefore had the right to expect patients to carry out certain obligations to their physicians, which included honesty, obedience, and eschewing quacks. But the Code did not make any mention of the rights of patients.

From its inception, the AMA worked intently to drive out rival alternative providers, such as midwives, herbalists, and water cure practitioners, and by the end of the nineteenth century it had mostly succeeded.[15] Yet private physicians could not take full responsibility for all the health needs of the community. Physicians relied on hospitals to house the most desperately poor and sick, and also to provide important training and educational opportunities for doctors and medical students. Doctors also counted on state and local governments to take care of certain types of patients who would otherwise fall through the cracks. Care of the insane, for example, was fully accepted as a state responsibility, and state asylums for the mentally ill were established throughout the nineteenth century. Private doctors and private hospitals seeking to maximize their fees and their reputations also preferred not to accept patients with long-term, chronic ("incurable"), or contagious diseases. Cities and counties took on increasing responsibilities for these kinds of patients, establishing hospitals and clinics specifically dedicated to tuberculosis, venereal diseases, and chronic diseases.[16] This separation of responsibilities between private practitioners and government institutions was a kind of rationing by health condition and one that greatly benefited many private doctors, who needed not be saddled with expensive, long-term, or stigmatized patients.

The hospital system practiced a similar division of labor between public and private. Private or "voluntary" hospitals had been established even before the nation's founding. Although, as already noted, early voluntary hospitals were primarily for the sick poor, as were their public counterparts, they quickly developed distinctive roles and served distinct parts of the population. The earliest voluntary hospitals, including Pennsylvania Hospital and Massachusetts General, were founded by wealthy members of the community and governed by voluntary boards. Starting in the middle of the nineteenth century, religious groups began opening their own hospitals to serve their members; by 1885 there were 154 Catholic hospitals in the United States, alongside hundreds of others representing Jewish or Protestant denominations. As historian Rosemary Stevens argues, the term "private hospital" is really a misnomer, since many private voluntary institutions also received some government support, such as cash grants or the donation of public land. In areas with no public hospital or extremely high patient demand, local governments sometimes provided subsidies to voluntary hospitals for indigent care (care for the poor).[17]

Whether or not they received government support, voluntary hospitals prided themselves on their charitable role and many admitted poor patients unable to afford their care. But even charitable hospitals had specific standards for admission, and no hospital would admit everyone. The tasks of assessing patients' qualifications for admission and excluding those who did not pass muster were part of the hospitals' mission. As a Catholic hospital administrator put it in 1932, "Every hospital has definite limitations—it cannot care for every sick person"; a "general hospital should carefully sort its patients" to exclude the contagious, the mentally ill, and the chronically ill. As for ability to pay, "no deserving poor person [should] be excluded simply because he is poor . . . [but hospitals] cannot receive all poor patients, much less all who ask for free care . . . Only the deserving ones need be accepted."[18]

Public hospitals, sanatoria, and asylums excluded patients too, especially those institutions designated for sufferers of particular diseases only. But in general, the existence of public medical care served as a safety valve that ensured private hospitals' ability to exclude.[19] Voluntary hospitals felt justified in turning away patients with chronic or contagious diseases, mental illnesses, alcoholism, and even severe injuries, in the belief that their care was properly the responsibility of government-funded institutions. The existence of public medical care also allowed private hospitals to limit the amount of care they provided to those unable to pay. The practice of what later came to be known as "patient dumping"—the transfer of seriously ill, injured, or even dying patients from private to public hospitals—has a long history (and will be discussed in detail in Chapters 4 and 8).

But the resources of public hospitals and other government-funded facilities were never great enough to meet the need. Overcrowding, waiting lists, and outright denials became central features of the US "safety net." At Chicago's Cook County hospital in the 1870s, "there was scarcely a day when there was a bed to spare." The *Chicago Medical Journal* described patients dying in the city's jails and police stations "because there is no room for the sick or wounded poor in the hospitals of this great city of Chicago."[20] Even as both public and private facilities expanded early in the twentieth century, severe shortages of care for the poor and for patients with undesirable conditions continued.

Hospitals excluded not just on the basis of ability to pay or medical condition, but also on the basis of race. Both private and public facilities practiced racial discrimination well into the twentieth century. Most hospitals in both the South and the North either refused blacks altogether, sending them to the local "Negro" hospital (if there was one), or placed them in separate wards. The county branches of the American Medical Association denied membership to nonwhite physicians, which meant that they could not receive hospital admitting privileges. Even hospitals that admitted black patients excluded black physicians from privileges. In 1895, African American doctors formed their own National Medical Association to fight against exclusion by the AMA. In response to the desperate need for hospital care, black doctors and philanthropists also raised funds to build hospitals solely to serve members of their own race, such as Provident Hospital in Chicago, Howard University Hospital in Washington, and Hubbard Hospital in Nashville; by the early twentieth century there were close to 200 such institutions. The federal government also sponsored all-black institutions, including Freedmen's Hospital in Washington, DC, and Tuskegee Veterans' Hospital in Alabama. The majority of black hospitals were "small, poorly financed, and ill equipped," historian Vanessa Gamble notes, and could not come close to meeting the medical needs of their communities. Racial discrimination, segregation, and a shortage of adequate facilities contributed to a "multitiered, unequal health system."[21]

Rationing by race limited the health care access of other groups as well. In Los Angeles in the 1920s, separate public health clinics were established for "Americans" and "Mexicans." In Tucson, Arizona, city, county, and even religious hospitals regularly refused to admit Indians, arguing that tribe members had the option of going to the federal Indian Health Service hospital—75 miles away. "Some of our members have died due to lack of attention. . . . We believe this is a great injustice," protested a Papago tribal leader in 1944. Again, public provision in one limited area (a hospital for Indians only) supported rationing and denial elsewhere in the system.[22]

Outpatient clinics, or dispensaries, were another means of access to medical care. These facilities, some of which had been around since the 18th century, could be free-standing or attached to a hospital, public or private, open to the public or serving workers from a particular factory or people with certain conditions only. Few clinics were "designed for service to the whole community."[23] Like hospitals, they had strict admissions requirements. Patients often had to undergo a "means test"—an investigation of their income and assets—in order to receive care at a clinic. Dispensaries hired professional social workers to conduct elaborate "budget studies" of patients and their families in order to determine their eligibility for care. Race, residency, health condition, and other factors determined eligibility for clinic treatment (as discussed in chapter 1).

Strict admitting practices kept clinic load manageable and within the resources of the facility, but another major reason for all the sorting and classification was to ease the fears of the local medical profession. Although many physicians volunteered at dispensaries and some clinic appointments were seen as highly prestigious, the average community doctor worried that patients would use clinics in the place of private physicians, even if they could afford to pay. Starting in the late nineteenth century, urban dispensaries became hugely popular. The working poor sought dispensary care not just because it was free or low cost, but also because of their belief that the doctors and equipment would be of high quality. The rising demand for dispensary care led members of the medical profession to denounce what they called "dispensary abuse," the use of dispensaries by patients not entirely destitute. Local medical societies accused clinics and dispensaries of unfair competition and demanded even stricter admissions standards and more stringent definitions of indigence. This opposition from the medical profession led to the closure of hundreds of dispensaries by the second decade of the twentieth century.[24]

Physicians' concern with "dispensary abuse" also extended to government public health activities that they saw as encroaching on the medical profession's territory. The sanitarian movement, which spread throughout the United States following the Civil War, led cities and towns to establish water and sewer systems, garbage removal, housing reform, workplace sanitary inspections, and other measures that greatly improved health and living conditions. The responsibilities of public health authorities increased after the turn of the century, sometimes in ways that seemed to step on the toes of the medical profession. Although many physicians strongly supported public health activities and some became leaders of the public health movement at the beginning of the twentieth century, local medical societies tended to oppose such measures as school health clinics (which they demanded provide only screening, not treatment, of medical problems in children), public vaccination campaigns, university health services, and rural health centers as unfairly competing with physicians.[25] "Hospitals, health centers, governmental agencies or bureaus and other similar organizations are merely accessory to the private physician," asserted the Chicago Medical Society in 1934, "and any form of competition set up by such organized groups against the private physician is contrary or inimical to the public interests."[26] Public health officials and clinic administrators mostly complied with physicians' demands for a clear separation of public health from the delivery of medical care, but such controversies would continue to rage throughout the twentieth century.[27]

Did patients have a legal basis to claim medical care? While the constitution remained silent on this, the answer from the courts was a resounding No. The voluntary hospitals' hybrid public / private nature worked to protect the rights of hospitals while precluding rights for patients. Voluntary hospitals received exemption from local taxes due to their status as "charitable institutions." Courts decided in the 1870s that, as charities, hospitals could also claim immunity from patient lawsuits. But at the same time that they affirmed hospitals' charitable status, courts also agreed that voluntary hospitals did not have to admit everyone and could continue to categorize and exclude patients.[28] In 1934, the Alabama Supreme Court ruled that it was legal for private hospitals to turn away emergency patients (see chapter 4).

Even as courts affirmed their "charitable" and tax-exempt status, hospitals increasingly behaved like businesses and sought the kinds of patients who would increase their incomes. With the rise of laboratory science, x-rays, and other technologies, and the growing importance of the teaching hospital following the 1910 Flexner Report on the quality of medical education, hospitals became viewed as places of medical science rather than custodial care for the poor. Wealthier people increasingly wanted the antiseptic surgeries, nursing care, and, later, childbirth services provided by hospitals. By the 1920s, US voluntary hospitals had shifted their emphasis to paying patients, greatly reducing the amount of free care they provided and relying on income from patient fees more than charitable donations.[29]

But not everyone had the money to pay for a hospital bed. The Committee on the Cost of Medical Care (CCMC), a group of public health experts, elected officials, and physicians who published a series of influential reports between 1927 and 1932, announced that wealthy people used hospital care far more than the middle class or people of moderate income. Rather than questioning whether hospital care was the best use of health care dollars, the CCMC instead asked how hospital care could become more accessible to the entire population.[30] As hospitals evolved into the centerpiece of the medical system, how would people be able to afford to use them?

Health Insurance: The Early Debates

Early in the twentieth century, one of the biggest economic worries of American workers was getting sick. This anxiety stemmed not from doctor or hospital fees, which were still quite modest, but from lost wages. Since employers did not offer what are known today as "sick days," the serious illness of a breadwinner could plunge the entire family into poverty.

Working people themselves initiated the earliest attempts to address this aspect of health insecurity in the United States. Immigrant organizations, unions, and neighbors came together to create mutual aid societies, in which members paid regular dues in return for a modest "sick benefit" to replace their wages if they became ill. Many nineteenth-century mutual aid societies also included some form of medical care in the sick benefit, and the larger ones hired their own physicians to care for their members (generating accusations of competition from local medical societies). But the system of mutual aid strictly rationed care and coverage because membership requirements were extremely narrow, confined to members of a particular occupation, gender, workplace, ethnicity, religion, or sometimes even to an immigrant group whose members all originally came from the same village.[31] During the Progressive Era, reformers argued that such a private and scattershot patchwork of coverage could never come close to offering true security to American workers, insisting that European programs of government-sponsored "sickness insurance" provided better models.

The first health insurance system had been created in Germany in 1883 by Chancellor Otto von Bismarck, who was trying to put down a socialist uprising in his country by offering new state benefits to working people. Under the German system, workers joined a local, government-regulated insurance plan, with the premiums divided between workers and employers, and received both sick pay and medical benefits. Other European nations followed in Bismarck's footsteps. By the 1910s, most Western European countries had adopted some kind of sickness insurance system, including Britain in 1911.[32]

When Theodore Roosevelt ran for president on the Progressive Party ticket in 1912, his party included "sickness insurance" in its platform. Roosevelt's defeat did not end the momentum, and bills to create state sickness insurance systems—also known as "compulsory health insurance"—were introduced in a dozen states. These proposals were supported by Progressive reformers, public health physicians, and some labor unions, especially unions representing female workers and immigrants. Reformers did not use rights arguments in advocating these proposals; instead, they emphasized both efficiency (businesses would benefit from healthier and more secure workers) and the concept of social or contributory insurance (both workers and employers would help fund the system through a payroll tax).

But employers, insurance companies, and state medical societies furiously opposed compulsory sickness insurance. Employers did not like that they would be required to pay for part of the coverage; insurance companies feared competition, since the bills included a life insurance benefit; and doctors argued that government involvement would take away the right of physicians to set their own fees and to practice as they saw fit. The American Federation of Labor, the country's largest and most influential labor organization, also opposed the bills. In contrast with the trade unionists who supported compulsory insurance, AFL leader Samuel Gompers believed workers should fight for higher wages and provide their own benefits, rather than turn to government and employers. The US entry into World War I in 1917 dealt the death blow to the sickness insurance movement, because looking to Germany as a model suddenly became very unpopular. Only the New York and California proposals ever came to a vote, and both were defeated.[33] The American Medical Association announced its official opposition to compulsory health insurance in 1920.

The battles over compulsory health insurance took place in the states; health insurance was never seriously discussed at the national level. But in the 1920s, high maternal and infant mortality rates in the United States led reformers to propose the Sheppard-Towner Act of 1921, which allocated $1.2 million federal dollars a year to states to establish infant and maternal health programs. Supporters of Sheppard-Towner, led by the staff of the federal Children's Bureau, argued that the government should be at least as interested in the health and welfare of the nation's babies as it was in the proper care and feeding of cattle (the United States spent millions on assistance to farmers for their livestock but nothing on human mothers and children). States used the funds to open maternal and child health centers, distribute educational literature, and bring visiting nurses into the homes of rural women and children. Because of opposition from the medical profession, Sheppard-Towner funds could not be used to provide physicians' services. But even the limited services under the Act represented too much government intervention for physicians. The American Medical Association, describing Sheppard-Towner as "tending to promote communism," successfully lobbied Congress to cancel the program entirely in 1929.[34]

In 1932, the Committee on the Costs of Medical Care published the results of its five years of work studying the American health care system. The report celebrated the growing efficacy of medical science, assuming that more medical care would lead to better health for all Americans.[35] The committee warned, however, that the social organization of medical care and payment lagged far behind medical science's rapid advance. In the United States, physicians, hospitals, and health departments "are not distributed primarily according to needs, but rather according to real or supposed ability of patients to pay for service. As a result, many communities are undersupplied with practitioners, hospitals, and other facilities, while others have a surplus." The committee described a system that distributed resources on the basis of ability to pay and that lacked coordination and planning. "Although medical service is as essential to the national welfare as public education," the report summarized, "the task of providing it to all the people has not yet been tackled in an organized and coordinated way."[36]

While the committee agreed on the desirability of medical care "for all the people," there was serious disagreement on the best methods to achieve this goal. The majority recommended two forms of medical organization, physician group practice and voluntary health insurance, to help rationalize medical services and distribute the cost of medical care more evenly. Group practice, in which physicians work in partnerships rather than as solo practitioners, had already shown its potential in the Mayo Clinic, founded in Rochester, Minnesota, in the 1880s. The Mayo Clinic had become world renowned by combining specialist physicians, surgeons, laboratories, and research under one roof. The Committee report argued that group practice was preferable to the traditional fee-for-service method of payment of solo doctors, which, they argued, encouraged physicians to perform unnecessary procedures and discouraged preventive medicine (since doctors could not make money from prevention).

Several physicians on the committee, however, dissented strongly from the majority view, arguing that group medicine threatened physicians' tradition and right of private, fee-for-service practice.[37] The dissenting physicians also opposed the report's other recommendation, for voluntary health insurance, because they believed that even private, commercial insurance would pave the way for national, compulsory insurance, as it had in England. The American Medical Association also denounced the CCMC's recommendations. Even though group practice and voluntary insurance were far less sweeping reforms than the Progressives had advocated two decades earlier, they were still seen as too radical and disruptive of traditional practice. Until the 1940s, the American Medical Association would remain opposed to even these moderate forms of medical reorganization.

The costs of medical care were rising without new methods to help Americans pay for them. The poorest of the poor could still pass a means test and receive some indigent or free care, and the affluent could pay for private doctors and hospitals, but those in between faced increasing problems with affordability. Then, when the Great Depression struck, many members of the middle class found themselves plunged into poverty. The health care system was utterly unprepared for a deluge of patients who simply could not pay anything. Who was responsible for their care became a most urgent question during the dark days of the economic crisis.

PART I

The Struggle for Health Care
in the Great Depression

CHAPTER ONE

A Crisis of Access

On a wintry Chicago morning in 1936, ten-year-old Vera Lahr began complaining of stomach pains. Suddenly, she doubled over and started vomiting "green stuff." Her panicked mother immediately called the charity clinic where she had been taking the children since their father lost his job. Now that the family was "on relief," they could no longer afford their former family doctor, but the clinic told Mrs. Lahr to call him anyway since there was nothing they could do for the sick girl. Mrs. Lahr phoned the doctor several times and even sent one of her other children down to his office. Hours passed, but "still he did not come." Later that afternoon, the doctor sent word that he would be over "after office hours." When he finally arrived, he immediately ordered the girl hospitalized. Shortly after surgery disclosed her burst appendix, Vera Lahr died.[1]

The Lahrs claimed that Vera lost her life because she was a clinic patient and her family was on relief. Her grieving father told an interviewer that he "blamed the doctor's indifference, and the lack of immediate medical care as the cause of his daughter's death." Although they had known the doctor for years and even considered him a friend of the family, the Lahrs felt that he was annoyed with them "because they had not been doctoring with him in recent years . . . they had been going to clinics where services were free."[2] The family believed that by accepting charity medical care they had lost their standing with their former physician—a loss that, in her parents' eyes at least, cost Vera her life.

Despite its unusual drama, Vera Lahr's story encapsulates many of the changes that ordinary Americans experienced when seeking medical care during the Great Depression. Like Vera's father, millions of breadwinners found themselves suddenly out of work and turning to relief in the form of government cash or work assistance. Relief checks were inadequate to cover a family's most basic expenses, much less medical costs, and local relief authorities' responsibilities did not include financing health care. Large numbers of families attended "free" or charity clinics or used public hospitals for the first time during the Depression. Public and charity facilities that had been designated for the poorest of the poor now overflowed with the newly impoverished—people who had previously been able to afford private doctors but could no longer do so. As the formerly employed and their families found themselves suddenly flung into medical indigence, the public-private health system struggled to accommodate the new demand.

With no coordinated system to care for them, the newly indigent had to navigate a complicated patchwork of rationed services: government and voluntary hospitals, charitable physicians, private and public clinics and dispensaries. Each service had different requirements for access or eligibility; a patient rejected for one type of care might be eligible for another, but the standards proved variable and sometimes mysterious. Facilities could be difficult to get to and far from each other, making transportation a crucial part of access—in Vera Lahr's case, a matter of life or death. If the Lahrs had been able to call an ambulance Vera might have made it to a hospital sooner, but Chicago in the 1930s had no public ambulances, and the city's 22 private ambulances were too expensive for people on relief.[3] No US city had a coordinated plan for emergency health services during the Depression, and the clinics on which the poor depended were not equipped to deal with emergency cases.

Access to private physicians depended on ability to pay or the doctor's willingness to provide care at reduced rates or free of charge. As the Lahr case illustrated, the Depression brought physicians' ambivalence about charity care to a head. Some physicians supported the expansion of charity and government clinics and hospitals to relieve the medical profession of the growing burden of free care, but others deeply resented free or low-cost facilities for luring away patients who had previously been willing or able to pay doctors' fees.

The health care system of the 1930s not only failed to guarantee access; it also offered no rights of recourse for people who were denied medical care. After the Lahrs lost Vera, they complained only to a social work student who interviewed them for her thesis on health care in their West Side neighborhood. There was no official way for patients to make themselves heard about neglect or poor treatment from doctors or hospitals. Even if the family had wanted to take their doctor to court, malpractice law offered no course of action for patients who had been denied medical care, since malpractice could occur only after treatment by the physician had begun.

The sudden increase in the need for affordable health care during the Great Depression directly challenged the ideology and institutions of voluntarism. Physician charity, private philanthropy, and voluntary hospitals and clinics, despite their best efforts, proved incapable of meeting the demand. As the economic crisis deepened, many leaders of voluntary institutions argued that the new conditions required an increase in government's responsibility to subsidize care of the indigent sick.

The role of government itself was undergoing massive change during the Great Depression. Workers, the unemployed, and the elderly joined together in vocal organizations demanding an increased federal role in the economy and in the protection of ordinary people's security. The programs of Franklin D. Roosevelt's New Deal embodied many of these new ideas about government responsibility. This was a time of talk about economic rights and security. It is no coincidence that the first explicit discussions of a right to health care in the United States began during the Great Depression.

One part of the story is well known (and will be discussed further in chapter 2): the President gave in to pressure from the medical profession and refused to include health coverage in the Social Security Act. Even so, the Great Depression transformed government's relationship to health care. By the end of the 1930s, the crisis of access had forced local, state, and even the federal government to play a greater role in health provision than ever before. New voluntary institutions, including private health insurance, emerged to challenge the state's encroachment into the health field, but the trajectory of government involvement begun in the 1930s would only gain momentum during the decades that followed. As this section of the book will show, however, new responsibilities for government did not at first translate into new health care rights for citizens.

Even before the economic depression threw millions into unemployment after 1929, the United States experienced a great disparity between impressive medical progress on the one hand, and unequal distribution of health and medical resources on the other. In the first three decades of the twentieth century, life expectancy for the average American increased from 47.3 years to 59.7, thanks to improved sanitation, vaccination for some contagious diseases, and new treatments for diseases like syphilis. Yet, notes historian John Duffy, "the advances in medicine and public health did not benefit all Americans."[4]

Even at the height of prosperity in the 1920s, "millions of families cannot afford to obtain any medical care," reported the Committee on the Costs of Medical Care. "Hundreds of thousands of cases of sickness needing medical attention are unattended; less than seven percent of the population have even a partial physical examination and less than five percent are immunized against some disease."[5] Although scientists and doctors were making great strides against scourges like tuberculosis, diphtheria, and venereal diseases, health reformers argued that these disorders remained far more common than they should have been because of the nation's uncoordinated and inadequate medical services.[6]

When the Depression struck in 1929, the age-old correlation between poverty and sickness became even more evident. Urban areas experienced increasing rates of illness during the early 1930s. A study of several large cities by the US Public Health Service in 1933 found that lower-income population groups experienced higher incidences of disabling illnesses, with the greatest increase among families who had a drop in income due to recent unemployment. Workers who lost their jobs and had to go on relief had higher levels of chronic disability and their children lost more time from school because of sickness than people with higher incomes.[7] "Unemployment means a greatly reduced standard of life," asserted an organization of the unemployed. "Long hours, low wages and bad working conditions when there is work, undermine health. Relief and poverty diets lower resistance."[8]

Rural areas continued to suffer high rates of "preventable or treatable diseases such as pellagra, hookworm, syphilis, tuberculosis, malaria, and typhoid . . . stark reminders," points out historian Michael Grey, "that rural America had been materially poorer than the rest of the nation for decades." Nearly half of all loan defaults among farmers were linked to sickness in the family. The devastation of the rural economy by drought and depression meant that by the early 1930s, doctors in the countryside were able to collect less than half of their bills.[9]

In both urban and rural areas, race played a part in sickness and health. While overall life expectancy was improving, African Americans' life spans fell increasingly behind those of whites. Black infant mortality in South Carolina, to give just one shocking example, was over 15 percent in the 1920s, meaning that 15 percent of black newborns would not survive their first year. In Chicago, the tuberculosis rate among blacks was five times as high as among whites.[10] Higher disease and mortality rates were always attributable to poverty and overcrowding, but also to overt racial discrimination. South Carolina had far fewer hospital beds for black tuberculosis patients than for whites, even though blacks suffered from the disease in far greater numbers. Blacks in Chicago were routinely sent to overcrowded Cook County Hospital instead of the closest hospital because of their race.[11]

Medical progress itself created a new challenge: the rising cost of health care. More Americans entered hospitals for serious illnesses, and in the 1930s childbirth began to shift from the home to the hospital. More doctors trained as specialists, raising the price of physician services. Technological advances, particularly improvements in anesthesia, also increased the cost of care. National medical expenditures in 1929 exceeded $3.5 billion (around $30 per capita)—less, noted the CCMC report, than annual expenditures on tobacco or automobiles, but increasing each year.[12]

The economic depression, coupled with rising physician and hospital costs, pushed medical care beyond the reach of many Americans. Sudden illness, chronic disease, childbirth—each could take a devastating toll on family finances. In a survey of medical costs in one Chicago neighborhood, a woman called it "disgraceful" that her daughter and son-in-law had just finished paying the doctor and hospital bills for their baby's birth—and "the child was past two years old!" For a diabetic, "all of her earnings ($50.40 a month) went for medicine, appliances and a special diet." An Italian immigrant had given up a visit to the "old country" in order to pay the doctors' bill of $313 to remove a breast lump. Her family "'hadn't had a doctor in their home for years—they 'couldn't afford to get sick!'"[13] Sometimes, people had to forego care altogether, like a woman who needed cancer surgery that would cost $100, but canceled the operation after her husband was laid off.[14]

Both the poor and the middle class went to private doctors less often during the Depression, and when they did go, they had a harder time paying. One national survey found that 66.6 percent of doctors' bills were delinquent in 1933. Although some doctors refused to see or limited patients who could not pay, many others continued to be "generous with their services and did a great amount of 'charity' work." The result was a dramatic drop in physicians' incomes of 47 percent between 1929 and 1933. "Many physicians, surgeons and dentists," lamented the *Chicago Medical Society Bulletin* in 1934, hovered "on the verge of privation because they could collect no money for the work they did."[15] The nursing profession also experienced severe distress, with 60 percent of all nurses unemployed by 1932–33.[16]

The economic crisis threatened hospitals, too. Admissions at private hospitals dropped during 1931–33, and the patients they did have were less likely to be able to pay. Charity patients—including those paying part of their costs on a sliding scale—accounted for 40 to 50 percent of all patients admitted to voluntary hospitals nationwide in 1933, an increase of 25 percent in three years.[17] In 1932, the total patient load in New York City's private general hospitals dropped 13 percent, but service in these hospitals to "free" patients nearly doubled as the Depression created an enormous increase in the demand for free medical care.[18] The following year, the city's public hospitals operated "at an average of 110% of their rated capacity," with "beds in the aisles, queues at the clinics."[19] Both government and private hospitals and clinics faced a major shortfall in patient fees, coupled with a decline in philanthropic giving. The many physicians willing to give care found themselves increasingly unable to afford to do so. Yet the health needs of the population continued to increase. Who was to care for the swelling ranks of the indigent sick?

Storming the Clinic Doors: Crisis in Chicago

In the summer of 1938, on the second day of the National Health Conference convened by President Franklin D. Roosevelt in Washington, DC, a woman named Florence Greenberg rose to speak. "Yesterday," she told the audience, "Dr. West of Chicago extended an invitation to the delegates . . . to visit the American Medical Association offices in Chicago to see its accomplishments. I, too, want to extend an invitation to the delegates present here to visit Chicago—but I want to show them another picture. I want to show them a sick Chicago, a Chicago of dirt and filth and tenements." Greenberg, a member of the Steel Workers Organizing Committee, spoke of how she had seen families devastated, first by unemployment, and then by sickness and lack of medical care.[20]

The Depression had hit Greenberg's city especially hard. Chicago was heavily dependent on manufacturing, and 50 percent of its factory workers had lost their jobs by 1933. A tax revolt left the city government bankrupt and forced public school teachers to go without pay for months. Chicago's large African American population suffered especially high rates of unemployment—a devastating 40 percent— exacerbated by job segregation and racial discrimination.[21] One historian describes Chicago early in the Depression years: "World War I veterans took to selling apples on Loop streets. Some found their way to the bread line sponsored by Immanuel Baptist Church. Here, 1,500 to 2,000 would line up two blocks long to receive bread, coffee, and on alternate days meat . . . Homeless men erected shanties on scattered vacant lots throughout the city . . . Hundreds of children came to school without breakfast, existing on one meal per day."[22]

Although not as famous a medical center as Boston or New York, Chicago was still better equipped than most cities (and all rural areas) to handle the needs of the indigent sick. The city boasted the fine medical schools of the University of Chicago, University of Illinois at Chicago, Northwestern, and Rush, and was headquarters to the American Medical Association and the American Hospital Association. Chicago had dozens of private, voluntary hospitals, including Catholic, Protestant, and Jewish hospitals as well as ones catering to the Swedish, German, and African American populations.

The city was also home to Cook County Hospital, one of the largest public general hospitals in the country. Before the Depression, most Chicagoans saw the county hospital as a place only of last resort. "Workers are afraid of going to 'Cook County,'" said Greenberg; "they look upon it as sort of a death house."[23] Some low-income people preferred to incur private hospital bills rather than enter County; one woman went to a Catholic hospital during a hemorrhage, even though she couldn't afford it, because "she was too sick to go through all of the necessary red tape before she could have been admitted to Cook County Hospital." (Her bills remained unpaid two years later.)[24]

But, the poor and unemployed generally had no choice other than "County," and more and more Chicagoans relied on the hospital during the Depression. Yearly admissions rose from 45,953 in 1930 to 68,014 in 1940.[25] At the same time, Chicago's private hospitals lost paying patients in droves; by 1934 half of all "pay beds" lay unoccupied, even as Cook County Hospital became vastly overcrowded.[26] And more than half of the patients who were admitted to Chicago's private hospitals in 1933 were classified "unable to pay."[27]

Even more than on the private hospitals, the weight of the growing numbers of newly indigent sick fell on Chicago's outpatient departments and clinics. Individuals not sick enough for inpatient care and unable to pay a private physician turned to the outpatient departments of the larger voluntary hospitals, or to freestanding clinics sponsored by a hospital or private agency.[28] Clinics treated working people and the poor for both acute and chronic conditions endemic among these groups.[29] The Clinic Section of the Council of Social Agencies (CSA), an umbrella organization of Chicago charities founded in 1914, oversaw Chicago's private clinics, dispensaries, and outpatient departments. Council leaders fiercely upheld the tradition of private charity and voluntarism in Chicago, but the Depression radically challenged their belief that private institutions could meet the medical needs of the population without help from the government.

As unemployment rose dramatically in the early 1930s, the character of clinic patients changed. Chicago's charity workers confronted a completely new category of medically indigent: "sick people who are not known to social agencies and who up to the present have been able to pay for medical services"[30]—in other words, people who had never before turned to charity or public services for help. By 1931, Chicago charity administrators saw a major increase in demand on the city's clinics. "The U of I clinic is working to capacity, 125,000 visits for the full current year; Municipal TB Sanitarium is averaging 25,000 visits a month," reported the CSA.[31] Visits to St. Luke Hospital's outpatient department had risen by 10,000 in just one year, and the hospital imposed "drastic regulations" to limit the number of free patients. In 1934, 95,000 individuals made 718,000 visits to Chicago's six largest clinics, representing "a city as large as Cincinnati."[32] In 1935 social workers declared that the Provident Hospital clinic on the city's South Side "has literally expanded to the curb and has to turn dozens away daily." The West Side's Central Free Dispensary "is taking 500 a day [about double the average rate in the 1920s] and has reached the limit of its capacity."[33]

The huge increase in clinic visits occurred despite the numerous barriers Chicagoans faced when they attempted to get care at such facilities. These hurdles illustrate the numerous forms of explicit and implicit rationing in the city's health care system.

Clinics rationed first by medical condition. Municipal clinics existed solely for patients with tuberculosis and venereal disease; patients with those conditions would be turned away from private outpatient facilities. Medical schools held clinics for specific conditions, such as heart disease or eye problems, only at the times that specialist doctors were able and willing to volunteer there. Several hospitals ran clinics solely for prenatal and maternity care. It was probably confusing for many patients, especially those using the clinics for the first time, even to figure out where they should attempt to seek medical help unless they had guidance from a knowledgeable welfare or relief worker.

Another form of rationing was by geographic location. Since the city's clinics and public facilities were concentrated around the wealthier downtown area, the majority of working and poor people had to travel significant distances to reach them. The *Chicago Daily News* described a woman who had to leave her home at 6 A.M. to get to a clinic by 9 A.M. to see a doctor once a week for heart trouble.[34] Travel difficulties often meant that no medical care was obtained at all; labor activist Greenberg described an "old man who can't see but has no carfare to go to the public hospital for eye treatment or to buy glasses."[35]

Red tape also created a significant barrier to care. No one could just walk into a clinic and receive aid. Patients were usually required to bring a referral from the county Bureau of Public Welfare (and, later in the decade, from the Chicago Relief Administration), so new, often very sick patients were required to make two journeys—from home to the welfare or relief bureau, and from the bureau to the clinic—before being admitted. Clinics would refuse admission to a patient who had previously been seen in another facility, unless he or she had obtained a written release from the first clinic. Similarly, clinics required a patient who had been treated by a private doctor or hospital to show a referral.[36] In the days before extensive phone service, these releases and referrals had to be obtained physically by the patient and presented in person at the registration desk.[37]

Long waiting times were the next hurdle. Many clinics did not offer appointments and simply required patients to wait to be seen on a first-come, first-served basis. Sometimes it was not possible to be seen the same day, or even the same week; these patients had to leave and return later, sometimes much later. Twenty-five percent of clinic patients in Chicago had to wait between one and four weeks before a physician would see them.[38]

The dispensaries' tradition of opening only for limited hours caused additional delays in treatment. Since physicians worked in clinics without pay, they could offer their services only a few hours a week. A few well-staffed facilities might be open 9 A.M.–5 P.M. with a break for lunch, but elsewhere hours of, for example, 9 A.M.–3 P.M., 9 A.M.–11 A.M., or 2 P.M.–4 P.M. were standard. Outpatient departments offered clinics for certain disorders only at designated times depending on the availability of specialists, perhaps every other week or once a month. And although a few facilities did offer limited evening hours—for example, two hours two evenings a week—most were open only during the work day, creating another major barrier to care. "I could not take the time away from my work," responded a former patient when asked why he never returned to a University of Chicago clinic for follow-up care. A working woman with a sick child left the dispensary before even completing her admissions interview. "Although she was told to return at a later date," staff reported, "she decided that she would be unable to wait long enough for the child to see the doctor." She ended up going to a private physician and owing him over a hundred dollars.[39]

Many Chicago clinics rationed on the basis of race. In 1934, six out of thirty-two city clinics "reported that they did not admit negroes."[40] Others had explicit quotas for African American patients. In a survey by the CSA, "Ten [unnamed] clinics reported that they are not limiting their negro patients and three reported that they are." Both the Central Free Dispensary and the University of Illinois clinic "restricted negro patients." Central Free also kept out nonwhite patients by narrowing its residency boundaries, a practice apparently followed by numerous other clinics. Suburban Evanston Hospital denied that it turned away patients on the basis of race, but a social worker at Children's Memorial clinic, which did not ration by race, "reports that she has been given to understand quite differently and that in fact a number of the children have come to them having been refused at the Evanston Hospital." Apart from the all-black Provident Hospital clinic, in 1937 "the proportion of Negroes to white patients varied from 35% Negroes in some clinics to practically none in other clinics." CSA leaders occasionally visited clinics to persuade them to "increas[e] intake of Negro patients," but their concerns did not lead the Council to adopt an official policy against discrimination by race during the '30s.[41]

Obtaining a referral or appointment—just getting in the door—was far from the last obstacle to access. Once they arrived at the clinic, patients faced long waits of several hours in crowded conditions. A reporter described waiting rooms "so crowded that [patients] must stand up" while waiting to see a doctor, and then they "must stand

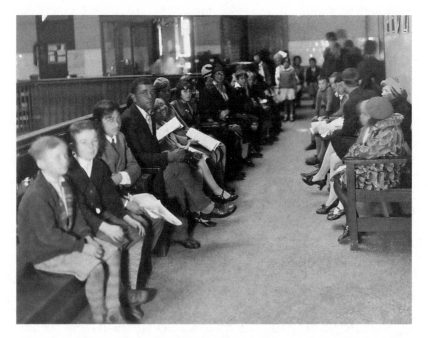

FIGURE 1. Hope Clinic, New Haven, Connecticut, sometime in the 1920s. Courtesy of Yale School of Medicine Library.

again, in a long, slow line" to get their medication prescribed. At one clinic, patients remained standing in line throughout the lunch hour, when the registration desk was closed, for fear of losing their place. [42] A headache patient gave up on her treatments because the clinic she attended "was always crowded, and she disliked having to wait each time she went."[43] One day in the waiting room of the Mandel Clinic of Michael Reese Hospital, a nineteen-year-old boy began screaming and demanded to be seen immediately. Admissions workers, amazed because such an incident was "without precedent in their clinic," later found out that the young man's pregnant sister had fainted after waiting four hours at Mandel's prenatal clinic.[44]

Finally, every patient faced the possibility of being rejected for medical care entirely. Applicants underwent an admissions interview—lasting from a few minutes to twenty minutes or more—to demonstrate that they did not have enough money to pay a private physician. In an updated version of the means test, welfare and clinic workers developed elaborate "budgets" to help determine patients' eligibility, and required candidates for care to fill out forms describing their incomes, housing and clothing costs, debts, and other financial information.

Some Chicago social workers urged clinics to be relatively lenient with budget determinations and to allow patients with more severe or chronic medical conditions to be classed as indigent even if their income was "over budget"—a recognition of the growing costs of medical care and also of the expanding definition of medical indigence. One study gave several examples of "over budget" cases admitted for clinic care because the patients required "frequent hospitalization and long-term medical care," including a "wage earner with carcinoma of rectum" who "became unemployable"; a person with a spinal cord tumor whose family could no longer afford the "expensive medical care needed," including x-ray therapy; a child with a cleft palate whose repeated hospital stays had put the family into debt; and a "neurosyphilitic" couple who had made 51 visits to a physician "and many more to come," and whose care, noted a social worker, "will extend over a period of years."[45]

More frequently, patients whose incomes classified them as "over budget" or who failed other eligibility requirements were rejected outright, regardless of medical condition. Chicago's largest clinics rejected a total of around 800 patients a month in the mid-1940s (comparable figures are not available for the '30s). The reasons given for rejection included "referred to own physician," "referred to other physician," "over budget," "known to other clinic," "type of care not provided," "geographical (residency) reasons," and "other reasons."[46] In 1935, Chicago clinics rejected nine patients because they owned cars.[47]

As the demand for clinic care increased throughout the Depression, facilities increasingly rejected patients not just for lack of eligibility, but for lack of room. By the summer of 1938, Chicago's Grant Hospital reported that its clinics "can accept no more cases in general medical or cardiac clinics, and the prenatal services have appointments scheduled into the fall." Mandel reported "appointments made two and three weeks in advance, and . . . patients are being rejected beyond these appointments." At Northwestern's clinics, "some 40 patients a day are rejected because clinic capacity ha[s] been reached."[48]

Different clinics handled rejection cases differently—Children's Memorial, for example, allowed rejected patients to see a doctor one time only, while others sent patients away immediately, with or without a referral—but no clinic made an attempt to follow up on rejected patients.[49] Clinics stated that they simply did not have enough staff to locate or ensure follow-up care for them.[50]

Some of the sickest patients never even reached the clinics. A federal study found that 30 percent of cases of serious, disabling illness among families on relief received no medical attention.[51] Chicago social workers reported that numerous people forswore medical care altogether, either because they were not aware of the existence of the free clinics, or because they were simply too sick to go out. A truant officer located a little girl who had been out of school for days; she was at home with a "touch of diphtheria." Her father had the sickness as well, which made them both too ill to leave the house.[52] The aged and chronically ill had to stay home as well. What the sickest poor needed most were home visits from doctors, but these became more difficult to get during the Depression. A family whose child had scarlet fever could not pay for her special diet or medicines, and the mother reported that "their own physician is reluctant to call because he knows they cannot pay him." She tried to obtain a county doctor—they did make house calls—but there were none available. Fortunately, she reached a social worker who sent a visiting nurse from the Chicago Commons settlement.[53]

Chicago newspapers decried the horrors of the clinic system. "If Ill and Poor, Be Very Ill," advised the *Daily News*, since the totally incapacitated would at least be taken care of promptly at the county hospital, while those remaining upright languished in outpatient departments.[54] But aside from an occasional screaming fit in the waiting room, ordinary Chicagoans left little evidence of their responses to the vagaries of clinic care. Clinic staff, hospital administrators, and charity workers, on the other hand, took their problems public as they grew increasingly frustrated with having to turn away so many, and with expecting little or no reimbursement for the patients they did treat. Even as they sought to preserve their private, rationed system, providers began demanding a larger role for government in financing care for those who could not pay. They did not argue for this on the basis of a right to health care for patients. Their demands instead were based on both growing need sparked by the Depression, and a different kind of rights claim—the right of doctors, clinics, and hospitals to reimbursement for care they had previously given without compensation. Governments had an obligation, providers insisted, to enforce this right by paying for indigent care. This could be accomplished by an expansion of public health care, and also by public subsidies for the private, voluntary system.

"We Need Help": New Demands on Government

In 1935, the Chicago Council of Social Agencies asked for "an adequate municipal clinic to relieve pressure on existing non-governmental clinics."[55] With this demand unmet, private clinics began to insist that they deserved government funding because they were serving the victims of the Great Depression.

Most prevalent was the argument that economic depression had created new responsibilities for government. In their quest for state subsidies, voluntary institutions insisted that expanded government funding would simply extend traditional notions of community responsibility for the indigent. If governments did not assist voluntary institutions in doing their duty, private hospitals and clinics would be forced to reject those in need and accept only paying patients. At a 1932 meeting of the American Hospital Association, for example, the head of an upstate New York hospital declared, "I think it is our duty to take care of all the people who come to our doors, regardless of whether they can pay or not, but we can only do that insofar as we are supported from some source, and if we are not supported I do not think we can be blamed for closing our doors."[56]

In 1934, the American Hospital Association (AHA) resolved that "local government funds should be used to pay for service in . . . voluntary hospitals" because "the care of the indigent sick is a fundamental responsibility of governmental bodies." They made sure to specify that this did not mean the AHA was advocating government-run facilities that would threaten their business: "governmental hospitals should be expanded only where other facilities are not available to provide for local needs," the resolution concluded.[57] In their arguments for state support, hospital leaders drew on the nation's tradition of government provision for the poor to insist that public responsibility now extended to the Depression-made indigent being treated in private facilities. A 1936 editorial in the industry journal *Modern Hospital* titled "We Need Help" asserted that the state's role in health care had historically been established through the creation of municipal, state, and county general hospitals; "the principle of government responsibility for the care of the sick has already been accepted," so the state's support of private hospitals was a natural extension of its traditional role.[58]

Many physicians also clamored for new public funding for their ancient obligations to the poor. "There is not a doctor in the US who does not feel that the indigent should be taken care of free of charge and well taken care of," opined the *Chicago Medical Journal*, "but that the economic responsibility of this load should not fall upon the physician, but is purely and justly a civic or community liability."[59] A doctor in downstate Illinois wrote to the state's relief commission asking for "some compensation for my time and services" caring for the unemployed. "They all want to transfer the load of caring for the sick on the drs. I am willing to do my part, but" it was unfair that "the whole thing is pushed on me."[60] The AMA argued that the depression had created a class of unemployed who "had been rendered indigent by society" and demanded "a recognition of the duty of society to care for their needs."[61] Members of the Medical Advisory Committee, a group appointed by Franklin D. Roosevelt to advise the framers of the Social Security Act, referred specifically to the clinic crisis in their arguments that doctors should be paid for services previously given at no charge: "The recently increased burdens of clinic service, and the reductions in medical income also due to the depression, have created a widespread demand for the payment of physicians for their clinic work." Payment would assure a higher quality of doctors in the clinics, committee members argued.[62]

Hospitals' and doctors' new demands came after the plight of millions of unemployed had already begun to greatly expand the role of government. First states and then, for the first time in history, the federal government became involved in dispensing direct funds, or "relief," to cities, organizations, and individuals. Early in 1932 the State of Illinois issued $20 million in bonds to create the Illinois Emergency Relief Commission (IERC). Chicago's clinics were among the beneficiaries of the new fund, but the need for relief in Illinois proved so severe that the IERC's $20 million was spent in three months. With Chicago's 750,000 unemployed still in desperate condition, in June of 1932 Mayor Anton Cermak went before the US Congress asking for "Relief or Troops"—without funds from Washington, he warned, riots of the unemployed would create total chaos. The federal Emergency Relief and Reconstruction Act of 1932, signed by President Herbert Hoover, authorized $300 million to the states for relief efforts.[63]

After President Franklin D. Roosevelt came into office and established the Federal Emergency Relief Administration (FERA) in 1933, relief funds from Washington almost completely supplanted state, local, and private dollars.[64] By the fall of 1934, the 13 Chicago clinics in the Council of Social Agencies had received $200,000 from the IERC, slightly less than one-third of their annual operating budgets; hospitals received twice that amount (from Cook County, not from FERA, which excluded direct funding for hospitals).[65] FERA also allowed relief recipients to use part of their grant to pay for medical bills.[66]

For some people, federal help made all the difference. A Chicago man told a neighborhood meeting, "My children were saved by the emergency relief when they needed medical treatment."[67] But FERA, as its name indicated, was intended as an emergency measure only. The Roosevelt administration far preferred work to cash relief for the unemployed, and announced in January 1936 that all direct federal relief to the states would end. The cutoff "dumped relief responsibility back into the lap of local authorities,"[68] leading to a second crisis for Chicago's clinics. Although they continued to serve patients with subsidies from the county, pressure on the clinics worsened as families lost federal cash payments.

Lack of food and loss of shelter exacerbated medical problems. Clinic workers reported cases of a man with cancer, one with asthma, and one with diabetes, all of whom were found to have no food in their houses because they had stopped receiving relief checks. Several patients faced eviction for nonpayment of rent, including a man with heart disease who was released from the hospital to find he had been evicted from his home; clinic workers reported that this cardiac patient, who needed full bed rest, "had been sleeping out of doors." Staff reported "caring for patients too ill to come to the clinic" who had been turned away for home visits by the County Physician Service. Workers at Cook County Hospital found themselves more overwhelmed than ever; a nurse reported that "the admitting department was simply swamped and did not know where to turn. She stated that she simply does not know how they will be nursed."[69] Following the cutoff of funds on July 1, desperate families gathered outside a South Side relief station seeking food and medical help. A tubercular woman said that she had eaten only bread for three days. A man whose daughter suffered from meningitis waved a prescription over his head and demanded to know "of all within earshot how he was going to have a prescription . . . filled when he had no money and no prospects of any."[70]

Pressure for subsidized medical care stemming from the growth in economic need showed no signs of abating. By 1938, patients crowded clinics to the point that some were unable to see patients without an appointment months in advance. Alexander Ropchan of the CSA complained bitterly about the inadequacies of Chicago's clinic system: "What justification is there for the community to depend upon this haphazard way of meeting the total problem of clinic services? . . . Public responsibility for medical care of the sick poor has been recognized" but "a deplorable lack exists in meeting this obligation."[71]

Ropchan's frustration was understandable. Apart from the short-lived FERA subsidies, some public health nursing services, and the clinics set up by the federal Farm Security Administration in rural areas (discussed in Chapter 2), no New Deal program directly paid for medical care. The major public works program that replaced direct relief, the Works Progress Administration (WPA), allowed workers to be taken to a public hospital if injured on a work relief project, but made no provision for other types of medical care, or any care at all for workers' families.[72] Charity and social work leaders complained that the WPA wage was far too small to allow workers to pay for any medical services. The American Public Welfare Association was furious that the WPA lacked "any recognition of the responsibilities for medical care, except as it came in lip service."[73] Only 3 percent of WPA funds went for any type of health activities, the majority of which were large-scale public health programs such as swamp clearance for the prevention of malaria, and the construction of new public hospital facilities, mostly for tuberculosis and psychiatric patients (the WPA did not fund construction of private hospitals). WPA workers also participated in mass inoculation and health education campaigns, and researchers paid by the WPA conducted the first National Health Survey in 1935. But the program emphasized traditional public health activities over the direct provision of health care.[74]

While welfare and clinic leaders were disappointed by the lack of federal commitment to providing medical care, the hospital industry succeeded in winning greatly expanded state funding (significant federal support for hospitals would not come until World War II). By 1935, the amount received by US voluntary hospitals from state and local tax funds ($25 million) had surpassed their receipts from charitable giving. An AHA report in 1937 confirmed that "the policy of supplying public funds for care in private hospitals or other than government institutions seems to be generally accepted."[75] Providers succeeded in winning rights to public funds, but the funding came with no new obligations toward the public. Hospitals continued to admit or exclude

on the basis of the ability to pay, medical condition, race, and many
other factors (see chapter 4).

Despite the modest resources that the New Deal devoted to health
care, during the 1930s publicly funded medical care touched large
numbers of Americans for the first time. Dr. Thomas Parran of the
Roosevelt administration estimated at the height of emergency relief
expenditures in 1934 that "during the past months . . . about 18 percent
of the population [have been] receiving from public funds all the necessities of life including medical care."[76] Many of these were people
who crowded into the free clinics of the nation's cities.

   For many who made it past the barriers and received free and subsidized medical care during the Depression, it was their first experience
of access to health care. As this chapter has shown, once clinic leaders, hospitals, and physicians got a taste of state funding, they argued
that government subsidy was now a necessity. Would patients react
the same way? Parran, who would be appointed Surgeon General in
1936, thought that the expansion of medical aid during the Depression might raise expectations and create new demands among working people. "Having accepted free and, in about a third of the states,
moderately adequate medical care—in many instances more freely
available than in their whole previous experience, and of better quality
than provided by the quacks and shysters so often patronized by those
in the lower income classes—will they, having experienced such care,
continue to insist upon it?" he wondered.[77] The AMA's Morris Fishbein,
a passionate opponent of government involvement in medical care,
thought that New Deal–funded medical programs would lead to more
demands for free care, calling them "a sort of insidious propaganda for
state medicine among the persons who received the benefit."[78] A Rockford, Illinois, newspaper editorialized that, following the provision of
medical care for people on relief, "there is no doubt that a trend in the
direction of socialized medical care is one of the stepchildren of the
depression."[79] But would President Franklin D. Roosevelt agree?

CHAPTER TWO

Social Security without Health Security

President Roosevelt did not believe in cash relief. The massive injection of federal funds in the form of FERA, much of which ended up directly in the hands of the unemployed and their families, was intended to be only temporary. With his New Deal programs, FDR sought not just to end the Depression but to prevent future ones—indeed, to save capitalism itself. Following the emergency relief, industrial regulation, and public works jobs programs of the early New Deal, the President turned to creating permanent federal institutions that would make the American worker—and the American economy—more secure.

Other governments that provided forms of security for their workers, like Germany and Great Britain, built their programs on three pillars: protection from unemployment, protection from poverty in old age, and protection from ill health. The enduring New Deal programs created by Roosevelt might have addressed all of these. Instead, old age security came first, followed closely by unemployment insurance. But health coverage ended up getting left out of the 1935 Social Security Act altogether, in part because the President wanted to avoid antagonizing the medical profession. By the time the United States entered World War II and the Depression ended, the opportunity to add protection against sickness to the Social Security system had been lost.

However, toward the end of his life Franklin Roosevelt came to believe in a stronger government role in health and even spoke of a right to medical care. His ideas resonated with those expressed in the nationwide upheaval of workers, African Americans, and the unemployed during the Depression. Following the exclusion of medical care from the Social Security Act, many of these groups began to call for national insurance and a right to health care. These vocal and explicit demands for health care rights met with opposition from the medical profession, hospitals, and others. But medical leaders could not ignore the public's desire for greater health security. In the 1930s and '40s hospitals and doctors began offering a new type of private insurance, called Blue Cross and Blue Shield, which would fill part of the health care hole left in the Social Security Act. They hoped to fill that hole just enough to derail demands for a universal right to health care.

The Emergence of Health Care Rights Demands

Organizations of American workers, the aged, and the unemployed during the Depression included medical care on their list of the essentials needed by working and poor people and called for government assistance in paying for it. Representatives of the unemployed, many of whom were organized into Communist-led Unemployed Councils, were particularly vocal in their demands for comprehensive security. In 1932, for example, the Chicago Workers' Committee on Unemployment announced a platform that called for cash relief, jobs, unemployment insurance, and "adequate medical and dental care."[1] The Workers' Alliance of Cook County (Illinois) announced a march on Chicago City Hall in July of 1936 to protest the cutoff of federal relief (described in chapter 1). Their twelve demands included a "Provision of adequate medical and dental service." "We propose," announced the Alliance, "that legislation shall be introduced in the Illinois State legislature, which shall set up in Illinois the proper machinery, operating in every community, for the medical, and dental care of all in need unable to provide it for themselves . . . to reduce the growing menace of disease and disability caused by the lengthening years of unemployment and inadequate relief."[2]

Calls for assistance with the costs of sickness were not confined to groups with communist or socialist leanings. The enormously influential Townsend Movement in support of old-age pensions, led by retired physician Francis E. Townsend, had two million members organized into 7,000 clubs nationwide. Many "Townsenders" were from small-town, conservative backgrounds, and their enthusiasm for the movement was due to their experience of poverty (or fear of it) and to Townsend's charismatic leadership, not socialist ideology. When Townsend supporters were surveyed in 1935 on how they would spend their proposed pension money, more respondents put "doctors" first than any other category of spending, including rent, mortgage, and home repairs.[3]

Mainstream labor unions joined the unemployed organizations in supporting the 1931 Lundeen Bill, a proposal in Congress to establish a comprehensive system of worker security. The bill, sponsored by Minnesota Farmer-Labor Party Congressman Ernest Lundeen, proposed far more sweeping measures than the unemployment insurance legislation backed by President Roosevelt. It included not only government insurance against unemployment, but also old age pensions and health insurance. When a more modest unemployment insurance bill passed instead, leaders of the national Unemployed Council objected that the new law included "no insurance for sickness, accident, old age, or maternity."[4]

Unemployed, elderly, and labor activists saw medical insurance or help with medical bills as essential components of economic security. However, they did not specifically talk about health care as a right until later in the 1930s. But rights language was beginning to appear in the speeches and writings of some academics, journalists, and even physicians. Sociologist James Brossard, speaking at a 1934 medical conference, said that the increase in state and local government support for medical care during the Depression had created "a new social attitude toward health and health services in the direction of regarding health and adequate medical service as a social necessity, and perhaps it is safe to go so far as to say, as a social right. The great mass of people, in other words, are coming to look upon medical service as they do upon education and police protection."[5] Like Surgeon General Parran, Brossard believed that Depression emergency measures were creating new expectations among the public, and that these expectations of access to health and medical services led to a belief in health care as a right.

"Certain epochs give birth to a whole crop of new ideas," wrote Atlanta physician Stewart Roberts in a 1935 issue of the usually staid *New England Journal of Medicine*. The "new idea" was the concept of health care as an "inalienable right." "The Negro plowing in the river bottom is as much entitled to adequate medical care as an inalienable right as any of us," wrote Roberts, a member of FDR's Medical Advisory Committee who had previously served on the Committee on the Costs of Medical Care. "The expectant mother in a two-room cabin has an inalienable right to medical care. The opposition to it will ultimately be as helpful as a small canoe in a great storm on the open sea."[6] Roberts' statement argued for civil rights as well as health care rights and denounced rationing both by race and by class: neither skin color nor income should determine an individual's access to health care. In August 1938, Kelly Miller, co-editor of the civil rights newspaper *Crisis*, also used the Declaration of Independence to make a case for health care rights. Miller wrote in his weekly column, which appeared in over 100 newspapers, "That public health would be made one of the chief objectives of the New Deal is essential to the fulfillment of its basic purpose. It is indeed but the concrete embodiment of the Declaration of Independence, which declares that all men are entitled to the inalienable right of life, of which health is the prime essential. Health is more essential than wealth, knowledge, culture and goodness; for without health none of these other human values would be very much worthwhile."[7]

These writers invoked the emergency of the Depression, the broad goals of the New Deal, the fulfillment of the Declaration of Independence, and the imperative of racial justice to support their assertions of a right to health care. Paul de Kruif, the most influential medical journalist of the time, made an impassioned plea for health rights on the basis of the rapid and stunning advance of medical science. The spreading belief in a right to health care, de Kruif wrote, emerged from the public's growing knowledge of the power of medicine. The people would not "rest content" to see medical science used to help celebrities like "the derelict Al Capone" (who had seen the best doctors for treatment of his syphilis) at the same time that babies continued to die of treatable diseases. De Kruif, a passionate supporter of the medical profession, called the right to access to medical science "The Fifth Human Right" after the right to food, clothing, shelter and fuel. The right to benefit from modern medicine should really come first, de Kruif argued, since it had become essential to the inalienable right to life. But he acknowledged with regret that New Deal legislation was putting medical care last, not first.[8]

Talk of the right to health care was everywhere. Yet President Roosevelt remained reluctant to use New Deal legislation to broaden access. There were several reasons why FDR did not prioritize health insurance as he pushed for Social Security. Old-age pensions stood at the top of his agenda, both because of the terrible poverty among the elderly and because of pressure from the hugely influential Townsenders, who demanded government payments of $200 a month to retired people.[9] And of course the immediate needs of the unemployed required the most urgent response. Although most organized groups during the Depression had something to say about health care, it was a priority for none of them. Unemployment, the rights of workers to organize, and the basic civil rights of African Americans understandably came first for people organizing during the Depression. As Surgeon General Parran put it, the public was less passionate about proposals for medical insurance because "immediate, tangible returns from health insurance seem slight in comparison with the other forms of social security more widely discussed of late."[10] No mass movement on the scale of the Townsend Clubs or Huey Long's "Share Our Wealth" movement emerged on behalf of access to health care. Such a large-scale, mass organization would have been necessary to counteract the force of the American Medical Association's opposition to including medical insurance in the Social Security Act, and to persuade FDR that such a battle would be worthwhile.

Roosevelt adamantly refused to antagonize the AMA. Despite his devastating misdiagnosis by an incompetent physician when he was stricken with polio, FDR deeply respected the medical profession and shared many of its leaders' beliefs. Two of his closest friends and advisors were doctors: White House physician Ross McIntire, who visited the President twice each day, and world-renowned brain surgeon Harvey Cushing, whose daughter was married to FDR's son James. In their book on presidential health care politics, David Blumenthal and James A. Morone note that FDR consistently sounded "deferential to the white coats" in the rare public remarks he made about health care. The President instructed his staff to reply to letters from doctors with the statement that physicians "can rest assured that the Federal Administration contemplates action only in their interest."[11]

In 1934 Roosevelt appointed five top members of his cabinet to a Committee on Economic Security (CES). The CES was charged with studying "the entire problem of economic insecurity" of the American people and with drafting a social security program to bring before Congress.[12] When FDR put together a Medical Advisory Committee of physicians to work with the CES on developing health legislation, he made Dr. Cushing chair, and appointed Dr. McIntire as the President's liaison to the committee. Cushing and McIntire represented the more traditional wing of the medical profession, and Cushing strongly opposed the attempts of his public health–oriented colleagues on the committee to push for an increased government role in health protection.[13]

Members of the CES divided over whether medical care should be included in the President's program of economic security, and the argument that health insurance would "doom the whole bill" won out.[14] In the end, the 1935 Social Security Act included old-age insurance (what we now call Social Security), old-age assistance for the poor, welfare assistance to poor children of single mothers (later known as Aid to Families with Dependent Children), and expanded maternal, child, and public health programs, but no medical insurance of any kind. The Act provided $3,800,000 in federal grants to the states to provide health services to poor mothers and babies and to "crippled" children, and another $8 million for state and local public health services. Since these activities did not interfere with private medical practice, they were deemed acceptable by the AMA.

Roosevelt had promised health insurance supporters in his administration that they could revisit the issue after passage of the Social Security Act. In 1937 they formed the awkwardly named Technical Committee on Medical Care of the Interdepartmental Committee to Coordinate Health and Welfare Activities. In contrast to the CES, this committee was firmly committed to pushing for a national health plan, although not all of its members agreed that national health insurance was the way to go. The committee's report, *The Need for a National Health Program*, called for expanded public health programs, hospital expansion, indigent care, and "insurance against loss of wages during sickness."[15] When the Interdepartmental Committee called an unprecedented National Health Conference in 1938 to discuss its proposed program, new voices entered a debate previously dominated by the medical profession. Committee members were aware that public support and mobilization, as well as the President's backing, would be crucial to secure health legislation, and with this in mind they invited a diverse array of people to the conference in Washington.

In the words of historian Alan Derickson, the National Health Conference of 1938 was a "wholly extraordinary event."[16] It was the first time that representatives of groups outside the medical profession were invited to the nation's capital to discuss health reform. The participants included the AMA, but also business leaders, members of the social work profession, the labor movement, farm organizations, and civil rights groups. President Roosevelt himself did not attend—he was on a cruise—but he sent a message to the delegates agreeing that "there is need for a coordinated national program of action." But FDR again declined to call for sweeping legislation, stating, "We cannot do all at once everything that we should do."[17]

Traditional opponents of national health insurance spoke at the conference and cautioned against government intervention. AMA President Dr. Irvin Abell acknowledged "certain local inadequacies and certain inequalities in the distribution of medical care," but argued that any plan emerging from the conference must operate under the control of the medical profession. The problems of medical care should be resolved by "your Family Physician," Dr. Arthur T. McCormack agreed. Dr. Morris Fishbein, editor of the AMA's journal, argued that Americans were "essentially a healthful people" and that health should not be a major national concern. Several physicians, including Hugh Cabot of the Mayo Clinic and famed physician Alice Hamilton, a pioneer in the field of industrial medicine, argued in favor of a comprehensive national program, but most statements from medical, hospital, and business representatives preached caution and further research, if not outright opposition to the Committee's proposals.[18]

But the National Health Conference put a new spin on old debates by including the testimony of both expert and nonexpert delegates from all over the country, describing in their own words the problems of the current health care system. Although they did not use the term "rationing," speakers noted the injustices created by the uneven allocation of health care by region, by income, and by charity means testing. A member of the Kentucky Farm Bureau objected to the imbalance in resources between the countryside and urban America, reminding the crowd that many rural areas had only one doctor for every 1,000 to 1,500 people. "In our opinion," he concluded, "the farm people are entitled to just as many doctors and just as good doctors in proportion to population as the people in the urban centers." Mrs. Henry W. Ahart, the wife of a California sheep rancher and spokeswoman for the American Farm Bureau women's auxiliary, pointed out that, even before the Depression, "four-fifths of the rural areas of the United States lacked any organized health service." The Farm Bureau was attempting to bring voluntary health projects and health insurance to the countryside, but Mrs. Ahart expressed frustration that "we are 60 years behind Europe in providing health insurance for the people of the United States."[19]

Other speakers condemned the tradition of charity medicine, with its accompanying moral stigma. As a representative of the American Legion put it, "I like to think of a woman being able in the future to take her ailing child . . . to a capable physician in the community, without downcast eyes and without scraping or dimpling or blushing or bobbing or bowing, or without any mental reservations that she will get the service and then will not be able to pay the doctor afterward." T. Arnold Hill of the National Urban League, the civil rights organization, was critical of the nation's meager medical services for the indigent. He emphasized the medical needs of transient and migrant workers during the Depression and how the residency-based system failed them: "If a man is sick and in need of care, his health should not be endangered by the red tape necessary to determine whether a certain State, city, or county . . . should ultimately have to pay the bill."[20]

Civil rights leaders demanded health measures to redress not just the conditions of the Depression but also continuing, long-term racial inequities and vicious discrimination. Dr. Louis T. Wright of the National Association for the Advancement of Colored People thundered, "Organized medicine has ignored the health of my people," adding that the NAACP "welcomes the intervention of the federal government . . . to the end that the inadequacy of hospitalization of colored people . . . will be overcome."[21] Both Wright and the Urban League's Hill asked that African Americans be included in any government health program as full and equal participants; "Any fundamentally sound program of health coverage must be based and administered per unit of health, and not arbitrarily per unit of population," said Wright, repudiating separation and rationing by race.[22]

The most explicit demands for a right to health care came from the labor movement, including a refusal to define health as a market good. "Health . . . is not a commodity, not an article of commerce," American Federation of Labor representative Joseph Padway told the conference. "We believe that health is within the realm of human rights and requires the protection of Government regardless of what other private agencies do or what protection, medical or otherwise, is offered to aid in the alleviation of the problem."[23] Florence Greenberg of the Steel Workers Organizing Committee, who had spoken so dramatically of shocking health conditions in Chicago, concluded her remarks with a rousing call for health care as an inalienable right. "My people are asking that our Government take health from the list of luxuries to be bought only by money and add it to the list containing the 'inalienable rights' of every citizen." Her speech met with enthusiastic applause.[24]

"To the President's summation that one-third of the nation is ill nourished, ill housed, ill clad, recent research has added evidence that one-third of the Nation puts up with inadequate medical service or none at all," stated the summary report of the National Health Conference.[25] The meeting did not, however, result in a consensus about how to address this problem. In fact, Roosevelt asked conference organizers to be circumspect about any possible next steps. The American Medical Association quickly convened its House of Delegates to reaffirm its members' opposition to health insurance in any form—including voluntary, private health insurance—and their opposition to government-subsidized care for anyone except the indigent.

Supporters of national health reform took the opposite message from the conference. "I really believe there is overwhelming sentiment for it," wrote New York Senator Robert Wagner, who had earlier introduced an unsuccessful bill for national health insurance. Wagner was a leader in proposing social welfare legislation during the Depression—in fact, he was far more active in doing so than the President. The Senator, who is most remembered for the 1935 National Labor Relations Act bearing his name, believed that sickness was "perhaps the single greatest cause of economic insecurity" and that health insurance was the "last remaining frontier of social security in America." Following the National Health Conference, Wagner introduced a new proposal for health reform in 1939. His bill did not call for medical insurance to be grafted onto Social Security, as administration reformers had hoped; instead it would have provided federal matching funds for the states to set up their own health insurance programs.[26]

Labor organizations continued to call for more government action on health care. The Chicago branch of the Workers' Alliance, an organization of the unemployed, announced at its 1938 convention that "the present Social Security program does not meet the health problem" and proposed a far-reaching "comprehensive" program for compulsory health insurance whose "cornerstone" would be "the *Prevention* of disease," including research and public health education. These Chicago activists thought they could enlist the public works programs of the Works Progress Administration in the cause of better health, and demanded the "immediate setting up of wPA Health Projects to inaugurate a program of adequate medical care."[27] Women's auxiliaries of industrial labor unions in Pittsburgh launched a "campaign for government-supported health clinics, free medical care and progressive health legislation." A delegation from the United Auto Workers union visited President Roosevelt in September of 1938 to encourage him to raise wPA wages and to expand the program to include medical care for wPA workers.[28]

At the 1939 congressional hearings on the Wagner bill, dozens of major national organizations, including the Farm Bureau, the Farmers' Union, the General Federation of Women's Clubs, both major labor organizations (the AFL and the CIO), and the National Association for the Advancement of Colored People, expressed support for the New York Senator's National Health Program.[29] Supporters included many mainstream organizations that would have been less enthusiastic about universal insurance, but approved of federal support for indigent care. But the AMA still deemed Wagner's bill too "socialistic." The doctors, of course, did not oppose government subsidy per se. The AMA House of Delegates announced its agreement with the "basic principle" that "tax monies be used to help care for the indigent sick," but deplored that in Wagner's proposal "Federal agents are given authority to disapprove plans proposed by the states. Federal subsidies mean federal control."[30]

FDR decided not to endorse the Wagner bill, instead proposing a modest federal program of hospital construction. (Aside from spelling doom for Wagner's proposal, FDR's decision also set another important precedent: the separation of hospital legislation from a broader, more universal health program.)[31] An incident related by medical writer de Kruif helps explain the president's reluctance to back national health reform. In 1939, de Kruif met with FDR's close advisor Harry Hopkins to persuade him to bring a plan for national public health legislation to the President's attention. De Kruif wrote that the meeting left him with the feeling that "amid the terrific issues of unemployment, the persisting economic tailspin, the threat of world war, our proposed fight for the nation's health and lives was . . . minor league stuff, strictly speaking."[32]

As the Depression brought to light new ideas about rights, it also brought about a corresponding opposition. The AMA had successfully opposed the inclusion of health insurance in the Social Security Act and helped defeat the Wagner health bill. The medical profession fought other types of health care reorganization as well, such as worker-run clinics and group practice. At the heart of this opposition was doctors' struggle to retain control over medical delivery in the face of new rights demands and increasing government involvement.

The Opposition to Health Care Rights

Like so many other Americans during the 1930s, medical professionals did speak increasingly of rights, but the rights of physicians, not patients. Physicians were to serve the public, they agreed, but the public did not—and would not—have enforceable rights to care.

As the Depression increased the demand for charity care, the medical profession's tradition of free service strained to the breaking point. The drop in physician incomes meant that fewer doctors could afford to continue charity practice. As a result, the medical profession began to call for physicians' right to reimbursement, even to the extent of questioning the continuance of the free care tradition. In 1933 the president of the New York State Medical Society said that "a physician had the same rights and responsibilities as all other Americans, such that he was entitled to a monetary return for his labor, experience, and knowledge that is commensurate with the services rendered"; free clinic and hospital service by doctors was thus "ethically wrong and economically unsound."[33] When Harvey Cushing insisted at a meeting of the Medical Advisory Board that doctors were eager to volunteer in clinics for prestige rather than pay, others argued that this notion was outdated. "I know it is becoming increasingly difficult in cities like Philadelphia and I think in New York to get competent men to work in clinics, for the reason that they won't work for nothing. That age is gone," said George M. Piersol of the American College of Physicians.[34]

The Depression only increased doctors' fear of competition. The medical profession had always been wary of potential competition from clinics and dispensaries, but as clinics received more government funding, they became an even greater threat to physicians' incomes. The Chicago Medical Society launched a study of the city's clinics in 1934, determined to find evidence of "abuse" of services by patients who could afford to pay. Clinic leaders secretly called the Medical Society's motives "selfish," but deferred to the physicians and promised to intensify admissions procedures to exclude patients able to pay a private doctor.[35] Organized medicine's opposition to clinic expansion became explicitly connected to fears that new forms of relief would lead the public to demand rights to health care. In 1934 Detroit's Wayne County Medical Society condemned what its members saw as a new feeling among the public that dispensary service was now available to people of all incomes, "a belief which seems to be spread by over-zealous, not well-trained welfare workers." This belief, according to the society's members, "is destroying the responsibility of many people well able to pay their own way and is causing them first to accept, next to ask, and finally to demand that government or private philanthropy give them free medical care."[36] A New York physician studied a public hospital in the Bronx in 1934 and found that over 40 percent of the patients receiving free services there were either "able to pay" or "possibly capable of paying." He claimed that when it came to free medical care, many New Yorkers "believe that usage has finally created a right."[37]

Physicians' concern about growing rights demands came from the soaring demand for clinic care, and also from the new forms of medical organization that began to emerge during the 1930s, both within the New Deal and in the private sector. The most prominent example was the experimental medical program of the New Deal's Resettlement Administration (RA) and Farm Security Administration (FSA). Rural doctors and patients knew that sickness was part of the vicious cycle of poverty in the countryside. The loss of crops and farms led to chronic malnutrition and acute diseases, making farmers and their families less able to work. Local officials reported farmers defaulting on federal loans and selling their remaining assets in order to pay doctors' bills.[38] The RA and its successor, the FSA, initiated a program of medical clinics and cooperatives in rural counties, mostly in the West and South. The clinics primarily aided transient farm workers, who only rarely, if ever, qualified as candidates for private medical care.

Far more controversial, the cooperatives organized farmers and their families into prepaid medical care plans. Unlike traditional fee for service medicine, in prepaid plans members paid a particular amount per year or month, no matter how much or how little medical care they used. Payment of physicians was by capitation (per number of patients enrolled in the plan) or by salary, rather than by individual service. Even though participation in these cooperatives by patients and doctors was entirely voluntary, and most local medical societies participated enthusiastically, the AMA increasingly saw the program as an opening to national health insurance, and successfully lobbied to discontinue the cooperatives by 1946.[39]

The AMA similarly opposed innovative health care experiments that were not initiated by the government, such as physician-run prepaid group medical practice. In prepaid group practice, doctors organized into teams providing primary and specialist care, and consumers paid a standard yearly fee to cover all or most medical services they would need. The AMA argued that prepaid insurance injected a third party into the doctor-patient relationship and violated the sacred principle of fee-for-service payment. So resistant was the mainstream profession to these alternative practices that the Los Angeles County Medical Society expelled the founders of the Ross-Loos Medical Group, which enrolled 60,000 members by the late 1930s and paid salaries to its physicians. The local medical society in Elk City, Oklahoma, attempted to end the career of Dr. Michael Shadid when he assisted farmers in setting up a cooperative hospital association providing prepaid hospital and medical care in 1929. Group practice plans organized by labor unions faced similar opposition from the medical profession.[40]

When the AMA tried to retaliate against the physicians of the consumer-owned Group Health Association in Washington, DC, they found themselves brought up on antitrust charges. In 1943 the Supreme Court ruled that the AMA was guilty of conspiracy in restraint of trade because it denied hospital privileges to Group Health Association doctors.[41] The ruling, however, did not end the AMA's attempts to curb cooperative medicine and group practice. Throughout the 1940s, physicians successfully pushed for laws against consumer medical cooperatives in 26 states.[42]

With the exception of the Kaiser health system in the West, which began in 1935 as a health plan for construction magnate Henry J. Kaiser's employees, prepaid group practice saw little expansion and would not do so until the 1980s. But another form of health care organization that was not threatening to the medical profession—prepaid hospital care—did take hold, and it spread like wildfire.

Blue Cross and the Origins of the Private Insurance System

Patients' inability or reluctance to pay their bills created a problem for hospitals even before the Depression. Hospital administrators constantly complained that many patients "will try to evade payment for . . . services. A patient will pay for his railroad or steamship tickets in advance but resents the hospital's equally logical request for an advance payment."[43] In the 1920s some hospitals had gone so far as to detain patients in their beds until they paid their bills—a practice challenged several times in court but upheld as long as the hospital did not engage in "the use of force or threat of force." In 1925, one Alabama hospital held a female patient "by threat of force from 9 in the morning until 8 P.M." According to the patient, hospital staff threatened to tie her to her bed until her parents arrived with a check. She later took the hospital to court and recovered damages "for the wrongful act as well as for nervousness resulting from her experience."[44]

Hospitals throughout the 1920s and '30s wrestled with the question of how best to persuade patients to settle their bills. Commonly, a hospital financial officer would pay a visit to the patient's bedside during the hospital stay. Some hospitals decided this was too heavy-handed and replaced bedside billing with the practice of assigning "a nurse, attendant or competent employee" to escort patients to the cashier's office upon discharge.[45] When fees could not be collected on site, "offering credit and riding hard on bad debts were two ways of keeping income up," writes historian Rosemary Stevens. In some towns, hospitals joined together to create their own collection agencies. Hospital journals regularly featured articles on the best ways to run a cashier's office, extend credit, collect bills, and, when all else failed, compose "dunning letters."[46]

In 1929, Baylor University Hospital in Dallas, Texas, attempted to ease its financial crisis by creating a hospital prepayment plan for city teachers, which charged members a monthly fee in exchange for coverage of hospital bills. By covering hospital costs only, and not doctors' or surgeons' fees, Baylor's plan circumvented any opposition from the medical profession. Because of the plan's success, similar individual hospital plans sprang up in several cities. In 1933 the American Hospital Association (AHA), the national trade group for voluntary hospitals, officially endorsed "the principle of insurance against the costs of hospital care.[47] The AHA created a Committee on Hospital Service, later named the Blue Cross Commission, to standardize and approve multihospital prepayment plans around the country. For a plan to be granted "the right to use the AHA insignia superimposed over a blue cross," it had to offer service rather than indemnity benefits (payment went directly to the hospital, not the patient) and it had to operate on a nonprofit basis.[48]

By 1938, the AHA had approved sixty Blue Cross plans. The largest one operated in New York City with 800,000 subscribers. At the end of the decade, total enrollment in hospital prepayment plans numbered four million, or about 9 percent of the population; most members were enrolled through the workplace.[49] Blue Cross was a success, and membership would rise even more dramatically in the next decade.

Blue Cross's popularity was due to its affordability to both employers and individuals, and its attractive offer of protection against high hospital bills. But even early on, the plans showed clear limitations. In

1935, the members of FDR's Committee on Economic Security wrote that "obviously insurance against hospital bills alone, without inclusion of professional services and other sickness costs, is an incomplete and unsatisfactory provision against the risks and losses of illness.[50] In many states, thanks to pressure from state medical societies, hospital service plans were actually banned from offering physician coverage. Blue Cross members would come home from the hospital believing that both hospital and doctors' fees had been covered, only to find a large bill for doctors' services. This led to numerous complaints and anger from the public.[51] In response, in 1939 the California Medical Association created a plan to cover doctors' fees, the California Physicians' Service. The coverage was indemnity only, and was limited to doctors' services in the hospital, not office visits. Similar plans, which came to be known as Blue Shield, sprang up across the country, all of them controlled by physicians and all of them limited to care in the hospital. Some employers began offering Blue Cross and Blue Shield together in their benefits packages.

Blue Cross and Blue Shield were controlled by the very providers whose services they covered. Their creation was both a response to the national discussion on health rights, and a way to forestall future reforms. As an alternative to national health insurance, the AMA cautiously endorsed Blue Cross plans following the National Health Conference of 1938. Blue Cross, Blue Shield, and other types of private health insurance would be bulwarks against government-controlled "socialized medicine" (see chapter 5).

With their limited benefits and provider control, Blue Cross plans were a far cry from the health rights demands of New Deal reformers and Depression-era protest movements. This new form of coverage was tied to employment (rationing by job status), covered hospital and doctors' bills separately (rationing by type of provider), and was not offered as a guaranteed right to anybody. By extending a limited form of medical coverage to millions for the first time, Blue Cross became an effective argument for voluntary, private solutions to the nation's health care crisis.

FDR and Economic Rights

In his State of the Union address in January 1941, President Roosevelt proclaimed the famous "four freedoms" that should be enjoyed "everywhere in the world": freedom of speech and expression, freedom of worship, freedom from want, and freedom from fear. The speech did not refer specifically to health or health care, although "freedom from want" did include, according to Roosevelt, a "healthy peacetime life" for all.[52]

This was more than just powerful rhetoric from a President about to lead his country into war against threats to freedom. Roosevelt insisted on including these principles in the Atlantic Charter, the document he produced with British Prime Minister Winston Churchill to lay out aspirations for the postwar world. And on January 11, 1944, FDR proposed an Economic Bill of Rights, which outlined rights that, the president argued, would be essential in guaranteeing the Four Freedoms. In this address, he declared the following rights to be "self-evident": the right to a job, the right to adequate food and clothing, farmers' right to a fair price, the right to free trade, the right to a "decent home," and the right to a "good education." Two of the economic rights he listed specifically included health care: "The right to adequate protection from the economic fears of old age, sickness, accident, and unemployment," and "The right to adequate medical care and the opportunity to achieve and enjoy good health." FDR put a strongly American spin on these rights: economic security was required to ensure freedom. "True individual freedom cannot exist without economic security and independence," the president insisted.[53]

As World War II spread around the globe, the president announced his commitment to a list of economic rights that would ensure freedom both for Americans and for people around the world. But implementation of this new bill of rights, Roosevelt conceded, would have to wait until after the war was won.

PART II

Prosperity and Exclusion, 1941–64

CHAPTER THREE

Health Care at War

Like every other aspect of American society, health care was enlisted for the war effort. Despite the horrifying carnage of the conflict in Europe and the Pacific, medical and surgical breakthroughs made World War II the most survivable war ever for combatants. The American military threw its massive resources into the medical care of its armed services, and the government made new investments in health care for military families and civilian war workers. With the war effort encompassing all aspects of American life, it seemed like an ideal moment to expand access to health care for all. And access *was* expanded, but not in the ways reformers envisioned. With new government intervention came a renewed opposition to any type of health care not controlled by the medical profession and hospital industry. For this reason, many of the most successful public wartime health programs were discontinued after 1945.

Still, World War II marked a turning point for ideas about the right to health care. After struggling through a war to end tyranny and oppression, Americans became more aware of deep-seated inequalities at home. The 1948 United Nations Universal Declaration of Human Rights listed adequate medical care as a right of all people. Soldiers' and veterans' claims to medical care became widely acknowledged, and some became embodied in permanent changes to the health system. Even Americans who benefited only temporarily from wartime health programs, such as farmers, defense workers, and military families, emerged from the war with stronger ideas about the importance of health care in their own lives; many would no longer be content with haphazard access and poor quality. These changes, along with President Harry Truman's failed push for national health insurance, set the stage for the two massive transformations of the postwar health system: the dominance of the hospital, and the spread of private insurance. Neither hospitals nor private insurance plans acknowledged health care as a right, and in most ways (as chapters 4 and 5 will show) they explicitly denied such a right, while also creating new forms of rationing. The possibilities for rights that emerged from the war were almost completely repudiated by the end of the 1940s, as the medical system poised on the brink of its greatest expansion.

Despite the ongoing Depression, when war broke out in Europe in 1939, Americans were enjoying major improvements in health conditions. Between 1920 and 1940, average life expectancy had risen from 51 years to over 60. Infant mortality had been cut from 100 per 1,000 live births in 1915 to 47 per 1,000, and maternal mortality had been reduced by more than half.[1] Better sanitation and nutrition could take most of the credit, but medical advances were also starting to make a difference, particularly with the discovery of sulfa drugs to fight infection.

But there was a troubling side to this picture of progress. The death rates of American mothers and infants were still much higher than in some European nations. Improvements in sanitation had not reached all communities; some small towns in the mid-1940s still had open sewers running through the streets.[2] Farm families still came down with highly preventable and treatable diseases because they couldn't reach a doctor in time.[3]

Because of the uneven distribution of medical care, much of the new medical progress simply was not available to people who could not afford doctors' visits, drugs, or transportation to a hospital. Patients died of newly treatable diseases because they lacked access to the treatment. Rural social workers reported cases like that of the 17-year-old son of a Missouri farmer, who was diagnosed with diabetes and anemia. "Insulin and a special diet were recommended. But how could they obtain these on the limited funds allotted the family . . . In two years the son died."[4] And although mortality had improved for all races, black Americans continued to experience death rates on average 60 percent higher than whites.[5]

Health and Medicine in Wartime

Wars have always been catalysts for transformations in health and medicine. World War II, the deadliest war in history, also came at a time of great medical advances. It used to be that microbes, not weapons, were the greatest killers in war; World War II was the first in which military deaths from combat exceeded deaths from disease. For the first time, physicians could not only identify the cause of diseases, but also prevent and treat them. Vaccination prevented typhoid, measles, and other scourges that had killed thousands of soldiers in previous wars. Spectacular progress in surgery meant that more wounded men survived than ever before.[6] Most dramatically of all, sulfa drugs and penicillin attacked and could even eliminate the killing infections that usually accompanied war injuries. But medical advances were slower to cross over to civilian care back home. Scientists rushed to mass-produce penicillin, but it did not become widely available to the public until after the war.

At first, war did more to unmask existing health problems in the US population than to address them. The entire nation was scandalized when the military draft uncovered shockingly bad health conditions among the nation's young men. By 1944, "more than 40 percent of the registrants were rejected as physically or mentally unfit." The biggest problems reported among recruits were venereal disease, tuberculosis, hernias, poor teeth, and "mental diseases."[7] The revelations of draftees' poor health led to an outcry. "5 Million Are Unfit for War," screamed a 1944 New York Times headline.[8] This revelation "removed any fond complacency we have had about the nation's health." Senator Claude Pepper of Florida convened hearings to uncover the causes of this national disgrace. Because so many unmarried young men were found physically or mentally unfit, "foreigners, scientists, students, and fathers of children had to be called upon for service." Venereal disease was so prevalent that the Army could no longer afford to reject all such cases and began to offer recruits treatment instead.[9]

The problem needed both an immediate and a long-term solution. President Roosevelt's suggestion for a massive health rehabilitation program for soldiers was scuttled after Pearl Harbor. Instead, the Selective Service created "prehabilitation," requiring inductees to see a local doctor and correct any defects before their military exam.[10] Health reformers raised the bar, declaring that draft rejections were a product of the country's failure to create a national health system. On the first day of the Pepper hearings, some medical experts called for a "concerted effort to use the information and experience of Selective Service examiners to prepare a national program of health for the future."[11] Most of the press and official commentary on the issue took for granted that some form of national health care would be a result of these wartime revelations, but figuring out exactly how to do it would have to wait until the war was over. In the meantime, soldiers and civilians had to be kept alive and healthy for the duration.

War made health more important than ever. Not only did effective fighting men have to be disease-free for the battlefield; civilian health also became crucial to the war effort. As one Harvard Medical School professor pointed out, "the armed forces must continually be replenished as the struggle proceeds," and workers in war industries had to be healthy to face "harder work and longer hours."[12]

But improving and even maintaining health standards would be difficult in the face of heavy new demands on the medical system. Military families and war workers flocked to communities that simply could not accommodate the health needs of thousands of new residents. Phoenix, Arizona, had 365 hospital beds for its 50,000 residents; during the war, its population swelled to 140,000. Wartime residents recalled how "ambulances and police cars with sirens wailing, roamed in vain through the night from hospital to hospital."[13] Los Angeles had to absorb 6,000 new people a month in 1943 because of its huge concentration of war industries, leading to a "critical" hospital shortage. The *Los Angeles Times* reported that city hospitals turned away 1,000 people in a two-month period. Not only was the situation dire for the sick, but "in the event of a bombing or other attack on Southern California," warned Mayor Fletcher Bowron, "there would be much suffering and loss of life because of this lack of facilities."[14]

In 1943, the *New Republic* magazine reported on devastating medical problems in war production areas with their "mushroom trailer camps and squalid shanty towns."[15] Military camps were opening in communities with no public health facilities, including "a Florida camp located in a county which does not have a single health officer . . . a Georgia camp occupying parts of three counties, none of which ever had a full-time health department, and . . . a camp in the midst of Louisiana malarial swamps."[16] Gibson General Hospital, in Coffee County, Alabama, had a voluntary hospital of 44 beds, previously sufficient, but had to ask the US Public Health Service for a new wing. "Most of the increased demand is from industrial accidents at Camp Rucker," reported the hospital administrator.[17]

Even areas that did not experience population growth faced new health care shortages as thousands of physicians and nurses entered the military. By 1942, more than 41,000 of the nation's 120,000 eligible physicians had joined the armed forces.[18] The "grab anything" recruitment policy (as the *New Republic* described it) decimated the ranks of civilian doctors, including even pediatricians and obstetricians.[19] A Senate manpower subcommittee warned of the dangers of "doctor

famines" to civilian areas. It described the military's recruitment policy
as "hoarding . . . unused doctors" and noted that underserved rural
areas were "contributing twice and sometimes four times their quotas
of doctors as cities, so that some counties in Southern States now have
only a single doctor for 7,000 persons."[20] Concerned primarily with
civilian health, the federal Children's Bureau questioned why the army
needed 45,000 medical officers. The disparity between civilian and
military nurses was just as severe; "six nurses per 1,000 men is a little
extravagant in view of the [civilian] nursing shortage," complained the
Bureau. Many nurses had been taken by war industries as well as the
military—not surprising, since both paid better than traditional nursing salaries.[21]

Although the public as well as the military enthusiastically endorsed
the improved care given to fighting men, there was still concern that
while soldiers were now getting the best care and the most doctors
and nurses, Americans on the home front were left wanting. The *Ladies Home Journal* reported that during the first three years of the war,
the state of Mississippi lost 3,000 men on the battlefront, but on the
home front in this same period, it lost "8,397 infants and 774 mothers."[22] By 1943, Chicago hospitals were operating with only 57 percent
of their usual medical and surgical staff levels, and the loss of interns
and residents to the military created a "serious shortage on emergency
staffs."[23]

In 1943, the *New Republic* went so far as to argue that this neglect
of civilian health "threatens the entire . . . war effort."[24] Others saw
the shortage as simply part of the sacrifice of wartime. "You can help
the war effort by conserving medical and nursing care," the magazine
American Home advised readers in 1943. Doctors, "forced by the present
emergency to carry three practices," could be helped by patients who
scrupulously followed their orders. To address the nursing shortage,
the magazine also suggested that parents encourage their daughters
to attend nursing school.[25] The Chicago chapter of the American Red
Cross began holding classes on home nursing for women, emphasizing
"the importance of home nursing knowledge, now that both nurses
and doctors are going by thousands into the fighting services."[26] Doctors who were older or otherwise ineligible for military service "these
days are not only working overtime," according to a 1943 report by the
Office of War Information, "they are—most of them—working practically all the time and in total disregard of their own health."[27]

The loss of medical personnel fell harder on the populations that already lacked good care. In the South, black doctors and nurses were supposed to treat only black patients (and in some Northern institutions as well, including Veterans Administration hospitals).[28] Early in the war, many black physicians were not allowed into the commissioned service and instead were drafted as "buck privates"; "frequently a small town was drained of its only Negro physician." Under pressure from an advisory committee that included African American physicians, the government agreed to stop drafting black MDs from rural areas with the greatest need and to offer a few more commissions to black doctors, assuring some maintenance of medical care for black Americans while also continuing Jim Crow in the armed forces.[29]

When it came to losing doctors and nurses, the public's tolerance of wartime health care rationing sometimes wore thin. One man wrote to the *Chicago Daily Tribune* that the drafting of medical personnel "will be a serious handicap to our hospitals and also deprive the public of needed physicians when so many doctors from private practice are taken by the army."[30] At the same time that wartime medicine offered its promise to all, the shortages continued to send the message that medical progress would not be distributed equally.

Government Health Programs during Wartime

The war emergency gave the US government an opportunity to expand its role in health services while avoiding accusations of socialism or foreign influence. Healthy soldiers and citizens, after all, were crucial to the war effort. Some World War II health programs had the potential to form the basis of a national health program or more generally expanded health services. But only one of the experimental federal programs—hospital finance and construction—continued after the war's end. The war presented a variety of promising options, from medical cooperatives to comprehensive maternal and child health care, but in the end only the voluntary hospital and employer-based health insurance emerged triumphant. The story of Americans' experiences with the new programs, and government's role and responses, helps explain the limitations of wartime health reform.

The war not only brought old health concerns to light; it created new ones. New problems included epidemics and shortages in the rapidly growing areas around military bases, and the problems of soldiers' families left behind. To address conditions in the overcrowded defense towns, the US Public Health Service (PHS) received major budget increases during the war, from $19.5 million in 1940 to $108 million in 1944, and grew from 9,592 to 16,000 employees. In response to concerns about wartime epidemics, the agency expanded its venereal disease programs and initiated rat control and mosquito abatement in military camps to control typhus and malaria. Tuberculosis was of particular concern in wartime, since migration and crowding made its spread more likely, and the Public Health Service began offering TB exams to the war labor force. The extensive movement of people throughout the country during wartime required a larger role for the federal agency, as most migrant workers were not eligible for local public health services because of residency requirements.[31] But the war years offered no direct challenge to the historic separation between public health and medical services. Apart from a program that paid for medical treatment for US civilians evacuated from war zones (discussed below), the PHS's role remained confined to disease prevention and control rather than the provision of health services.

Concern over the nation's health extended to the White House. President Roosevelt created the Office of Scientific Research and Development to fight the "war of science against disease." The US Public Health Service had been involved in medical research since the nineteenth century, but this new office transformed and expanded the government's role to include funding private sector research. The results were spectacular, including the 1944 discovery of how to mass-produce penicillin.[32] The 1944 Public Health Service Act further increased federal commitments to medical research, and helped set the stage for the United States to become a scientific powerhouse after the war.

Roosevelt also took note of the crisis in the supply of doctors and delivery of medical care. In September 1941 he ordered the establishment of an Office of Defense Health and Welfare Services within the Federal Security Agency (the post–New Deal umbrella agency for health and welfare). The office ran the Procurement and Assignment Service for drafting doctors, as well as medical care programs for civilian defense workers and for American civilians injured overseas. "Total war means a war affecting civilians as well as the military," noted a Senate report. The most deserving civilians were those making major contributions to the war effort; their sacrifices were to be rewarded with access to health care. Defense workers and farm workers were seen as especially deserving. A Civilian War Benefits program reimbursed 400 civilian defense workers per month for medical treatment.[33] Although anti–New Deal conservatives in Congress cut the budget of the Farm Security Administration, they agreed to continue its medical care programs for migrant farm workers (described in chapter 2) as essential to the war effort.[34]

In 1943 President Roosevelt ordered the creation of a Civilian War Assistance program for US civilians being repatriated or evacuated from war zones. The program included an Emergency Medical Service, which offered medical care with no means test to returning civilians with war-related disease or injury, including the most "serious cases" which "have come from war-ridden areas and prolonged imprisonment in enemy concentration camps." The program also paid for the treatment of "repatriates financially unable to secure medical care for a condition developing subsequent to arrival in the US." Of the 11,500 repatriates and evacuees in 1945–46, a total of 16 percent received medical treatment under the program. Civilian War Assistance, long since forgotten, was the first federal disability program in the nation's history, before Social Security expanded to cover disability in 1956.[35]

All of these programs rationed services by applying only to civilians who were seen as especially deserving because of their contributions to the war effort. In addition, they were all temporary, for the duration only. The federal government's most lasting involvement in civilian health care during World War II was its hospital building program. In 1941 Congress passed the Lanham Act for the construction of "community facilities," including hospitals, "where the absence or inadequacy of such facilities would impede the war effort and where the community itself could not provide them without unreasonable financial burden." Financed and run by the Federal Works Agency, the Lanham Act carried on the public works tradition of the great New Deal programs, but with a new emphasis on hospitals. During the program's existence (1941 to 1946), $121 million in federal funds built 874 hospitals and "related projects."[36]

Although the program was temporary, it helped lay the groundwork for the 1946 Hill-Burton Hospital Survey and Construction Act (discussed in the next chapter), which built up the nation's hospital infrastructure enormously. Its ideological impact was significant; as historian Rosemary Stevens writes, "the Lanham Act established the important precedent of allowing federal aid to private nonprofit hospitals as well as local-government institutions."[37] Public funding for private entities would become a crucial component of the postwar US health system.

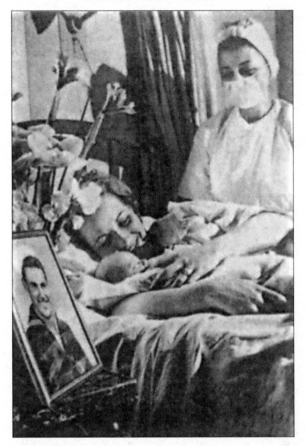

FIGURE 2. "Mrs. Mulligan and her Navy husband, John, do not have to worry about the high cost of parenthood. Under EMIC (Emergency Maternity and Infant Care), all medical bills for their new son, Robert Curtis, are paid by the government. 'I have had the best care,' she says." Photo by Ann Rosener-Fix. *Collier's*, August 4, 1945, 19.

"Uncle Sam Is My Baby's Godfather":
The Emergency Maternity and Infant Care Program

A newspaper photo shows a smiling woman who lovingly cradles her newborn baby under the protective watch of a masked and gowned nurse. Propped on the bedside table is a large framed photograph of a young man in a military uniform. "Mrs. Mulligan and her Navy husband, John, do not have to worry about the high cost of parenthood," states the caption, because "all medical bills for their new son, Robert Curtis, are paid by the government."[38]

In 1943, Congress created a large program to cover the medical costs of childbirth and infant care for families of servicemen in World War II. Described at the time as "the biggest public health experiment ever conducted in this country," the Emergency Maternity and Infant Care program was unique. "Never before has the government assumed responsibility for civilian medical care on so grand a scale. Never before have the nation's doctors agreed to participate in such a far-reaching program of 'government medicine,'" gushed *Collier's* magazine.[39] But, even though the program was a smashing success and popular with both participating doctors and their patients, hopes that it would form the basis for a comprehensive national health program ended when Congress let the program expire in 1947.

Although Title V of the Social Security Act had allocated funds for maternal and child health examinations and preventive services (totaling $5,820,000 in 1941), states could not use the grants to provide medical care to mothers or babies. Following US entry into the war in 1941, camp hospitals found themselves "overwhelmed with the problem of providing maternity services for the wives of servicemen."[40] All members of the military received medical care through the armed forces system, but the system made no provision for soldiers' dependents. Families received a cash allowance of only $50 a month. Pregnant wives, left behind as their husbands were shipped overseas, were a particularly vulnerable group. Because it was now possible to almost guarantee improved maternal and child health through good medical and hospital care, it seemed unfair for soldiers on the front to worry about their families lacking such care, or about medical bills when they returned.

Early in the war, 30 state health departments received permission to start small programs to pay for the medical care of pregnant wives and newborns of soldiers. These state programs reached about 6,000 women by 1943. Since the demand was estimated to be much greater, officials from the federal Children's Bureau argued that a national program was needed. Children's Bureau leaders Martha Eliot and Katherine Lenroot, pioneers in maternal and child health[41] and outspoken supporters of national health reform, saw in the war emergency an opportunity to expand the reach of maternal and child health care, and to allow the federal government to pay for direct health services.

The Children's Bureau called the program Emergency Maternity and Infant Care (EMIC), and requested congressional funding and authorization in 1943. It received almost unanimous support; what little Congressional opposition there was stemmed from the fear that EMIC might be a precursor for the national health insurance bill sponsored by Senator Robert Wagner. Even the AMA withdrew its initial opposition when it became clear that "the bill was wildly popular with Congress and the public."[42] Congress authorized $1,200,000 to meet existing requests from the states, and promised $6 million a year to continue "for the duration of the war and six months thereafter."[43] President Roosevelt then signed the bill into law.

Why were the President and Congress, normally opposed to national health insurance, so quick to support what was, in essence, a radical program for direct government payment for health services? Most observers attributed EMIC's success to the "emergency" nature of the program—emergency was in its very name, after all. Opponents of Wagner's bill were assured by the Children's Bureau that the program would end when the war ended. EMIC did not require a means test of income or any other restrictions on eligibility, with an important exception: families of soldiers in the top three pay grades of the military were excluded. Supporters pointed out that this was in itself an automatic means test (rationing by income). Even more important, lawmakers were told that EMIC was not a program of indigent care, but an "expression of gratitude" to soldiers on the front lines. After this point was made, "there were no further references by the members of Congress to a means test."[44] Reported Martha Eliot proudly, "The Congress has . . . made it clear that this is not a so-called 'charity' service, but that it is to be provided as the right of any wife of an enlisted man in the lower grades of the military."[45] There was also no residency requirement for the program—important since military families might have to move at short notice, and because pregnant wives whose husbands were overseas often moved from military bases back to their home towns to deliver their babies.

EMIC was immediately popular. The Children's Bureau publicized the program effectively, placing articles in major women's magazines and slipping notices in servicemen's pay envelopes.[46] (By advertising to the soldiers as well as their wives, the Bureau emphasized that the program was for the morale of the men as much as for the health of the women.) The demand for EMIC's services far exceeded expectation, and the Children's Bureau had to go to Congress for more money. Katharine Lenroot, asking for $29 million for fiscal year 1944, explained that the Children's Bureau had calculated the costs of the program correctly but "we underestimated the number of mothers that would use it." Forty thousand women a month were receiving medical care through EMIC and, to the Bureau's delight, "about 85 percent of eligible women are applying for the service."[47]

Cards enclosed with the monthly allotment check sent to servicemen's wives advertised EMIC as a right to health care, regardless of income, race, or residency. "The care will cost you or your husband nothing," read the cards. "No questions are asked about your income. Your race or color does not matter. Nor does it matter how long you have lived at your present address. *The service of your husband to our country gives you and your baby the right to this care wherever it can be provided"* (emphasis added).[48] Maternity care at home was essential to victory abroad; as Lenroot put it, "There is one casualty which no responsible nation should ask a fighting man to face. The casualty is the preventable injury of his wife or child back home."[49]

National magazines and newspapers portrayed EMIC in glowing terms. The coverage especially emphasized the peace of mind brought to the serviceman and his family. "'Uncle Sam is going to be my baby's godfather,'" began a 1943 piece in the *New York Times*. "Though her husband is training at an Army camp 2,000 miles away, Mrs. Jones is knitting tiny garments almost as placidly as her grandmother did. The worry of financing a baby's arrival on a serviceman's dependency allowance of $50 a month is now lifted from her shoulders by the Federal Emergency Maternity and Infant Care program." Adding to her peace of mind was the simplicity of the paperwork required to enroll. In New York, "There are now more than a hundred places in the city where the wife of a serviceman can pick up an application blank for maternity aid. If she can't go there, she can request one by mail." And the application itself was easy to fill out.[50] "EMIC administrators do not stand on ceremony in the face of emergencies," reported *Collier's* magazine. "If a baby is sick, the mother may take him to any approved hospital immediately, without even waiting to fill out an EMIC application." The program would accept applications up to a week after the baby's admission to the hospital.[51]

Servicemen's wives appeared in the media as stoic, even heroic, bearing their babies as their men faced the gravest dangers. But pregnant women also had a keen interest in their new right to health coverage. A New York EMIC program director described a young woman who "looked at me calmly and said: 'I'm due in six weeks. My husband has been reported missing in action. Will the government still pay for my confinement?'"[52] The answer was yes, the government would pay. (Her husband, the paper reported, was later found.) EMIC coverage also continued after a soldier's discharge or separation from the military, as long as the child had been conceived during his enlistment.

Popular as the program was, tensions and controversies still emerged. The biggest obstacle to EMIC's success was a shortage of participating physicians, due both to the war and to doctors' reluctance to accept fees set by the government. A woman wrote to a *Chicago Daily Tribune* advice column, "My husband is a private in the army overseas, and I am expecting a baby in June. Our family doctor doesn't want to take care of me under the government plan, but indicates he is willing to care for me and put his bill on the shelf until my husband returns." The columnist replied that it was quite common for doctors to propose this option, "presumably because they did not feel the payment provided is adequate." Federal regulations said that practitioners under EMIC had to accept the fee set by the state ($50 in Illinois), and were forbidden to accept additional payments. "Service men's wives who are finding their doctors 'reluctant' to help them out" were advised to contact the Chicago Medical Society or their local medical society, which would put them in touch with doctors "willing to cooperate."[53] Difficulty finding a participating physician was the most commonly mentioned drawback of the EMIC program for women.[54]

Although the AMA had officially endorsed EMIC, the program's maximum fees violated the medical profession's fiercely defended control over fee setting. Doctors' groups preferred to have the government give servicemen's wives cash grants to pay a doctor of their choice, who would also be free to set any fee. But it was difficult for physicians to attack the program as socialistic when its intent was so solidly part of the war effort. The New Jersey Medical Society "registered objections" to EMIC for setting payment levels, but in a carefully calculated announcement its members offered to cut their own private fees 50 percent for servicemen's wives "in need" (which was also a repudiation of EMIC's lack of means testing).[55]

In a great blow to the Children's Bureau, the American Academy of Pediatrics made a highly publicized split with the agency in 1944. With EMIC, announced the Academy, the Children's Bureau had gone beyond its original mission and had become "an active factor in the practice of medicine throughout the United States, dictatorily regu-

lating fees and conditions of practice." The pediatricians demanded
that "all health activities" be taken from the Bureau and put under the
direction of the US Public Health Service, which was traditionally
more cooperative with the AMA.[56]

Supporters rushed to the defense of the Children's Bureau and the
EMIC program. A professor at Yale Medical School wrote the *Journal
of Pediatrics* to oppose his colleagues' condemnation of the Children's
Bureau, fearing that "the public may conceive of pediatricians as more
interested in preserving certain professional mores than in promoting the welfare of mothers and babies."[57] Martha Eliot defended the
Bureau's record, reminding physicians that maternal mortality rates
had been cut in half, and infant mortality had been cut by one-third,
since the creation of Title V's maternal and child health programs.[58]
The *New York Times* argued that the EMIC program actually served
doctors' professional interests, because it encouraged mothers to see
physicians rather than midwives.[59] Although they might recognize its
health benefits and its contribution to the war effort, organized physicians still saw EMIC as a threat on a par with the Sheppard Towner
Act twenty years earlier. "Many doctors who cheerfully accept EMIC
because there's a war on, would kick mightily if anybody attempted to
extend it after the war," noted *Collier's* magazine.[60]

No one really tried. EMIC ended on July 1, 1947. The program had
funded 1,203,500 births—at its height, one in every seven babies
born in the United States. It had paid $63,500,000 to hospitals and
$50,500,000 to doctors. Under EMIC, announced the Children's Bu-
reau, "an all-time record was set for hospital births in this country.
More than ninety-two out of a hundred babies born under the program in 1945 were born in hospitals." Only 68 percent of mothers had
hospital births before EMIC. "Many were from population groups that
ordinarily had their babies at home, and sometimes had not even a
doctor, but only an untrained midwife in attendance."[61]

Since even the most ambitious Children's Bureau leaders had always
described EMIC as temporary, the program ended without much fan-
fare or opposition. The rights enjoyed by soldiers' wives and families—
including freedom from a means test and the freedom to choose a
private doctor—quickly evaporated. The growing veterans' medical
system was designed to care for the men, not their families. Shortly after EMIC's demise, servicemen's pregnant wives were again dependent
on the military's limited health care options, and American mothers

were once again on their own when it came to paying for maternity care.

Eliot of the Children's Bureau attempted to continue EMIC's precedent by working with Senator Claude Pepper for a nationwide program of expanded maternal and child health.[62] However, postwar plans for national health insurance for working Americans quickly eclipsed this agenda. EMIC did create some permanent changes—most importantly, it put federal backing behind the move of childbirth from the home to the hospital. But EMIC's broad vision of a right to comprehensive health care for mothers and babies was cut short with the war's end. Once again, as with the Lanham Act, a government program's most powerful and lasting impact would be its encouragement of (increasingly expensive) hospital use, further convincing Americans that the private hospital was the most important institution in improving health.

World War II and the Right to Health Care

The war changed Americans' ideas about rights. The struggle against fascism abroad made injustice at home more difficult to accept. When African American soldiers returned from the fighting front and confronted segregation, their belief that they had won the right to full citizenship helped create the civil rights movement. Women of all colors continued to exercise their right to enter the paid workforce. And the powerful defense of individual rights was increasingly joined by claims for social and economic justice. As noted in chapter 2, President Franklin D. Roosevelt in his "Four Freedoms" speech included "Freedom from Want" alongside the traditional constitutional guarantees of freedom of speech, freedom of religion, and national defense. The full employment of the war era gave American workers new ideas about their rights on the job, and their right *to* a job.[63]

But what about health care? Did their World War II experiences encourage Americans to see health care as a new social right? Although the currents of the time inspired the dream of rights for all, wartime health programs did not. The new rights to health care these programs conferred were temporary and emphasized categorizing and separating rather than universal access. Beneficiaries' deservingness was always at issue, whether through military service or a means test. While Americans were so often united in the war effort, there was also tension between civilian and military rights and needs. This tension emerged clearly in the prioritization of military medical care over civilian services and the resulting doctor and nurse shortage. The expansion of rights for some always seemed to mean a loss of access for others. Although rarely labeled as such, rationing by various categories continued as the norm for the distribution of medical care.

Still, for those touched by wartime health programs, the World War II era changed expectations of what medical care could offer and who should have access to it. As health care analysts Herman and Anne Somers wrote, the war "put the vast armory of United States medical resources and skills at the disposal of the humblest Army private, while millions of military families and civilian war workers, for the first time in their lives, had access to good medical care on a non-charity basis and learned what it could mean to them."[64] An Army doctor, quoted in *Harper's*, remarked that the war had "shown our patients a different type of medical service. Twelve million men and women have been given medical care without direct cost to them . . ." While the sick civilian "not only loses his paycheck but has to pay doctors' fees and hospital bills as well . . . not so in the Army. No one hesitates to report in at sick call for minor ailments, thus averting serious complications. There are no doctors' fees, no hospitalization costs, and no interruption of income." The physician concluded that former members of the military "will demand that good medical care be available to everyone, regardless of economic position."[65] Even Americans not directly helped by wartime health programs were affected by them: the American Public Health Association believed in the case of EMIC that "many mothers whose husbands were not in service learned from EMIC patients what to expect in the way of good medical care . . . They learned for the first time what good health supervision and medical care for an infant really is."[66]

Wartime rights expansions led some people to expect that benefits should be continued after the war and extended to more people. Health care had been offered to servicemen, their wives and children, and veterans; one Virginia woman wanted to know in 1946 whether there was also "direct medical assistance from the government available to the *parents* of servicemen." (There was not.)[67] In a small poll conducted of EMIC mothers, a majority wanted to pay for their own medical care after the war, but 32 out of 40 answered yes when asked if a plan like EMIC should be continued in peacetime. "If you can't afford it, you are entitled to maternity care just as much as a serviceman's wife is," said one mother. Another argued, "The country should provide health care for all. Sickness happens in families, and all need health care."[68]

The wartime experience was also transformative for some physicians. Unlike in private practice, regular, salaried pay, more standardized schedules, and higher levels of organization were the norm for physicians in the military. According to one returning MD, these experiences led many younger doctors to consider group medical practice. "In such groups the doctor has security, regular hours, and the stimulus of criticism from his colleagues," Dr. John Gibbon wrote in *Harper's*. Since the war was over, "we doctors are regaining our individual freedom . . . But we are leaving the security of steady incomes with good hours and working conditions and the opportunity to practice medicine for medicine's sake unhampered by economic factors. And these are freedoms too."[69] An AMA poll taken during the war showed that a majority of military physicians wanted to go into group rather than solo practice on their return to civilian life.[70] But, however much military practice may have succeeded as an "experiment" in socialized medicine (as Gibbon described it), the AMA would continue to vigorously oppose organized medical practice under government sponsorship.

The great advances of wartime medicine led to new rights claims. For the first time in history, doctors could cure deadly infections. It now cost $5 to save the life of an adult using sulfa drugs, $2.50 for a baby or child, and "who dares tell the voters that $5 is too much to spend?" asked medical writer Paul de Kruif. "Here is the entering wedge that the people can use in their demand for a national health program." New York Mayor Fiorello LaGuardia, announcing that a city clinic would begin distributing free penicillin in 1944, "declared that every one had the right to medical care."[71]

Many of the public's expectations about greater access to the benefits of modern medicine would be addressed by the great postwar expansion of hospitals and health insurance. On one central count, however—a universal right to health care based on citizenship—there was only retreat. Every wartime expansion of rights was accompanied by the caveat that it was temporary and intended solely for victory or as a reward for military service. EMIC was not an entitlement of mothers but a nod to the sacrifice of soldiers. Postwar medical benefits were offered to military veterans (with strict eligibility rules) but not to their families or to civilian war workers. General Omar Bradley, head of the Veterans Administration, refused to support Truman's proposal for comprehensive national health insurance because he feared it would take resources away from programs solely for veterans.[72] Farm Security Administration clients were given care at migrant health clinics but, at the behest of the AMA, other community members were excluded. The farmers' medical cooperative, wrote *Chicago Defender* columnist Charley Cherokee, "was a form of group health but was never called that because money-mad doctors faint at the word . . . For poor Negro workers it was the one and only chance for medical care." Disregarding the pleas of supporters, in 1947 Congress eliminated the entire FSA medical program, along with EMIC.[73]

A right to medical care for honorably discharged military veterans, including veterans with non–service-related illness or disabilities, had been established in 1924 by the World War Veterans' Act. As part of the outpouring of thanks to returning veterans that included the G.I. Bill, after WWII Congress authorized funds to expand the Veterans' Administration (VA) medical system and improve its quality. The VA built new facilities, hired more doctors and nurses, and created formal affiliations between veterans' hospitals and medical schools throughout the country. By 1950, the VA operated 138 hospitals. Despite this, the emphasis on acute hospital care maintained the shortage of ambulatory (primary care) facilities, and many veterans lived too far from VA facilities to receive regular access to care.[74]

Even as wartime health programs were cut and dismantled, the concept of a right to health care still held a prominent new place in public debate. The phrase appeared everywhere in reformer and press discussions of health after the war. "Because the doctor's services are purchasable and yet almost beyond price," said Dr. Alan Gregg, Medical Director of the Rockefeller Foundation, in 1946, "they are coming to be regarded like life, liberty and the pursuit of happiness—a civic right, a public necessity."[75]

Some countries had already begun to put the principle of a right to medical care into practice. In 1944 Tommy Douglas was elected premier of Saskatchewan, Canada, on the promise of free health care for all, and began a program of hospital building and public hospital insurance in the province. In Britain, public sentiment in favor of government-guaranteed health services had been mounting since before the war. Polls showed large majorities favoring public-supported hospital facilities and physician practices, with "benefits to be obtained as a right and without a means test."[76] Britain's Beveridge Report, calling for a system of economic security for all citizens "from the cradle to the grave" (originally FDR's phrase!) made front page news in the United States. The *New York Times* noted that the Report "is the first program yet devised to turn 'freedom from want' from a phrase in the Atlantic Charter into a practical reality."[77]

Although he did not live to witness it, Franklin D. Roosevelt's declarations of economic and social rights would strongly influence postwar international agreements. The United States ratified the 1946 World Health Organization constitution, which included a statement of the "fundamental right" to the "highest attainable standard of health." Two years later, the United Nations General Assembly adopted the Universal Declaration of Human Rights, with its right to health language in Article 25: "Everyone has the right to a standard of living adequate for the health and well-being of himself and of his family, including food, clothing, housing and medical care and necessary social services, and the right to security in the event of . . . sickness."[78] The prominent place of economic and social rights in the UN Declaration was due in part to the participation of Eleanor Roosevelt, who insisted that her late husband's goal of "freedom from want" be included any document the UN produced. "Freedom without bread," she wrote in her daily newspaper column, "has little meaning."[79]

Although the drafters of the UN Declaration were in full agreement on the inclusion of economic and social rights, they bitterly split over how such aspirations could actually be put into practice by nations. On this issue, the United States would not take a leadership role. Eleanor Roosevelt announced that, although her country gave "wholehearted support" to economic and social rights, it did not agree to "an obligation on government to assure the enjoyment of these rights by direct government action."[80] While the United States signed the Declaration of Human Rights, it never ratified the later Covenant on Economic, Social, and Cultural Rights. Similarly, when the United States in 1948 joined the World Health Organization (WHO), which had also declared health care to be a right, Congress insisted that the United States would "in no way be committed to any legislative program approved by the WHO."[81]

It is impossible to say whether Franklin Roosevelt, had he lived, would have done more to transform the ideal of economic rights into a concrete reality. But Roosevelt's 1944 declaration of a right to adequate medical care clearly inspired his successor, Harry Truman, who would vigorously take up the cause of health care for all. As one of Truman's very first acts in office, he declared a right to health care and called for a national system of medical coverage.

Harry Truman's Campaign for National Health Insurance

During the war, discussion of universal health coverage had been kept alive in Congress mainly through the efforts of Senator Claude Pepper's Committee on Wartime Health and Education, which concluded in favor of a national insurance plan in 1943, and through the Wagner-Murray-Dingell bill for national insurance, also introduced in 1943. The American Medical Association was so alarmed by the bill that it opened its first Washington lobbying office that year. Once again without President Roosevelt's support, the Wagner-Murray-Dingell bill "went nowhere."[82]

After Roosevelt's death in 1945 and the Allied victory in World War II, President Harry Truman took a leading role in reviving the call for national health insurance. Unlike FDR, Truman did not have to be persuaded to see health care as a central component of social security. According to presidential historians David Blumenthal and James Morone, Truman's interest in health care dated back to several episodes in his career. As a soldier in the First World War, he was dismayed to see how many young men were rejected for service because of their poor health. As a county commissioner in Missouri, Truman saw families devastated by medical bills and people "turned away from the big hospitals in town to die, just because they did not have the money to get in." As a Senator during the Depression, he became deeply committed to the New Deal and the idea that government guarantees of protection against sickness and unemployment were "a basic right, an essential part of citizenship."[83] Truman's conviction that fairness should be a goal of government action appeared in the name he gave his domestic legislation proposals, the "Fair Deal."

One month after the Japanese surrender, Truman presented an ambitious plan for postwar reconstruction in a special message to Congress. He proposed an expansion of Social Security, a minimum wage raise, a program of full employment, a broad new housing program, and a comprehensive national health plan. In his message, Truman reaffirmed FDR's Economic Bill of Rights, including "The right to adequate medical care and the opportunity to achieve and enjoy good health." Two months later Truman again went to Congress and asked it to pass a national insurance plan and other health measures.[84] Opinion polls that year showed 75 percent of Americans in support of the idea of national health insurance.[85]

Health insurance was only part of Truman's comprehensive health plan, which also included hospital construction, public health expansion, and federal funding for medical training and research. Not surprisingly, national insurance proved to be the most controversial piece. In 1946, Truman's efforts on behalf of the reintroduced Wagner-Murray-Dingell bill, which would have added health insurance to the Social Security system, failed in the Republican Congress, although lawmakers did pass the Hill-Burton hospital construction act (see chapter 4).

But Truman refused to let the matter drop. During his famed 1948 "whistle stop" campaign tour, the President repeatedly hammered on the message of national health insurance. The Democrats regained control of Congress, and the newly elected Truman asked Oscar Ewing, head of the Federal Security Administration, to draft a comprehensive national health insurance proposal. Ewing's plan, like Wagner-Murray-Dingell, proposed a new payroll tax to add medical care insurance to Social Security.

In April 1949 Truman went before Congress to ask for adoption of the health bill. The President acknowledged that private health insurance was covering more Americans than ever before, but argued that it was incapable of meeting the medical needs of millions. Only universal national insurance, Truman told Congress, "will mean that proper medical care will be economically accessible to every one covered by it, in the country as well as in the city, *as a right and not as a medical dole*."[86]

But then, Truman suddenly fell silent on the issue. National health insurance faced the opposition not only of Congressional Republicans but also of Southern Democrats, who feared a universal bill would force racial desegregation on the South. With so many other divisive issues before him—from civil rights to accusations of Communist infiltration in his own administration to a looming war in Korea—Truman relinquished the lead in the fight for health insurance. Without vocal support from the President, lobbying and publicity on behalf of the bill fell to a citizens' organization, the Committee for the Nation's Health (CNH), founded in 1946 by longtime health reformer Michael M. Davis. The CNH included such luminaries as former first lady Eleanor Roosevelt, philanthropist and public health advocate Mary Lasker, liberal businessman Gerard Swope (former president of General Electric), William Green of the American Federation of Labor, and Channing Frothingham, twice president of Massachusetts State Medical Society. Although seeming to represent business, labor, and the medical profession, the group really functioned as a committee of experts and made no effort to mobilize broad support among their constituencies or the wider public. As historian Alan Derickson points out, even the labor participation in the Committee was confined to top officials who did nothing to include the voices of the rank and file.[87]

Opponents of Truman's proposal were far more organized, well-funded, and ruthless than its supporters, and they had a strategy to mobilize grassroots support. Following Truman's election in 1948, the American Medical Association led a blitz against the national health proposal that was unprecedented in the history of lobbying. The AMA assessed $25 from each of its members to create a war chest in opposition to the president's plan. The physicians' organization then hired a public relations firm, Whitaker and Baxter of Los Angeles, to mount a national campaign against health care reform. Posters of a famous painting depicting a doctor at the bedside of a child were emblazoned with the slogan "Keep Politics Out of This Picture" and displayed in 65,000 physicians' waiting rooms around the country. The AMA led coordinated campaigns of letter and editorial writing to local newspapers—highly effective since many physicians knew the editors personally.[88]

Opponents' objections to Truman's plans rang familiar: national insurance would involve too much government control, destroy physicians' autonomy, and erode the quality of American medical care. Again, the specter of socialism was invoked, and opponents relentlessly labeled the plan Soviet-style "socialized medicine," despite Truman's insistence that it was nothing of the sort. Accusations of socialism or foreign influence went back to the very earliest days of health insurance debates in the United States, but in the context of the early Cold War they took on an even more menacing tone. Conservative Senator Robert Taft called national health insurance "the most socialistic measure that this Congress has ever had before it." Taft proposed his own health program that consisted of federal subsidies for private insurance companies to cover the indigent.[89] Dr. Edward H. Cary, chairman of the National Physicians Committee, called national health insurance "a dangerous move to foist an alien and collectivist mechanism on the people of this country."[90] Although it is difficult to measure the effect of this Cold War rhetoric on the public's perception of health reform, it undoubtedly served to sow confusion and distrust of the measure and to wear down supporters, and perhaps contributed to Truman's reluctance to advocate vocally for his proposal.

Opposition to Truman's plan was not just ideological but also economic. Physicians' incomes, which had risen dramatically during and since the war,[91] were under threat, opponents insisted. The anti-insurance forces emphasized the new taxes the plan would impose. Dr. Ernest E. Irons, president of the AMA, warned, "When the American citizen learns that the regimentation of war, to which he willingly acquiesced as a patriotic duty, is to be renewed and extended in peace time by a compulsory tax to pay for something he does not want, he will assert his own right to choose his doctor and his medical service."[92] A "Laborer," in a letter to the *Chicago Tribune*, complained that "you'll pay that [payroll tax], regardless of your probability of sickness; regardless of the size of your family, and you'll pay from now on," as opposed to the current system under which "I'm still a free man, can choose my doctor, and can carry insurance if I like when I need it most."[93]

Public opinion in favor of national health insurance dropped dramatically, from 75 percent in 1945 to only 21 percent in 1949.[94] The AMA's well-financed and carefully orchestrated campaign against Truman's plan undoubtedly played a major role. But the poll numbers are also hard to separate from Truman's disastrously declining popularity overall, due to foreign policy debacles in China and Korea, massive labor strikes at home, and the backlash against the New Deal. Democrats lost six Senate seats in the 1950 election, primarily because of the AMA's campaign to target Senators who supported national insurance. Truman also faced the enmity of Southerners in his own party who were furious at the President's support for modest civil rights legislation. It may be that Truman's failure to speak out in favor of the bill or to mobilize more supporters played a role in its defeat,[95] but his unpopularity was so great that presidential backing might not have helped. When Truman, who claimed to hate being President, declined to run for reelection in 1952, national health insurance fell by the wayside once again.[96]

World War II opened up new opportunities for expanded health care rights. Military medical care, the Emergency Maternity and Infant Care program, and hospital and public health expansion touched millions of lives during the war, and could have laid the foundation for more universal programs afterward. International declarations and postwar governments in Europe and Canada set the stage for implementing rights to medical care. When Harry Truman introduced his health insurance plan to the American public, he pitched the program as part of postwar reconstruction, arguing both that universal health protection was essential for the nation's economic security and prosperity, and that medical care was a right belonging to all Americans. But by 1950, visions of universal access to health care had been shut down. Programs that during the war had promised new rights, such as EMIC and the FSA cooperatives, were cancelled. The United States would not agree to implement the social and economic rights of the Universal Declaration. And, of course, Truman's national health insurance plan landed on the trash heap. All of these programs were repeatedly labeled socialistic and alien by influential opponents in and out of Congress.

This was more than just a political defeat for the right to health care. In Congress, and within the health care system itself, ideas about universal rights were pushed back in favor of the ideology and practices of US-style rationing. The system continued to separate and categorize people on the basis of race, income, region, military status, health condition, and many other factors. As the following chapters will show, the postwar health care system grew tremendously while maintaining traditional practices of rationing and creating new ones. Hospitals and private health insurance would bring more and better health care to more Americans than ever before, but their benefits would not be provided to all, nor would they be provided as a matter of right.

CHAPTER FOUR

Rights to Refuse: The Triumph of the Hospital

On a wet and cold February day in 1929, a car screeched to a halt in front of Baptist Hospital in Birmingham, Alabama. In the back seat, two-year-old Geraldine Crews lay coughing and gasping for breath. Her father, Earl, wrapped her in his arms and sprinted through the cold rain toward the door marked "Emergency." A nurse took one look at the child's blue lips and called for a doctor to administer diphtheria antitoxin. Diphtheria, a deadly childhood sickness, kills its victims with a poison secreted by the bacteria. The antitoxin can save a life if given in time.[1] Geraldine immediately received an injection of the drug, and somebody placed an oxygen mask on her face for a few moments. But then, the doctor turned to her father and told him to take her home. Birmingham Baptist, he explained, did not accept cases of contagious disease. Earl Crews obeyed the physician's orders, put his little girl back into the car, and drove as fast as he could through the pouring rain. Fifteen minutes after they arrived back home, Geraldine died.

The ejection of a dying child from the emergency ward was not a common occurrence at Birmingham Baptist Hospital, at least according to the nurse who was there and saw it happen. When called to testify in the wrongful death lawsuit brought by Earl Crews, the nurse burst out, "I was at the hospital for three years [and] I never did see any two and a half year old baby given forty thousand units of diphtheria serum or any other serum and oxygen, and five minutes afterward taken out and put in an automobile and in the wet and cold sent home, when they were in the serious condition that I saw that child in."[2] A Birmingham jury agreed with the nurse and the Crews family that the hospital was negligent when its physician discontinued treatment. But when the case reached the state supreme court in 1934, the Alabama justices ruled that not only was the hospital not violating any law when it sent Geraldine home, but that private hospitals had no obligation to

admit anyone, ever. In the words of the Court, "Private hospital owed
public no duty to accept any patient not desired by hospital, and was
not required to assign reason for refusal to accept."[3] Hospitals' right to
refuse patients even in an emergency, sometimes called the "no duty"
rule, would be upheld by state courts nationwide until the 1960s.

The right to refuse remained in place even as the hospital system
underwent a complete transformation after World War II. In 1946,
the federal government embarked on a massive expansion of the nation's hospitals. Thanks to the Hill-Burton Act, billions in taxpayer
dollars were used to build the world's most modern health care system,
putting a hospital in nearly every community and bringing hospital
care within the reach of more Americans than ever before. But, as the
persistence of the "no duty" rule shows, patients' legal rights to care
did not keep pace with the health care system's growing technical and
medical capacity. In fact, lawmakers and hospital and medical leaders
worked to make sure that the system's expansion did not lead to an
official, universal right to access.

The Hill-Burton Act came about because of a powerful alliance between the hospital and medical lobbies and sympathetic politicians.
This alliance ensured that control of hospital activities remained in
private hands even as the Act increased the flow of taxpayer dollars
into the system. Private, local control meant that a federally subsidized
hospital system would not lead to a right to hospital care.

The legislation required hospitals to offer some charity care and to
provide services to all, but in practice, local control meant that both
of these requirements could be given short shrift or defied altogether.
Most starkly, Hill-Burton left intact and actually expanded the racial
segregation of hospital care in the South. Later, in the 1960s and '70s,
Hill-Burton would be used to push for hospital desegregation and ensure some care for the indigent. But through two decades and billions
in taxpayer dollars, American hospitals successfully resisted increased
government control, maintained racial segregation, and limited charity care.

Hill-Burton both expanded and restricted access in other ways as
well. The law represented the federal government's support of the
shift from doctor's office to hospital. The choice to centralize medical care in the hospital made health care more expensive. Hospitals
were—and still are—the most costly part of the health care system,
with huge requirements for resources, facilities, technology, and labor.
Before Hill-Burton, the largest part of national health expenditures

went to physicians; after Hill-Burton, hospitals took the biggest slice of the spending pie. Hill-Burton's emphasis on hospitals overshadowed potentially cheaper and more comprehensive alternatives, such as local health clinics, expanded primary care, home care, prevention, and public health activities.

Finally, hospital expansion represented the ultimate repudiation of government control because it offered a political alternative to national health insurance. Hospital expansion was the only part of Truman's national health program approved by Republicans and Southern Democrats. Truman's opponents knew that they had to do something about health care, and hospital expansion was ideologically and politically palatable to them. Other opponents of Truman's comprehensive plan, including the American Medical Association, also approved of hospital construction using taxpayer dollars.

The hospital boom greatly expanded hospital care, but not citizens' right to receive it. Other countries that built up their hospital systems after World War II created national health programs to help citizens pay for hospital care, but in the United States, hospital expansion actually served as a barrier to more comprehensive health reform.[4] Hill-Burton's funding of segregated hospitals meant that rationing by race was sanctioned by the federal government. The program's weak requirements for free care ensured the continuance of rationing by ability to pay. Hospitals' right to choose and to turn away patients, affirmed by common law in *Birmingham Baptist Hospital v. Crews*, was reaffirmed by Hill-Burton's insistence on private, local control of hospitals even as the federal taxpayer dollars flowed. The result was an immense, prosperous hospital system, reaching more Americans than ever before, extending the benefits of modern medical science to areas previously underserved—but with exclusion and rationing built in, and rights to access kept out.

Hill-Burton and the Hospital Boom

At the end of World War II, the hospital was a very different institution than it had been at the beginning of the twentieth century. Once seen as houses of death, hospitals had been transformed into centers for new technologies and lifesaving treatments. Spectacular wartime advances in surgery and the discovery of antibiotics made millions aware of the new possibilities of modern medicine, possibilities that, it increasingly seemed, could be realized only in the hospital.

Hospitals boomed amid the nation's postwar mood of hope and

unlimited possibilities. The United States had emerged from the war militarily triumphant and economically prosperous. Thanks in part to federal investment in scientific research, for the first time in its history the United States had surpassed Europe as the leading center of medical innovation and progress.[5] The baby boomers were born in hospitals, and a new generation of Americans was introduced to the institution and became newly aware of its importance. And, Americans were increasingly able to pay for hospital care, because of both increased general prosperity and the rise of Blue Cross hospital payment plans.

In the mid-1940s, discussion in popular and medical literature simply assumed that more hospitals equaled better health. Americans were "borne along on a wave of optimism as to what science could do," as historian Rosemary Stevens writes, and they "looked to doctors and hospitals increasingly (and often unrealistically) for instant cures for all conditions."[6] Hospitals, "Our Forts Against Disease,"[7] represented the future. The American romance with the hospital was partly a product of the undeniable medical progress it represented, but its almost complete triumph over other alternatives also resulted from deliberate political choices made by private and public actors.

The first step in achieving hospital expansion was the widespread acknowledgment of a hospital shortage. Hill-Burton's supporters argued that the hospital was the weak link in US health care. The Depression had slowed hospital construction to an almost complete halt. Despite some building under the Lanham Act during the war, in 1945 forty percent of US counties, with some 15 million residents, had no hospital at all.[8] Lack of hospitals meant a lack of medical care in general. The hospital shortage was inextricably connected to the physician shortage in the countryside because doctors now felt that "X-ray, radium and expensively equipped laboratories are essential to good practice." Younger MDs who hailed from rural areas could not be persuaded to return to their home towns to practice because of the lack of hospital facilities.[9]

The *Ladies' Home Journal* reminded the public that the hospital shortage could lead to personal tragedy. "Perhaps you belong in one of the thousands of communities where 'If only we had a hospital . . .' is an oft-spoken wish, Or perhaps you're in a family where, 'If the hospital hadn't been so far away . . .' brings bitter memory of tragedy that might have been avoided."[10] "In a nation where there is a supermarket on almost every other corner and many villages boast an airport,

15,000,000 people are too far away from hospitals for real health and safety," the magazine reported in 1947. Not only were there too few hospitals, but "a shocking majority of existing hospitals are antiquated in design, constructed with inadequate fire protection, and pitiably short of beds." One hospital in Mississippi had cots "lined head to foot down corridors, in sun parlors, three beds in a room meant for one, jammed so closely together a nurse can hardly squeeze through," and trauma patients were forced to wait three days for a hospital bed.[11]

Newspaper and magazine coverage of health issues during the mid-1940s simply equated health with hospitals. Typical was language in *Collier's* magazine: "It seems obvious that until we can get the whole country properly equipped with hospitals, and the clinics that go with them, we shall not have all the necessary bases from which to wage all-out war on disease and ignorance about matters medical."[12] Nowhere was a systematic attempt made to connect hospital facilities with health outcomes; as sociologist Paul Starr writes, the benefits of hospital expansion were considered "too obvious to establish."[13] The *Illinois Medical Journal* pointed out that the Illinois counties lacking hospitals were the same ones with "the highest death and morbidity rates from controllable causes," but this was a correlation always assumed, never tested.[14] An Alabama doctor wrote to Senator Lister Hill that in his poor rural district "50% of our children are under nourished. This under nourished condition lowers resistive force and renders them susceptible to any disease that lurks around." The solution to what sounded like a nutrition crisis? "I think there should be a hospital located in every Congressional district of the state, equipped with Doctors, nurses, and ambulances."[15]

There may have been good (if unproven) medical reasons for wanting more hospital care, but there were political reasons as well. The hospital lobby and other opponents of national health insurance led the successful charge to define the private or voluntary hospital as the sole arena for expanding health spending. Voluntary hospitals, the American Hospital Association (AHA) exhorted, provided "a quality of service higher than ever attained in a nation with a compulsory insurance program."[16]

In 1944 AHA executive secretary George Bugbee assembled a Commission on Hospital Care, funded in part by the W. K. Kellogg Foundation, the Commonwealth Fund, and the US Public Health Service, to study the nationwide need for hospitals.[17] Bugbee also registered in Washington as a lobbyist to push the AHA's plan for hospital expansion, and quickly enlisted the support of the two Senators from Ohio, Harold Burton and Robert Taft. Burton was already well acquainted with Bugbee, who had been a hospital administrator in Cleveland, and Taft, a powerful senator known as "Mr. Republican," was eager for legislation to circumvent calls for compulsory health insurance. Taft was also planning his own run for the Presidency—"I need a health bill," he told Bugbee—and hospital construction suited him perfectly.[18] On the other side of the aisle, Alabama Senator Lister Hill led the Democratic support for hospital expansion, and a bipartisan bill, now named the Hill-Burton Hospital Survey and Construction Act, was passed by the US Senate in December 1945 and the House in July 1946.[19]

The Hill-Burton Act provided federal funds for states to survey their hospital facilities and to determine how far they fell short of the goal of 4.5 general hospital beds per 1,000 persons. (This figure was originally intended to be a ceiling, but then, as Paul Starr notes, it became a target.[20]) Spurred by Lister Hill, Congress's formula for allocating federal funds ensured a large amount of hospital construction in rural areas by allowing a higher bed ratio per person in "sparsely populated states."[21] This ended up, as Hill intended, disproportionately benefiting the South. The legislation also required localities to provide two-thirds of the financing, raising the possibility that the program might assist primarily wealthier communities, even within the poorer states.[22]

The legislation did include some attention to public health. The nation's public health infrastructure was even more inadequate than the hospital system; experts estimated that less than 10 percent of local public health departments had sufficient facilities. The Hill-Burton bill proposed one public health center to centralize public health activities for every 30,000 people. Not surprisingly, such centers could be located in hospitals. The bill also provided for specialized beds for tuberculosis, mental health, and chronic disease hospitals, and included significant aid for public, government-run hospitals.[23]

The hospital lobby deftly navigated the contradictions between voluntarism and massive federal aid; after all, for decades they had focused on retaining private control while winning government funds. As one hospital administrator had said back in the Depression, "If we welcome governmental assistance to aid us in rendering help, but never permit Government to control us, then we can be assured that the voluntary hospital will go on to do even bigger things than it is doing today."[24] Hill-Burton made specific provision for government dollars without government control. Section 203(c) stipulated that "no department or agency of the United States shall exercise any supervision or control over any hospital or other place for care of the sick" receiving government funds, nor "affect its administration, personnel, or operation."[25] This pleased not just the hospital industry but also the American Medical Association, which backed Hill-Burton while vigorously opposing Truman's more comprehensive national health plan. George Bugbee also recalled convincing the AMA leadership to "reluctantly" support hospital construction legislation because "they had been so against everything that they essentially said they needed something to be for."[26]

Stones, Not Bread: A Defeat for Critics and Alternatives

Hill-Burton was a juggernaut, seemingly bulletproof. How could anyone be against hospitals? Opponents of Truman's national health program backed the Hill-Burton Act because it tackled health care shortages without inviting government intervention, and national insurance advocates also supported it because they had included hospital construction as a plank in the reform platform as far back as 1938. Criticisms of the hospital that are common today—its high costs, its focus on technology over people—were yet to emerge. Still, a few dissenting voices spoke out. The Children's Bureau's Edith Abbott had pointed out in 1940 that "Hospitals Are Not a Health Program." Questioning FDR's modest hospital construction initiative, Abbott had cried, "we are to have . . . not a health program but a series of hospital shells. . . . Mr. President, we asked for bread and you are giving us stones!"[27]

A few critics noted that too many hospitals could be almost as bad as too few, and that hospital funding without national planning or oversight might lead to "the irresponsible building of hospitals" (which later in the century would be called "overcapacity"). The *Atlantic Monthly* magazine cited one such example, in which a hospital built a brand new obstetrics wing while several other hospitals in the same town were closing obstetrical units due to lack of demand.[28] The absence of overall planning in the Hill-Burton Act fit with the tradition of haphazard rationing in the United States.

Even fewer questioned the assumption that hospitals equaled better health. There was little attention paid to the quite common phenomenon of hospital-based illness. Epidemic diarrhea, for example, had killed 800 newborn babies in New York City hospitals in a twelve-year period, and in 1946 New York's Commissioner of Health warned that increasing institutional care could exacerbate "certain of the infectious diseases, which may become acute problems in hospitals."[29] But the possibility that hospitals could spread as well as cure disease was never mentioned in the press coverage or in congressional testimony on the Hill-Burton law.

A few others echoed Edith Abbott's concern that hospital construction created new facilities without creating new ways for people to get access to them. Senator James Murray of Montana, cosponsor of the Wagner-Murray-Dingell national insurance bill, argued that Hill-Burton was of only "limited value" without a comprehensive plan for paying hospital and medical costs; hospital expansion could not succeed with lack of provision for "care of needy persons" and lack of insurance for hospital care.[30] In Marin County, California, where locals grew angry over the high fees charged at the new Hill-Burton hospital, one "disgruntled taxpayer" was quoted as saying, "Well, it's nice to have plenty of hospital beds even if we can't afford to use them."[31]

Hill-Burton's adoption was a victory for the narrowest possible definition of medical care—temporary residential care for acute conditions. The legislation did not address contemporary calls for an expansion of the hospital's role into preventive medicine or home care.[32] Some public health advocates were disappointed that Hill-Burton reinforced the "unnatural and undesirable" separation of preventive and curative medicine. "Unfortunately," complained New York's public health commissioner, "relatively few hospitals have assumed any great social responsibilities to the community, at least in the field of preventive medicine. We are wasting time, effort and money when we devote our entire energies to the care of the sick to the exclusion of all preventive activities."[33] Although nursing and medical care in the home reportedly cost only one-fourth as much as a hospital bed, and experimental home care programs were widely applauded, Hill-Burton did not include funding for this option.[34]

The Hill-Burton legislation won the support of private interests when its sponsors agreed to allow federal funding to hospitals without federal control. While the physician and hospital associations praised this aspect the most, critics warned that a lack of government oversight could create new problems. Senator Murray argued against giving so much authority to the states in constructing taxpayer-funded hospitals. "Everything essential to assure wise use of Federal funds is left to the States," said Murray. "This is a dangerous and unwise proposal, considering how inadequate—and, in many cases, nonexistent—State control of hospitals has been in the past."[35] A *Washington Post* columnist criticized Hill-Burton as "private" legislation that would put millions in federal dollars under the control of the "hospital crowd."[36]

The program provided buildings and facilities but not the personnel to staff them. Supporters argued that new hospitals would attract physicians or keep them in rural areas, but the law did nothing to distribute practitioners or address specific manpower shortages. This was to ensure the support of the medical profession, which did not want government having any authority over the supply of doctors. Critics faulted Hill-Burton for this omission, arguing that "it does not go far enough" to ensure an adequate distribution of physicians.[37] Given Hill-Burton's failure to address access, American Federation of Labor leader Matthew Woll, who was a member of the Commission on Hospital Care, approved of hospital construction but concluded that support for compulsory national insurance was "the more advanced position" when it came to improving the nation's health care system.[38]

Hospital Care for the Poor: Required or Optional?

Through Hill-Burton, states were supposed to be able to provide hospital care "for *all* their people." But what about people who could not pay hospital charges? Would it be enough to rely on the voluntary hospitals' tradition of providing some free or reduced-cost care at their own discretion? Or should federal funding lead to an obligation to serve all, regardless of ability to pay? Other countries had adopted the latter policy; Canada, for example, had since the 1910s required hospitals receiving government funding to "admit patients according to demonstrated medical need." In 1946 Britain brought its voluntary hospitals into the National Health Service and hospital care became free of charge to all.[39]

Rather than creating a new obligation and therefore a right to access, US lawmakers carefully protected hospitals' discretion in providing free care. In its final version, the Hill-Burton Act authorized the Surgeon General to require, as a condition of approval of federal funding for a hospital building project, assurances that the hospital provide a "reasonable volume of services" to "persons unable to pay therefore."[40] This condition, which became known as the "uncompensated care" clause, was a nod to congressional advocates of universal access, while preserving hospitals' traditional prerogative to choose how much free care to provide, and to whom.

Critics such as Senator James Murray feared that the requirement could be easily disregarded by the states and hospitals. The law did nothing to define a "reasonable volume" of care, nor to stipulate how the requirement would be enforced. An American Hospital Association official later said that the free care regulation was "a very casual thing," intended to give psychological assurance that hospitals would continue to serve as community-oriented institutions.[41] State agencies were supposed to monitor compliance with the regulations, but no agency ever did so until the 1970s.[42] As the *Nation* magazine reported in 1952, "most states simply ignored [the free care] clause"[43] —and were able to do so because hospitals were free to spend federal money without federal oversight. Furthermore, because the law required hospitals to be self-supporting after receiving federal funds, hospitals had a financial incentive to provide the lowest possible amount of free care.

The amount of free care provided by Hill-Burton hospitals before the 1970s is impossible to determine because of the lack of reporting requirements. However, it is clear that there was an overall decline in the amount of charity care provided by hospitals in the two decades between Hill-Burton and Medicare. The spread of Blue Cross and rising hospital costs undoubtedly led to less provision of free care.[44] Voluntary hospitals increasingly shunned charity cases, the *Chicago Tribune* admonished in 1948, because they were becoming "'money mad' and have lost sight of their service responsibilities to the community."[45] Apart from the public hospitals and some "safety net" voluntary hospitals, which continued to provide large amounts of free care, the amount and availability of charity care varied widely, on the basis of the resources and commitment of individual hospitals rather than on need or a right to care.[46] Hospitals retained the right to privately ration their services. In the 1970s, advocates for the poor would rediscover the Hill-Burton uncompensated care clause and demand its enforcement (see chapter 7).[47] But for the first twenty-five years of the program, federal funding did not ensure access to hospital care for those who could not afford to pay.

Building the Jim Crow Hospital System

At a 1946 meeting of the Commission on Hospital Care to formulate recommendations for hospital legislation, Commission member Sarah Blanding, president of Vassar College, urged that the group's report take an "enlightened stand" against discrimination. "It seems to me that in a country which professes the philosophy of democracy,"

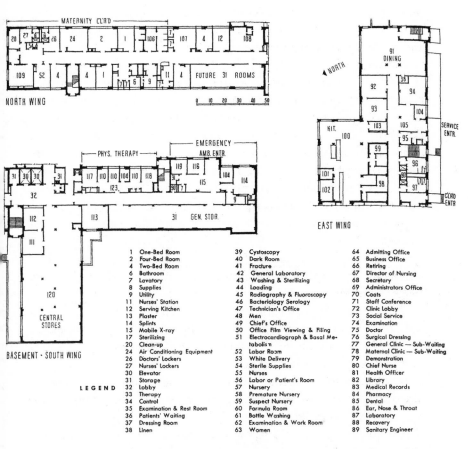

FIGURE 3. Partial floor plan of George H. Lanier Memorial Hospital, Langdale, Alabama, the first hospital completed using Hill-Burton funds, designed by Robert and Company, Atlanta, Georgia. The plan shows segregated "colored (c'lrd)" entrance and maternity ward. *Architectural Record* 107, (June 1950):148. Reprinted with permission of Robert and Company.

Blanding stated, "we would be in an untenable position if our report glossed over this question of Negro segregation in hospitals." However, the Commission's director, Chicago hospital administrator Arthur Bachmeyer, cautioned that "we must be careful in drafting our rec-ommendations . . . so as not to antagonize the white population in the southern states, but rather to encourage them to provide facilities for Negroes." Although commission member Albert W. Dent, president of historically black Dillard University, criticized this stance as "the easy way out,"[48] Bachmeyer's approach prevailed.[49] The Commission's final report recommended an end to separate black and white hospitals wherever possible, but encouraged the establishment of separate black and white facilities within the same hospital.[50]

Alabama Senator Lister Hill, Hill-Burton's powerful cosponsor, supported greater access to hospital care for black Southerners but insisted that it be provided within the framework of segregation. Hill-Burton's emphasis on local control allowed Hill to vigorously promote the bill as a states' rights measure. "That the principle of states' rights and local initiative be preserved and encouraged is essential to the success of any health program," Hill told a Senate committee.[51] Some African American leaders, termed "pragmatists" by historian Karen Kruse Thomas, also argued that a "separate but equal" policy could bring immediate improvements to the health conditions of Southern blacks by allowing segregated facilities within the most technically up-to-date white hospitals, as the Commission had recommended, as well as the modernization of all-black facilities. Northern Senators Wagner and Murray supported this approach as a compromise, since "a direct assault on segregation would doom passage of any proposed legislation." In this view, segregated facilities were better than no facilities at all, especially given the devastating lack of access to medical care suffered by African Americans.[52]

In the end, the Act included both a nondiscrimination and a "separate but equal" provision: all facilities applying for federal support (applicants) "will be made available to all persons residing in the territorial area of the applicant, without discrimination on account of race, creed, or color, but an exception shall be made in cases where separate hospital facilities are provided for separate population groups, if the plan makes equitable provision on the basis of need for facilities and services of like quality for each such group." Hill-Burton thus gave official federal sanction to maintaining and expanding Jim Crow.

The exception for Southern hospitals dismayed civil rights advocates. W. Montague Cobb, head of the National Medical Association (NMA), the organization of African American physicians, said that "separate but equal" facilities "would prove again to be a myth. . . . We wish to declare emphatically for the elimination of the entire racial separation practice in the construction of any new facilities." "How adequate can health programs become when developed in the procedural patterns of racial separation?" asked Atlanta's Urban League. A writer to the NMA's *Journal* criticized the "many 'so-called liberals' and well-meaning whites and appeasing Negroes who will enthusiastically

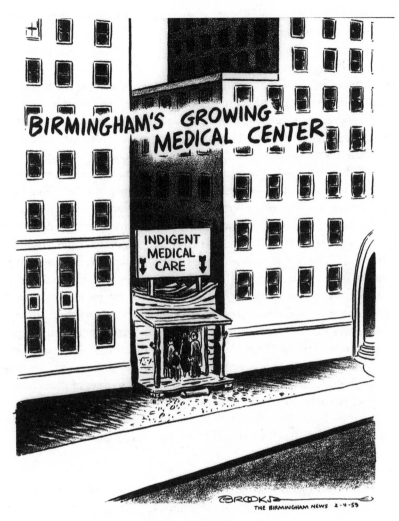

OUR SHAME

FIGURE 4. This cartoon contrasts the shortage of care for the poor in Birmingham, Alabama, with the city's gleaming new hospital complex built using federal funds. *Birmingham News*, February 4, 1959. Artist: Charles G. Brooks. Reprinted with permission of the *Birmingham News*.

collaborate in the establishing of segregated hospitals, erroneously believing that we are happy within segregated walls."[53]

Because of both Lister Hill's influence and the law's bed-ratio formula favoring rural areas, half of all hospitals built with Hill-Burton funds were in the US South. In its first decade the program greatly increased the number of hospital beds available to African Americans in the segregated wards of new and expanding white hospitals, thus increasing blacks' access to hospital care overall.[54] But greater access combined with segregation did not lead to "equality" in facilities or care. White hospitals still treated black patients differently, segregating them to separate rooms, wards, and bathrooms, and labeling hospital equipment "white" or "colored." One Maryland hospital admitted nonwhite patients to a white ward "in rare instances," but would draw a curtain around the black patient's bed to keep him or her out of sight.[55] The new, modern hospitals with segregated wards may have admitted black patients, but nearly all still did not allow black physicians to practice there.[56] Because of the lack of any enforcement mechanism, some new hospitals continued to exclude blacks altogether. In 1963, a delegation from the National Medical Association met with President Kennedy in the White House and reminded him that "the effect of the [Hill-Burton Act] as written . . . has been to permit entrenchment of old segregative and exclusion practices in new, modern plants built with the help of everybody's tax money."[57] And rationing by race, coupled with the "no duty" rule, meant that black patients could be turned away because of a shortage of segregated facilities (discussed later in this chapter).

Six months after Hill-Burton's passage, in his State of the Union Address, President Harry S. Truman reminded Congress that hospital construction was intended to be the beginning, not the end, of a comprehensive national health program: "I urge this Congress to complete the work begun last year and to enact the most important recommendation of [Truman's national health] program—to provide adequate medical care to all who need it, not as charity but on the basis of payments made by the beneficiaries of the program."[58] But national health insurance was not to be realized. Congress gave Americans a hospital system, but not a way to pay for their care.

Critics of Hill-Burton warned that the new hospital program fell far short of comprehensive health care for all Americans; that it slighted public health and prevention; that it was haphazard rather than planned; that it would lead to inefficiency and overcapacity; that it funded buildings but not doctors and nurses; and most of all, that federal funding without federal control allowed hospitals to exclude patients on the basis of race, the ability to pay, or any other factors they wished. But these critical voices were few. Thanks to Hill-Burton, the federally subsidized, locally controlled hospital became the centerpiece of America's health care system. Over the next 25 years, Hill-Burton funded close to one-third of all hospitals built in the United States. National spending on hospital care quadrupled between 1950 and 1965. And by the 1980s, 60 percent of all US hospitals had received some form of federal Hill-Burton funding.[59]

The number of hospitals in the United States rose from 4,445 in 1946 to 5,735 in 1965. By 1960, the annual rate of hospital admission— 120 per 1,000 people—was twice what it had been in the 1930s. Hospital stays were shorter, but the overall increase in hospital admissions meant that by 1959 total days of hospitalization annually was far greater than it had been before the hospital boom.[60]

Americans flocked to hospitals because of the promise of lifesaving treatments within them. A pamphlet distributed by the American Hospital Association in 1953 captured particularly well the transformation of hospital care since the war. It described a family whose father had come down with pneumonia in the early 1940s. He had spent weeks in the hospital, a time marked by "the awful waiting . . . life hanging in the balance," and full recovery took months. Now, twelve years later, their young son Jimmy was hospitalized with the same condition. "But for Jimmy, pneumonia was to be a different experience from his father's. In little more than a week the near-magic of powerful antibiotics, along with highly-specialized medical and nursing skills, had done their job."[61]

Hospitals' specialized care, and the promise of better health and longer life, cost money. "You're safer. . . . You live longer!" announced AHA public relations material in 1953. "When you or a member of your family goes to the hospital now your chances of complete recovery are at an all-time high. In time of sickness, you want and must have the best that science can offer. You can't buy it at cut rates."[62] But hospital costs were rising beyond the ability of the average American to pay the full charges out of pocket. The public should be prepared "to pay what the hospital needs to provide good care. The easy way to do this is to enroll in Blue Cross or another plan for prepaid hospital care."[63] Since doctors were quicker to hospitalize patients with insurance, more hospital coverage contributed to the rapid growth in hospital admissions (further discussed in chapter 5). And increasingly, Americans sought access to the miracles of modern hospital care through the doors of the emergency room.

The Rise of the ER

Few hospitals before the 1940s had full-fledged emergency rooms, which were also known as accident rooms, emergency wards, or emergency departments. Hill-Burton dollars allowed many hospitals, for the first time, to create distinct emergency areas with their own entrances. Already existing hospitals used Hill-Burton funds to add new emergency rooms or to expand their emergency facilities. In a 1940 sampling of hospitals, the average floor space given over to emergency care in US hospitals was 63,000 square feet; by 1955 it had more than doubled to 159,280 square feet.[64] The emergency room became an expected feature of new hospitals built with the help of federal funds. Expected, but—given the lack of government oversight and absence of central planning in hospital expansion—not required.

The nation's growing emergency care system had to make room for growing numbers of patients. In the postwar decades, visits to hospital emergency departments grew spectacularly. A major study in the *New England Journal of Medicine* found that emergency room visits increased 400 percent from 1940 to 1955.[65]

Observers puzzled over the reasons for this stunning growth in demand. In some ways it seemed a natural result of a swelling population, new facilities, and rising public expectations of medical care.[66] Rates of accidents and trauma had risen since the war, mostly because of automobile crashes and industrial injuries, but these could account for only part of the increase; in several ERs studied in the early '60s, accidental injuries accounted for only about one-third of emergency room visits.[67]

One explanation that hospitals repeatedly mentioned for the rise in ER usage was "the orientation of the public to the hospital as a place where one can receive aid at all times."[68] The public's willingness to use the emergency room could not have come without wide awareness of the ER's role as an around-the-clock resource for care—an awareness that was promoted by the hospitals and providers themselves. Hospitals aggressively advertised their emergency capabilities. An AHA radio spot in 1949 touted "Night and day . . . 'round the clock . . . the hospitals in [your area] stand ready to serve your every health need."

The hospital association assured the public, "When the windows of homes and stores are dark and the whole city seems to be sleeping, a light can be seen behind a door marked 'Emergency Entrance' in your hospital."[69] "The light over the emergency room door is the most trusted and comforting light known to the American public," gushed the journal *Medical Economics*. "It spells security."[70]

Hospitals wanted patients, but their public relations campaign on behalf of ERs was perhaps too successful. By the late 1950s, it was becoming evident that many of the patients coming through the doors did not have an emergency condition at all. A 1960 study in *Modern Hospital* commented that the emergency room "has now become a sort of a community health center to which many patients come for care of non-emergent illnesses."[71] By 1965, professional journals and popular news media featured "sensational" headlines announcing a "great emergency room emergency."[72] Patients were using the ER for nonurgent care in such large numbers that the nation's shiny new emergency wards were transformed into overcrowded purgatories staffed by overworked nurses and physicians, where patients waited for hours, and people with the common cold took attention away from those with true emergencies.

The percentage of ER visits classified as "nonurgent" or "nonemergency" in the late 1950s and early '60s was substantial, in some cases much greater than today. Hospitals reported rates of nonemergency visits ranging from 42 percent to as high as 70 percent of their total caseloads. At one Indianapolis emergency room, *84.5 percent* of visits were of a "less than urgent" or "nonemergency" nature.[73]

Many patients were drawn to emergency rooms simply because they wanted to see a doctor. After World War II, because of greater mobility and an increasing shortage of primary physicians, fewer Americans had a family doctor. But many patients crowding the ERs were middle-class people who *did* have private physicians. It turned out that these patients could not get their doctors to see them on weekends or in the evenings. "It's a good thing we have the ER these days," said a relative of one patient, surveyed while sitting in the waiting room. "It's getting so that if you want a doctor in private practice you have to be sick by appointment."[74] Also, fewer doctors were making house calls; by the 1970s, the practice was almost extinct.

Physicians themselves were encouraging emergency room use, instructing their office staff to direct patients to the ER when the doctor was unavailable. Private doctors also sent patients to emergency rooms because more kinds of routine care, especially care for injuries, had been moved out of doctors' offices and to hospitals.[75] As noted, increasing numbers of Americans in the 1950s and '60s had hospital insurance, which paid for visits to the hospital—including the ER—but not visits to the doctor's office. Some MDS admitted they were more likely to send patients to the hospital knowing that they were covered for such care but not for doctor's fees.[76]

The public pressure on the nation's emergency rooms indicated a growing rights consciousness regarding emergency care. As hospitals advertised their ER's availability to the community, emergency wards became places where "they can't turn you away." US-style rationing led to this new rights claim. Hill-Burton built up the hospital system while primary care declined. Patients turned to the emergency room when their doctors were not available, or when they had no doctor, or when their insurance covered hospital but not physician fees. The belief that ERs should be open to all would eventually lead to the establishment of the legal right to emergency care in 1986 (see chapter 8). In the meantime, hospital practices did not always meet public expectations.

Emergency Patient "Dumping": Hospitals' Right to Refuse

Hospitals advertised that their emergency rooms were always available, that their doors never closed. The reality, however, proved different. The law did not prevent hospitals from rejecting any patient for any reason, including emergency cases. Of course, hospitals did not open emergency wards, and physicians and nurses did not staff them, with the goal of turning patients away. Many hospitals struggled valiantly to provide aid to all. But the lack of a legal right to access, along with US-style rationing, meant that hospitals did refuse emergency care more frequently than is recognized.

A 1949 exposé in *Collier's* magazine denounced "the buck-passing voluntary hospitals" that "prefer to dump all troublesome and expensive emergency patients on overworked public institutions." The article listed case after case of hospital rejections: patients dying in Washington, DC, because "no voluntary or private hospital likes to take a gunshot case"; a baby who died of intestinal obstruction after being rejected from three New York area hospitals because they feared a contagious disease; a child who died from choking on a peanut because the hospital's x-ray equipment was locked up for the night. In California, "State highway patrolmen rushing victims to hospitals were so often refused admission" that "they asked the legislature to make acceptance compulsory." The governor vetoed the measure.[77]

This magazine piece gave rare attention to emergency refusals; hospital and medical journals had next to nothing to say about the phenomenon, which later became known as "patient dumping." Professional associations remained equally silent. But one organization did work to bring public attention to a particularly widespread kind of dumping: patients refused emergency care because of their race. The Southern Conference Educational Fund (SCEF), an interracial civil rights organization based in New Orleans, documented and publicized incidents of hospital refusal in the late 1940s and '50s. They found that race had been a common reason for emergency refusal at least since the 1930s, and an unconscionable number of black patients were dying because they were "dumped" from the ERs of hospitals in both the South and the North, even after the Hill-Burton Act. Deploring this practice, a 1952 editorial in the *Afro American* newspaper stated, "Many who might still be alive today have come to untimely graves. This exclusion is another form of lynching by proxy."[78]

Emergency Care Denial Based on Race

In the fall of 1930, George S. Moore Jr., a black man, was in a car crash outside of Huntsville, Alabama. No hospitals in Huntsville were "available for Negroes," so hospital staff sent him more than ten miles away to the segregated black hospital, but he died en route. In 1931, Juliette Derricotte, Dean of Women at Fisk University, and a student named Nina Johnson were in a car crash in Dalton, Georgia, and died after being denied care at whites-only Hamilton Memorial Hospital. When Mrs. Sinia Donaldson was refused care at Memphis's John Gaston Hospital in 1951, she gave birth to twins on her front porch. One baby died, strangled by the umbilical cord.

These cases appeared in a 1952 pamphlet produced by the Southern Conference Educational Fund titled *The Untouchables*, describing a long history of racial refusal by hospitals. The pamphlet listed many additional cases that had been documented by the *Crisis* newspaper and civil rights organizations from the early 1930s through the early 1950s.[79] It included stories of patients who died after being turned away from emergency wards because of their race not just in the South, but also in the North. Hospitals in Chicago, Washington, DC, and New York City had rejected critically ill or injured black patients,

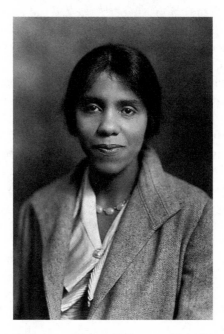

FIGURE 5. Juliette Derricotte, Dean of Women at Fisk University, was severely injured in a 1931 car accident and died after being refused care at a segregated hospital in Chattanooga, Tennessee. Courtesy of Fisk University Special Collections.

including "a 17 year old Negro girl with a bullet wound in her head" taken to Sibley Hospital, Washington, in 1932; the wife of jazz musician W. C. Handy, turned away from Knickerbocker Hospital in New York suffering from deadly cerebral hemorrhage (1937); and Trinidadian author Eric Hercules, badly injured in a car accident, who died after being transferred from Chicago's private Woodlawn Hospital to Cook County Hospital (1949).[80]

After publication of *The Untouchables*, which ran to 25,000 copies (Eleanor Roosevelt devoted one of her syndicated columns to it in 1952), the SCEF continued to gather examples of hospital refusal. The civil rights organization compiled newspaper clippings from papers around the country documenting such cases. They included two burned men wheeled into a Pittsburgh hospital on gurneys only to be told by the nurse on duty, "Hey! We don't treat Niggers here"; a baby who died after transfer from a private hospital in New York City to the public hospital 40 blocks away; a woman in a coma who died after being refused admission at Sedonia, Missouri's white hospital; and a

Galveston, Texas, man found dead in an alleyway after being sent away from the ER with skull and pelvic fractures and internal injuries.[81] An Oklahoma hospital superintendent told the SCEF, "I would refuse hospitalization to a Negro in an emergency regardless." (He had never had the opportunity, because blacks were forbidden by city ordinance from staying overnight in his town.)[82]

Although the SCEF devoted its efforts to ending Southern segregation, many of the emergency dumping cases compiled by the organization took place in the North. The SCEF documented additional refusals resulting in death in Pittsburgh, New York, Detroit, Philadelphia, and Chicago.[83] "Negroes in Chicago are not much better off for hospitalization than they are in the South," a local branch leader wrote to SCEF headquarters. "I am happy to know that Negroes are beginning to fight this evil."[84]

The increasing number of "Negro" hospital beds built with Hill-Burton funds may have alleviated emergency refusal in the South, but they did not end the problem.[85] Where hospitals generally admitted black patients into segregated Hill-Burton facilities, emergency dumping still occurred when black beds were full, even if white beds were empty and available. Duke University Hospital in North Carolina was proud of the number of segregated beds it had available, but still refused admission to Nonnie Clark, with burns covering 85 percent of her body, because its "Negro" beds were full. Emma Dangerfield, a black woman, died in the waiting room of Jefferson-Hillman Hospital in Birmingham, Alabama, in March 1951 after being denied admission. The hospital administrator "said officials denied Dangerfield access because of lack of space. He said Jefferson-Hillman had 27 beds for blacks and that 47 people were in the ward."[86] Jefferson-Hillman Hospital, later renamed University Hospital, received significant funding from Hill-Burton, but through the early 1960s, administrators required the hospital's emergency department to turn away "colored obstetric" patients, including those in labor, who had not paid a substantial fee in advance. This policy led to a notorious case of a woman who gave birth on the front lawn of the hospital after being denied admission due to her race.[87] As late as 1967, the parking lot of Hill-Burton–funded Maria Parkham Hospital in North Carolina was referred to caustically as the "black obstetrical unit."[88]

In addition to the Southern Conference Educational Fund, a few organizations around the country fought hospital segregation. The best-known was the Committee to End Discrimination in Chicago

Medical Institutions, founded in 1951 by African American and white physicians and community activists in the city to combat the frequent practice of local hospitals refusing black patients. By 1955, the Committee succeeded in getting Chicago to pass an ordinance against racial discrimination in hospital admissions, but it had little effect.[89]

Hospital discrimination committees also existed briefly in Knoxville, Houston, Wilmington, Hollywood, Detroit, and San Francisco, but were not able to make inroads against racial exclusion.[90] The only local movement that managed to win a state law against racial dumping took place in Louisville, Kentucky. A coalition of NAACP and church activists organized the Kentucky Interracial Hospital Movement (IHM) after a young black man died on a hospital waiting room floor in 1951.[91] Activists got the state legislature to consider a bill banning all racial discrimination in hospital services, and in 1952 Kentucky's Hospital Licensing Law was amended to state that "no person shall be denied emergency care solely because of race, creed or color." But the IHM was "dismayed" that "the words 'emergency treatment' had been inserted, and so the bill in its final form provides only for emergency treatment where we had called for hospital care without reservations of any kind."[92]

Thanks to the leadership of W. Montague Cobb, MD, anatomist, anthropologist, and civil rights leader, both the NAACP and the National Medical Association launched campaigns against hospital discrimination. Cobb, in a speech at the 1953 NAACP convention, denounced the Hill-Burton Act for "foisting on generations unborn the entrenched ghetto hospital system, through the construction of segregated hospitals."[93] Four years later Cobb, along with Louis T. Wright of the NAACP and physician Paul Cornely, organized the first national conference on hospital discrimination. Arguing that the *Brown v. Board of Education* school integration decision rendered hospital segregation unconstitutional, conference delegates unanimously approved a resolution demanding the removal of the separate-but-equal clause from the Hill-Burton Act.[94] In 1957, Congressman Adam Clayton Powell introduced a bill in the US House of Representatives that would have prohibited federal funding for any institution that practiced segregation. It was defeated 123–70. In the early 1960s, both the American Hospital Association and the Catholic Hospital Association passed resolutions calling for the elimination of the Hill-Burton "separate but equal" clause, and Senator Jacob Javits introduced a bill to that effect in 1962, but it died in committee.[95]

That same year, an African American dentist named George Simkins brought suit against segregated Moses H. Cone Memorial Hospital in Greensboro, North Carolina, for refusing to admit one of his patients. The plaintiffs argued that Hill-Burton's separate-but-equal provisions were in violation of the Fifth (due process) and Fourteenth (equal protection) Amendments to the Constitution, and the case went all the way to the Supreme Court, which ruled in favor of Simkins.[96] *Simkins v. Cone* (1963) ushered in the beginning of the end of official hospital segregation by race. The Supreme Court, by ruling that federal Hill-Burton funds brought the hospital under the purview of the Fifth and Fourteenth Amendments, set a precedent for full desegregation via the Medicare program just a few years later (see chapter 6). However, it did not bring an end to emergency refusal by hospitals.

Emergency Care Denial for Reasons Other than Race

We know about many cases of racial "dumping" because of the efforts of the Southern Conference Educational Fund and other civil rights organizations to document them. World-famous dramatist Edward Albee even wrote an acclaimed play on the subject. "The Death of Bessie Smith," which opened in New York in 1960, explored the 1937 death of the famed blues singer from the perspective of the white nurse who turned her away from a Memphis hospital following her auto accident. That the story was not literally factually (Smith was actually taken to the all-black hospital in Clarksdale, Mississippi, where she died of her injuries) made Albee's denunciation of a segregated health care system no less powerful.[97]

But there were other types of emergency refusal that were probably common but only rarely recorded. Patients could be and were refused emergency care on the basis of their health condition, their mental health status, their insurance status, how busy the hospital was, who their doctor was, their place of residence, and especially their inability to pay.

Hospitals had good reason not to keep records of emergency care denials. Emergency dumping cases for reasons other than race generally appear in the historical record only if the patient or family brought a lawsuit, as in the case of Geraldine Crews in Birmingham, Alabama, or if the case received newspaper attention.[98] Also, patients could bring suit for negligence only *after* a hospital or practitioner had begun treatment. Therefore, there was no legal recourse at all for patients refused care entirely, and little or no chance of documentation. Most patients or families who did attempt to bring court cases most likely had them dismissed early in the process, or could not find a lawyer willing to assist them, making a record of the incident even more unlikely. Finally, it is probable that most patients who were denied care were from low-income groups, and did not have sufficient resources (financial or otherwise) to even approach an attorney, or to gain attention from the press.

It may be that the small number of recorded examples means that emergency dumping was rare. However, given hospitals' legal right to refuse emergency care and the strong financial incentive for refusing or transferring undesirable patients, as well as the limitations on sources outlined above, it seems more likely that the surviving recorded cases stand in for many others.[99] As prominent a figure as Harry S. Truman spoke publicly of emergency refusal as a perennial, common problem. Remembering his days as a county commissioner in Missouri, Truman wrote in his memoirs, "I saw people turned away from hospitals to die because they had no money for treatment. We know that there has been considerable progress in many cities and towns in taking care of the sick and injured, but even in those communities the patient must prove ability to pay or qualify as a charity patient."[100]

In the decades of hospital expansion, transfer or direct refusal of emergency patients in serious condition might occur on the basis that the hospital was not equipped to deal with the patient's health condition, or could not accept contagious cases (as in the case of Geraldine Crews), or if the hospital did not have an available bed or if the staff was too busy. In New York City in 1951, Helen Jones, a victim of a knife attack, was brought to the ER of the Hospital for Joint Diseases. An intern gave her cursory treatment but then ordered her transferred, even though he had diagnosed her with a "penetrating stab wound of the abdomen." Jones died during surgery at the second hospital. The New York Supreme Court concluded that Jones's death occurred because of the transfer and that the intern had made the decision to discontinue care solely "for the convenience of the hospital."[101]

Patients who arrived in an emergency room showing symptoms of alcoholism or mental illness were routinely refused or transferred. For the mentally ill, "jails [were] used for emergency care" in communities that were short on specialized facilities; a jail cell was deemed a sufficiently "safe and comfortable place" for such patients.[102] Alcoholics or alleged alcoholics might also be moved straight from the ER to a jail cell, without medical treatment. In September 1954, Nicholas

Bourgeois was found unconscious and taken to the emergency room of Jackson Memorial Hospital in Dade County, Florida. The intern did not take a history or x-rays because the patient "reeked of alcohol." Discharged as a drunk, Bourgeois was put by police into a jail cell on a metal cot and left by himself. He was found dead the next morning, his lungs pierced by nine broken ribs.[103] Men appearing drunk or incoherent were turned away so frequently from Cook County Hospital in Chicago in the early 1950s that an outraged judge ordered one such man brought into his courtroom comatose on a stretcher, and invited newspaper photographers to view him. Dr. Ole Nelson, medical director of Cook County, defended the hospital's practice, telling the *Tribune*, "We do not have the space to treat drunks and alcoholics."[104]

The growth of health insurance coverage in the 1940s and '50s, described in the next chapter, greatly expanded access to hospital care. However, like other areas of health-system growth, health insurance expansion created new types of exclusion and rationing, one of which was emergency care refusal based on type of health coverage. In one such case, a New York man showing classic heart attack symptoms died after being turned away from Montefiore Hospital because he was a member of the Hospital Insurance Plan, a type of coverage that Montefiore did not accept.[105] Another reason for emergency refusal was that a patient was already under the care of a personal physician. This happened in the case of Darien Manlove, a four-month-old baby who died of pneumonia after the emergency room of Wilmington General Hospital in Delaware sent him home with his parents to wait for the family doctor's office to open.[106]

One common reason for refusal was the patient's place of residence. Municipal and county hospitals were authorized to treat only local residents who could show proof of address. This created a particularly difficult problem for migrant workers, travelers, and vacationers. In one 1952 case, a young man on vacation in Chicago was struck with acute polio and then refused admission to several contagious-disease hospitals in the city because he was not a resident. He had to return to his home in downstate Illinois for hospitalization.[107] Residency requirements were frequently used to exclude migrant workers and immigrants from all types of care, including emergency care.[108]

The type of refusal most emblematic of the US health care system—and one that still occurs today—was exclusion based on inability to pay. Refusal of care often took the form of transferring patients from private to county or other public hospitals. In New York City in the late 1930s, "scores" of accident victims were transferred "every week" from private hospitals to municipal ones.[109] In Chicago, the drivers of police emergency vehicles had "verbal orders to remain at the hospitals to which accident victims have been taken until the hospital has checked the financial responsibility of the injured person." Private hospitals routinely transferred indigent patients, black and white, to Cook County, sometimes in critical condition.[110] Even some "charity" hospitals, including Catholic hospitals, engaged in this practice. In 1957, a child named Angel Rivera choked to death on a balloon after being refused emergency treatment at a private Catholic hospital in Milwaukee. He was kept waiting for 20 minutes before a receptionist told his father to take him to the county hospital.[111]

Receipt of Hill-Burton funds did not deter hospitals from rejecting patients on the basis of inability to pay. A Missouri man with frozen feet requiring amputation was turned away from a Hill-Burton hospital in 1961 because administrators did not believe he would be able to pay his bill. In this case, the patient sued, but the Missouri Supreme Court noted that "the receipt of public funds under the Hill-Burton Act did not alter [the hospital's] status as a private hospital or create a duty to admit plaintiff."[112] The court did not even mention Hill-Burton's uncompensated care clause.

In rare instances, emergency refusal led to public outcry. In 1954, a severely burned five-month-old named Laura Lingo died after being transferred from the emergency room of Chicago's Woodlawn Hospital to Cook County because her mother, the wife of a factory worker, could not pay the $100 admissions deposit. The baby's parents went to the press, and the story received nationwide coverage. Laura had been scalded when she kicked over a boiling vaporizer. She received first aid at Woodlawn and was apparently stable when her mother, unable to pay the deposit, put her back in the car for the drive to County, which took 90 minutes because of traffic. The baby died there the next morning. *Time* magazine reported Mrs. Lingo crying at the coroner's inquest, "She was my only baby . . . I'll never forget this."[113] The national press picked up the story because Chicago's outspoken health commissioner, Herman Bundesen, publicly denounced Woodlawn's negligence, as did the county coroner. After sensational headlines and raucous public meetings, the county tax authorities removed Woodlawn from the tax-exempt list—one of the few examples of a hospital being punished for emergency refusal before 1986.[114]

The public outrage at this case of a patient being turned away because of inability to pay offers evidence of belief in a right to emergency care. Certainly Chicago politicians found the Lingos to be a popular cause to champion. But the case did not lead to additional laws or regulations governing emergency rooms; if anything, it led to a backlash against institutionalizing a right to emergency care. The Chicago Medical Society was infuriated at the attention the case received. The Society conducted its own investigation and "absolved" the hospital of blame.[115] The *Chicago Tribune*, while reporting frequently on the story, editorialized against the "hullabaloo" and "great howl" raised by the health authorities, and argued that "if the hospital was entitled to [tax] exemption before the baby incident, it is still entitled to it."[116]

The numerous rationales for emergency refusal described above help explain the persistence of "patient dumping" even after the Supreme Court ruled hospital segregation by race unconstitutional in 1963. Unlike public schools, hospitals were still allowed to let in only people who could pay. "I am all for attacking Jim Crow wherever it exists," said a prescient letter writer to the journal *Southern Patriot* in 1951. "However . . . even though segregation were abolished, persons without cash in hand would continue to be denied admission to hospitals. The elimination of segregation would mean for the majority of Negroes equality in being denied admission to hospitals for lack of funds, and its achievement would be more moral than material."[117] The ongoing relationship between racial and economic inequality meant that African Americans would continue to be subject to emergency refusal disproportionally in the decades following the civil rights movement.

Rationing based on ability to pay was and is a hallmark of US health care. Even when other justifications for exclusion were attacked and began to erode, economic refusal by hospitals remained acceptable, unchanged by Hill-Burton regulations or civil rights agitation. This ongoing reality was reflected by a Missouri hospital administrator who was asked in the early 1950s whether his hospital denied care on the basis of the race of the patient. He was happy to report that it did not: "We are here to take care of sick folks. The color of their skin or eyes makes no difference to us, as long as they pay their bills. . . ."[118]

CHAPTER FIVE

Rationing by Coverage: The Rise of Private Health Insurance

After the defeat of President Truman's national health insurance proposal, private or "voluntary" hospital insurance became the main solution proposed to rising medical costs. The hospital service plan known as Blue Cross had been invented in Texas in 1929 and became increasingly popular throughout the 1930s and '40s. The American Medical Association, which had early in the century opposed any type of third-party insurance, grudgingly came out in favor of voluntary health insurance plans in 1938, so long as they were controlled by providers. Soon after that, medical coverage became an important part of the benefits package of many American workers. Encouraged by federal tax laws, increasing numbers of employers began offering health insurance to workers during and after World War II, and labor unions embraced health benefits as an important aspect of collective bargaining. After the war, the growth of both nonprofit Blue Cross and for-profit private health insurance took off. By 1960, 125 million Americans had some form of private health coverage — close to 70 percent of the total population.[1]

Present-day commentators look back on this period as a time of generous medical coverage for most Americans. One influential health policy expert has described the era of private insurance before managed care as the "limitless, fairyland health care [system] in which most Americans had been reared since World War II." In this "fairyland," consumers had "completely unfettered access to a luxurious, open-ended health system, with few questions asked and no rationing at all."[2]

However, if we look at the actual extent of coverage and the actual experiences of Americans with private insurance after World War II, it becomes clear that a land of limitless health care never existed. While more people had health insurance than ever before, mostly through their employers, many could not obtain coverage at all. The workplace-based insurance system rationed coverage by occupation. Few low-wage workers, farmers, African Americans, disabled people, employees of small businesses, or senior citizens were covered by employers, and members of these groups could not afford to buy insurance on their own. The inability of private health insurance to cover so many people, especially the elderly who needed health care the most, paved the way for the creation of Medicare and Medicaid in 1965—paradoxically, as Paul Starr writes, "pushing the system ultimately toward some form of government intervention."[3]

The private insurance system left out too many people, but just as important, it did not offer true health security to those it did cover. Few Americans with health insurance in the decades after World War II were protected from the full cost of sickness. Most health plans were so limited and covered so little that in 1960, when the majority of Americans had benefits, insurance in total paid for only about a third of the cost of sickness in the country, and only 40 percent of the health expenditures of people *with* health insurance.[4]

After World War II, Americans came to believe in health insurance and the promise that it would protect their incomes and give them access to care in times of sickness. But their hopes for what health benefits could do for them clashed with the goals of the insurance industry, whose imperative was to treat health care like any other aspect of its business. As a result, most of the private system rationed health care by building on traditional insurance principles of limitation, selection, and exclusion. To defend these principles required strong resistance to the idea that health care and health insurance should be treated as rights.

Why did so much insurance cover so little? One reason is that most private insurance in the 1950s and '60s provided hospital coverage only; families still had to pay out of pocket for doctors' visits, drugs, screenings, lab tests, and care for chronic and long-term conditions. Blue Cross had been created by hospitals for hospitals—its goal was to ensure payment for hospital care only—and the private insurance system continued to reflect this bias in favor of hospital coverage. In 1968, after the greatest expansion of health benefits in history, still only 42 percent of *insured* Americans had coverage for doctor's visits outside the hospital.[5] Some types of health plans, known as major medical insurance, included both hospital and non-hospital care, but only after a steep deductible. All plans had caps on total coverage. For people not covered by employer group insurance, insurers refused to cover existing health problems, or refused to sell policies altogether to patients with preexisting medical conditions. Insurance companies could cancel a policy after a policyholder got sick, or when the policyholder got older and needed more health care.[6] Because of deductibles and copayments, people with large families, chronic illnesses, or sudden catastrophic health costs found themselves shelling out hundreds and even thousands of dollars a year for their care. Limitations, exclusions, copayments, and deductibles dashed many Americans' hopes that insurance coverage would buy them peace of mind in times of sickness.

The gap between public expectations and the reality of limited coverage led to discontent and, eventually, a new understanding of the possible rights of people with insurance. Beginning in the 1950s, many Americans, and the labor movement in particular, became increasingly unhappy with the narrow limitations of their health plans, and a movement arose calling for "comprehensive coverage." The very idea of comprehensive health coverage horrified the insurance industry, which feared that it would lead people to use too much health care, and thus drive prices so high that only government could afford to pick up the tab. Insurance companies in the postwar United States fought to defend the exclusionary principles of their business against demands for more comprehensive, universal coverage. They were largely successful, and their victory continued to shape the US system of rationing by insurance coverage into the twenty-first century.

Although the private health insurance industry grew to be a vast multibillion dollar enterprise, insurance companies initially hesitated to get involved in health coverage. Early in the twentieth century, the life insurance business was extremely profitable, but health insurance seemed a much more risky proposition. Insurers began selling some limited individual health plans in the 1930s, but they were expensive "indemnity" plans, which meant the insured had to pay the hospital up front, and then wait to be reimbursed later by the insurance company. Blue Cross attracted customers by offering "service benefits" rather than indemnity benefits. Under service benefits, the hospital billed Blue Cross, not the patient. This appealing feature, along with its nonprofit status, made Blue Cross very different from traditional insurance.

Blue Cross (for hospital care) and Blue Shield (for physician care in the hospital) initially dominated health coverage in the United States, but after 1945 they faced greater competition from commercial group indemnity insurance. Commercial insurance spread rapidly, more than doubling the number of policies within just a few years. By 1949, commercial companies covered 29 million people, closing in on Blue Cross's 31 million. By 1953, 29 percent of Americans carried commercial coverage, and commercial insurers had pulled ahead of Blue Cross, which covered only 27 percent.[7]

The growth of commercial health insurance resulted from employer rather than popular preference. Health coverage became an important part of the workplace benefits package starting in World War II, when the National War Labor Board instituted a wage freeze and a no-strike agreement but encouraged labor-management negotiations for fringe benefits. Although labor unions generally preferred Blue Cross, believing that service benefits would provide better health protection for their members than indemnity benefits, employers (as historian Jennifer Klein has shown) fought instead for commercial health insurance that they could control.[8]

All types of private or "voluntary" group insurance, whether Blue Cross or commercial, served some common purposes. Employers benefited because negotiated health packages helped them develop and keep a stable workforce. Hospitals benefited because Blue Cross and commercial coverage brought millions of dollars and new customers into the hospital system. Physicians benefited because insured patients had more money for doctors' bills after their hospital bills were covered. And all three groups shared another benefit of widespread private health coverage: the weakening of public demands for universal, government-sponsored health care.

Insurance against Socialized Medicine:
The Political Nature of Private Health Coverage

Republican President Dwight D. Eisenhower had strongly opposed Truman's national health insurance initiative. Upon taking office in 1953, Eisenhower promised to "defeat any move toward socialized medicine" during his presidency. The reformers and experts who had advocated universal health programs throughout the Roosevelt and Truman administrations no longer had a place in Washington. Eisenhower argued that Americans' medical needs should instead be met by "private and local institutions"—but not without some help from the government. In 1954 he put this belief into practice by sponsoring the

Revenue Act, which extended the wartime tax breaks for employer-sponsored health benefits.[9] This crucially important law made permanent the troubled relationship between employment and health insurance and cemented the rationing of coverage based on job status in the United States.

The President also proposed a plan called "reinsurance," in which the federal government would provide financial backing for private insurance companies who were willing to insure high-risk populations, such as people over 65.[10] Although the reinsurance proposal failed—the proposed subsidies were too modest to convince insurance companies to let the federal government get involved in their business—it foreshadowed the enthusiasm of future administrations for public subsidies to private insurers.

Private health insurance was not just an alternative to national, compulsory insurance, but also a way of preventing such a system from becoming possible. Champions of a private system of health coverage had their own economic interests in mind, but they also firmly believed in the superiority of "voluntarism" over "compulsion," or, in other words, the "American Way" over socialism. Ideology and private interest were hard to separate. Without the spread of private insurance, said Arthur C. Stevenson, MD, president of Arizona Blue Shield, "I feel positive the federal government would have been able to have socialized this element of our lives already. If Blue Cross / Blue Shield has done nothing else, it has alerted the nation to the dangers of such a system [national insurance] usurping our democratic patterns and our freedoms."[11] E. J. Faulkner of the Health Insurance Council spoke with even more conviction: voluntary health insurance was "in the very vortex of the world-wide conflict between individualism and collectivism."[12]

One organization, the Health Information Foundation (HIF), exemplifies how the public relations campaign for voluntary health insurance benefited private interests while pursuing the political and ideological goal of keeping government out of health coverage. Founded in 1949 by pharmaceutical leaders, HIF quickly signed up "130 drug and chemical manufacturers" to support its mission of conducting research and educational campaigns about health. The group also worked closely with leaders of the American Hospital Association and Blue Cross. HIF insisted on its neutrality as a purveyor of health care "information," as its name indicated, and "pledged to do no lobbying, to present its findings impartially."[13] But in the organization's early days, a clear agenda guided its research; as the group's own publicity stated, "private methods of paying for medical care should be the prevailing force shaping the development of health services." HIF's President, W. H. P. Blandy, a retired Admiral who had served in both World Wars, believed that "socialized medicine would be harmful, if not indeed destructive, to a free America, and in particular to free enterprise in the medical profession and the drug industry," and that HIF's goal of improved health facilities and increasing access to health care would "render socialized or nationalized medicine unnecessary and unwanted."[14] Former President Herbert Hoover served as HIF's honorary Chair. Speaking of Blue Cross in 1956, Hoover declared, "Here is an inspiring example of the ability of a free people to carry on great welfare activities outside of the Government."[15] (In order to distinguish private health insurance from "compulsory" or universal, government-sponsored health insurance, HIF used the phrase "voluntary health insurance" to describe all kinds of private coverage.)

In the early and mid-1950s, the Health Information Foundation became a public relations powerhouse for voluntary health insurance. With funding from the pharmaceutical industry, they retained the major ad agency J. Walter Thompson to design the campaign. HIF sent letters signed by former US President Hoover to 50,000 business leaders throughout the country, asking them to "spur the nation's business leaders to take positive action in encouraging health insurance coverage for employees, their dependents, and everyone in their communities."[16] The organization produced and distributed "health information films" and TV and radio programs, including films and programs on the benefits of private health insurance.[17] One HIF campaign featured a turban-wearing cartoon character named "Second Sight Sam" who almost broke into his son's piggy bank to pay for hospital bills until the boy says, "Pop, there's a better and easier way . . . VOLUNTARY HEALTH INSURANCE!"[18]

The rise of employer benefits, helped along by the public relations campaigns of HIF, the AHA, and Blue Cross, made health insurance a household word in the space of just a few years. By the mid-1950s, 45 percent of Americans had joined some sort of health plan, mostly through their employer.[19] A decade after the end of World War II, Americans were becoming accustomed to having part of their health costs covered by private insurance. "Investment in health coverage is no longer an experimental, novel thing," reported a 1956 Blue Cross study. "Both through experience and hearsay of friends and co-workers,

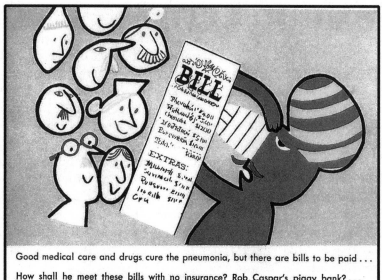

Good medical care and drugs cure the pneumonia, but there are bills to be paid . . .

How shall he meet these bills with no insurance? Rob Caspar's piggy bank? . . .

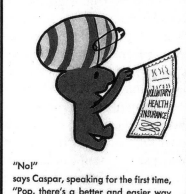

"No!"
says Caspar, speaking for the first time,
"Pop, there's a better and easier way
to meet unforeseeable medical bills—
VOLUNTARY HEALTH INSURANCE!"

☞ YOU too

Must Remember

Even Second-Sight Sam

Cannot Foresee

Costly ILLNESSES

And ACCIDENTS

Get VOLUNTARY

HEALTH INSURANCE

Today

FIGURE 6. "Second Sight Sam, The Prophesyin' Man" is counseled by his son to get voluntary health insurance in these excerpts from a Health Information Foundation pamphlet from the early 1950s. Center for Hospital and Health Care Administration History, American Hospital Association Resource Center. Reprinted with permission of the Center for Health Care Administration Studies, University of Chicago.

people are quite firmly convinced that this kind of investment pays off."[20] Another survey in 1959 found 81 percent of respondents "favorable" toward the idea of health insurance; of those who already had health insurance, 75 percent were satisfied with their current coverage.[21]

The 1959 survey asked Americans why they thought it was important to have health insurance; 76 percent said the main reasons were "to prevent worry over bills from illness" and "to avoid using up savings during a severe or prolonged illness," and 68 percent agreed that insurance was needed "to be sure of prompt medical attention."[22] The Blue Cross study found that "even those who have had little need to utilize the service are nonetheless convinced that it is a source of security and protection well worth paying for. . . . Health plans have done much to relieve feelings of helplessness in the face of illness."[23]

But the security and protection promised by health insurance was just that—a promise. Because the health coverage provided by both the Blues and commercial insurers was so limited, people with insurance still had to pay for most of their medical needs out of pocket. Only 43 percent of respondents in the 1959 study said that their present insurance "adequately covered the types of expenses most likely to be incurred," and families with the most health problems reported that they were covered for only 38 percent of their costs. Those families expressed a desire for more comprehensive insurance that would cover a greater portion of their medical bills.[24]

Not only was coverage limited, but also it could be canceled at any time (a practice known as "rescission"). In individual insurance, this was especially common when policyholders turned 65, even if they had been paying premiums for many years. Frank McLean of Jacksonville, Alabama, wrote to his senator, Lister Hill, in 1954 to express concern about this practice: "What this means is that those people who pay, year in and year out, for protection in time of illness, can be, and are likely to be, cut off with no protection at all in their old age, when money is less abundant and health hazards are greater." McLean could not understand why President Eisenhower insisted that commercial insurance would offer adequate help to the public when it "will do nothing to protect the very people who insure themselves in the hope of having old age coverage."[25]

By the end of the 1950s, most of the American public saw health insurance as desirable, although many were unable to obtain it because of age, income, job status, or other factors. But even those who had coverage, whether Blue Cross, Blue Shield, or commercial insurance, were far from secure. Typical employer plans, which still focused almost entirely on hospital care, did not cover the majority of Americans' health costs. And private insurance excluded not just certain kinds of medical care, but certain health conditions too.

Claims Denied: Health Insurance Exclusions

"Exclusion" is the literal term used by the insurance industry for conditions that are not covered by a policy. For example, health plans with a "cancer exclusion" will not cover cancer care. Exclusions are central to the insurance principle — necessary, according to the industry, to guard against the "moral hazard" of people purchasing insurance knowing they were going to use it. As one insurance executive stated in 1954, "We cannot insure the man who knows darn well he is on the way to the hospital. We have got to avoid that guy, and he wants insurance. . . . You cannot insure the diabetic without insuring the diabetes."[26]

In the 1950s and '60s, numerous exclusions became standard. Many health plans excluded not only "nervous ailments," but also "care in nursing homes, insanity, alcoholism, and narcotism [sic]," among many other conditions.[27] Insurers also refused to cover entire categories of people, such as individuals with mental or physical disabilities.[28]

Another major type of health insurance exclusion was the "preexisting condition" clause. These clauses stipulated that certain medical conditions existing before the insurance policy came into force could never be covered. As one industry group explained, "covering preexisting conditions . . . would be like issuing fire insurance on houses already on fire."[29] Again, insurers created preexisting conditions clauses to address moral hazard. They *could* then insure the diabetic, but only with the stipulation that any medical care arising from diabetes would not be paid for. Insurance companies had latitude to define "preexisting" any way they wished. If a policyholder developed a disease after purchasing the policy, the insurer might raise the premium or cancel or refuse to renew the policy.[30]

Ironically, given the earlier popularity of EMIC, one of the most common exclusions in all types of health insurance in the postwar period was maternity care. Insurers saw "normal maternity" as a classic setup for moral hazard — they actually called it "the maternity hazard," assuming (wrongly) that pregnancy was usually a planned condition. Until the late 1970s, many health plans did not cover hospital or medical care for childbirth or the postpartum period. Plans that did include maternity care had a nine-month waiting period before the insured became eligible for coverage.[31] The maternity exclusion became one of the main reasons for public criticism of traditional health insurance.

The private insurance system discriminated against women in both subtle and direct ways. Working women were less likely than men to have health insurance through their employers because they were concentrated in lower-paying, non-unionized industries that offered few or no benefits. Since the majority of American women remained outside of the paid workforce, those with health insurance usually received it as "dependents" on their husbands' insurance. For coverage of family members, workers had to pay the additional premiums out of their own pockets. Dependents were also subject to a waiting period before coverage kicked in.[32]

Insurance companies unapologetically charged women more than men for individual health policies, reflecting a long-held assumption that women used more medical care than men (not even counting maternity). Insurance executives put their belief in this stereotype on full display at a series of meetings held by the Health Information Foundation in 1953–54. According to one insurance executive, women were more expensive to cover because they were like his wife, who "spends a lot more money in the department stores where she has charge accounts."[33] The insurers used gender as an argument against offering more comprehensive care. Health plans that covered office visits would run up their expenses because, according to one delegate, so many women "liked to see their doctors in the afternoon." HIF President Admiral Blandy agreed that women liked to meet "socially every afternoon in [their doctor's] office."[34] Such attitudes helped insurers justify setting rates by gender.

Insurance coverage also differed by race. In 1957, 74.5 percent of whites had private health insurance coverage, compared to 52 percent of blacks. The insurance industry had a long tradition of excluding or charging higher rates to nonwhites. One insurance official stated as late as 1960 that "the underwriting problems involved in attempting to insure members of more than one race would be considerable owing to differences in physique, temperament, habit and environment."[35] Even when policies were available to African Americans, their premiums ran much higher. Occupational segregation and discrimination played an even bigger role in preventing racial minorities from obtaining health insurance, since the job categories in which most black

Americans found employment at the time—agricultural and domestic work—rarely provided benefits.[36]

Although Blue Cross offered very limited coverage, in general it was less exclusive, which helps explain its continuing popularity, especially among labor unions. Blue Cross was founded on the principle of "community rating." Community rating is a term for the broad pooling of risk. It involves insuring as large a group as possible and charging each member the same premium, under the assumption that the healthier members will subsidize those who get sick (this is also the principle behind "social insurance"). Commercial indemnity insurance, on the other hand, was based on "experience rating"—dividing groups into smaller segments on the basis of their purported risk, and charging high-risk groups or individuals more and low-risk ones less.

Experience rating was central to the "insurance principle" and helps explain insurance companies' elaborate efforts to evaluate and categorize different people and groups (known as underwriting). It also helps to explain the practices of exclusion; excluding people or conditions identified as high risk (known as "cherry picking") helped keep premiums down for low-risk individuals and groups.[37] Commercial insurance leaders adamantly opposed community rating, believing (correctly) that community-rated plans could not compete with experience-rated ones, which skimmed off the healthiest clients. And again, there was an ideological basis for experience rating. According to one industry group, proposals for community rating or nondiscrimination in insurance premiums "are really proposals to transfer income from one group to another. . . . They could not be put into effect so long as free competition exists in the health insurance field."[38] The logical outcome of the principle of community rating would be universal coverage.

Companies that used experience rating became more attractive to healthy people because they would be charged lower premiums, encouraging them to leave Blue Cross for cheaper commercial insurance plans. This led to rapidly growing costs and rate hikes for Blue Cross and Blue Shield. By the end of the 1950s, in order to compete with commercial plans, the Blues increasingly relied on experience rating as well, a stark departure from their original principles.

A few types of health plans operated on models different from Blue Cross and commercial insurance. Group practice, prepayment schemes, and cooperative health plans gave their members more comprehensive coverage and greater income protection. The existence of these alternative plans posed direct competition to the Blues and commercial insurers. They also threatened to become a gateway to government health insurance. In the 1950s, HIF and other groups opposed to "socialized medicine" took deliberate steps to push back against the challenge presented by these alternative types of health plans and the growing public demand for comprehensive coverage.

Alternatives

Alternative forms of medical organization, particularly group practice and prepayment, had become increasingly important in the 1930s and '40s. Such plans challenged the tradition of fee-for-service medical practice, and were actively opposed by the American Medical Association. The Farm Security Administration medical cooperatives were terminated after the war, but other forms of group medical practice and prepayment continued to thrive. By the 1950s they presented a threat not just to the AMA, but also to private insurers.

These plans operated on three principles that made them very different from commercial insurers: first-dollar coverage, comprehensive benefits, and preventive medical care. First-dollar coverage meant that members did not have to pay any costs up front before receiving care. Comprehensive benefits meant that doctors' visits, maternity care, lab tests, and other basic services were covered along with hospital stays. Preventive care meant coverage for vaccinations, annual checkups, and chronic conditions.

Kaiser Permanente was one of the most successful examples of a type of health care organization that fit neither the Blue Cross nor the commercial insurance model. This health plan, originating in a group practice plan for employees of California industrialist Henry Kaiser and opened to the general public after World War II, offered prepaid comprehensive medical care and built and ran its own hospitals. In 1955, it had half a million members. Kaiser's comprehensive coverage and emphasis on preventive care attracted labor unions, which put pressure on employers to offer Kaiser or a similar plan as an option in their benefits package. Preventive care was important not just to keep people healthy, Kaiser boosters argued, but also to reduce rates of hospitalization, saving insurance plans money and keeping premiums low. Physicians in prepaid group practices hospitalized their patients far less frequently than those in Blue Cross / Blue Shield plans, again leading to lower costs.[39]

The AMA had somewhat softened its opposition to group practice and prepayment by the 1950s, but private insurers and Blue Cross / Blue

Shield saw alternative plans like Kaiser as direct competition to their businesses. At a meeting called by the Health Information Foundation in 1953, both commercial and Blue executives agreed that prepaid group practices were so popular among subscribers that they threatened to spread across the country and "take over." Plans like Kaiser Permanente, commented one insurance executive, had "a tremendous psychological appeal that is very hard to wipe out of the minds of ordinary people." Another retorted, "Does not the fact remain that if Blue Shield and Blue Cross would get their house in order and do the job that they should be doing, that Permanente would not be flourishing the way it is?"[40] The question of what health coverage "should be doing" was exactly what was at stake. How much coverage, and how much security, should the public expect from health insurance?

Every Damn Thing under the Sun:
The Debate over Comprehensive Coverage

The narrow scope of the Blues and commercial insurance—exclusion of, for example, doctors' visits, tests, maternity care, and prescription drugs—meant that the coverage they offered was anything but "comprehensive." Beginning in the early 1950s, consumer groups and labor unions increasingly criticized these limitations and demanded more comprehensive insurance. In the words of one union leader, "It is high time, I believe, that we stop emphasizing insurance against the high cost of neglected health and devoted more of our efforts to developing more of a system of insurance or pre-payment which would give the American people a greater access to the kind of health care which prevents illness or nips it in the bud."[41]

Increasingly, public and medical opinion began to match labor's sentiments in favor of more comprehensive health benefits. In 1952, after a popular women's magazine ran an article titled "Are There Holes in Your Health Insurance?" the Cooperative Health Federation received 492 letters from members of the public, "all of them ask[ing] about comprehensive care."[42] A 1956 study asking Blue Cross/Blue Shield members how their coverage could be improved found that "by far the most frequent suggestion was that doctors' charges for office and home care be covered more fully."[43] As for doctors, one 1958 survey found that 65 percent of physicians questioned agreed that more comprehensive coverage "would be a good idea."[44]

Both the Blues and commercial insurers wrung their hands as criticism of their limited benefits mounted. At the end of 1953 and the beginning of 1954, the Health Information Foundation sponsored a series of meetings in the New York area to discuss the challenge (or threat) of comprehensive private health insurance. These meetings, which were by invitation only, provide a rare glimpse into the frank discussions of both commercial insurance and Blue Cross / Blue Shield leaders as they confronted public demands for greater coverage and access.

Participants at the meetings expressed distress over the rise of comprehensive prepaid plans that covered doctor's office visits, preventive care, and maternity. One hospital leader even referred to "this horrible word 'comprehensive.'"[45] HIF President Admiral Blandy mocked comprehensive plans for "offering every damn thing under the sun in the way of benefits" and blamed them for encouraging "a considerable trend . . . particularly on the part of the labor unions—to get everything that they can placed in the insurance package."[46] Dr. Charles Hayden of Massachusetts Blue Shield, a member of the AMA House of Delegates, complained about the "forces on the other side—the labor leaders, Kaiser . . . the New York Times," who were calling for more comprehensive care. Another participant referred to the "bleeding heart fraternity . . . that tries to impress the people that they need full coverage."[47]

Participants at the HIF meetings were so opposed to comprehensive care first of all because they thought that it would be too expensive. Blandy warned that the cost increases brought about by demands for comprehensive care could mean "the defeat of voluntary health insurance."[48] If the private insurers could not give the public what it wanted at a price it was able to pay, then government would step in to fill the coverage gaps.

Blue and commercial insurance leaders also agreed that, aside from the cost, comprehensive coverage violated the basic principle of insurance, which was meant to cover only unexpected events. Because doctors' office visits, diagnostic tests, and (sometimes) maternity were routine and planned, including such services would encourage "adverse selection" and moral hazard—in other words, people would purchase insurance knowing that they would use it. The insurance executives argued that ordinary policyholders, who cared not at all for the principle of insurance, would over-use their new comprehensive benefits in order to feel that they were getting their money's worth. One delegate asserted that "John Public . . . gets quite a boost out of getting that one doctor's visit paid for or those one or two days he spends in the hospital paid for."[49] The group did not discuss the possibility that comprehensive insurance might *discourage* overutilization by encouraging preventive care.

The Blues and commercial insurers, initially opposed to each other, found themselves in agreement about the nature of health coverage. As Paul Starr writes in his classic *The Social Transformation of American Medicine*, "the competition between commercial insurers and the Blues produced a tendency toward convergence."[50] Both types of insurers acknowledged that they faced a common enemy in the public demands for more comprehensive health benefits, which threatened their industries and raised the specter of government health insurance.

Calls for comprehensive coverage made the AMA equally apprehensive. One MD echoed insurers' fears of moral hazard: "Can we provide coverage for the individual with a tension headache, who under ordinary circumstances would obtain adequate relief from two aspirins but who, in the presence of an insurance program, believes he is entitled to visit a doctor?"[51] Arthur Kemp of the AMA Bureau of Economic Research advised that if the public wanted comprehensive insurance, they could purchase a Blue Cross / Blue Shield plan plus a major medical plan (see below for more on major medical). "Indeed," he said, "it seems to me that the outstanding achievement of the health care financial mechanism developed in this country is precisely this great variety of plans which are available for people to buy . . . thus providing for their own well-being in the purchase of health care." Organized medicine also opposed comprehensive insurance for the same reason private insurers did: the belief that it would erode their business and bring on government medical care. "Insistence on comprehensiveness can lead only to one end, and that is the destruction of the voluntary mechanism by any definition I would consider realistic," Kemp declared at a national meeting on prepaid medical care in 1960. "In many cases, I think this is precisely the reason some people insist on comprehensiveness — to destroy the private practice of medicine."[52]

Labor and consumer groups continued to insist that private insurance must become more comprehensive. In response to arguments that comprehensiveness would lead people to use too much medical care, Jerome Pollack, a researcher with the United Auto Workers, asserted that the problem was too little, not too much. "We now (1960) have roughly one-fourth of the total private health bill covered by insurance," Pollack declared. "There is no doubt that we could easily double the scope of present protection without seriously straining the upper limits of insurability. The question is how to get there, not how to avoid overinsurance."[53]

The insurance industry, the medical profession, and employers were acutely aware of demands for more comprehensive coverage. To defend against both government involvement and competition from comprehensive prepaid health plans, insurers and employers created "major medical" insurance. This type of insurance covered more types of services than traditional hospital plans up to a maximum limit, but only after the policyholder had already spent a specified amount on medical care out of pocket (the deductible—see below). Because it was designed to cover only major, sudden expenses rather than minor or chronic conditions, major medical has also been called "catastrophic" health insurance. Major medical plans emerged in the late 1940s, and employers adopted them so eagerly that by 1954 almost 7 million people had this type of insurance.[54] But even as private insurers began to offer coverage of services beyond the hospital, they reiterated their commitment to traditional insurance principles and continued to fight against truly comprehensive coverage, insisting that limitations and exclusions remain a central principle of health insurance. To major medical they also added a new type of limitation: the deductible.

Cost-Sharing: How Much Should the Consumer Pay?

One thing that the insurance industry disliked almost as much as comprehensive policies was "first-dollar" coverage. Many nonprofit prepaid health plans, as well as Blue Cross in its early days, did not require any cash payment to see a doctor or enter a hospital; the care was covered from the "first dollar" spent. This was anathema to the insurance principle, since policyholders would have one less reason to stay away from the doctor's office or hospital. Additionally, insurers thought first-dollar coverage encouraged small claims (or "sniffle claims" in industry parlance) that people could otherwise afford to pay for on their own, such as checkups or care for minor illnesses. "Sniffle claims," they believed, would drive up overall costs. Insurers insisted that major medical plans offering coverage outside of hospital care must include deductibles.

A deductible is a specified amount of money the insured must pay out of pocket before coverage kicks in. Deductibles had been part of auto insurance coverage since the 1920s. Early health insurance did not include deductibles, but insurers adopted the concept in response to the comprehensive coverage debate, and to fears of rising costs. In addition, deductibles, also known as cost-sharing, were intended to address perennial concerns about moral hazard. Insurers believed that deductible requirements would "curb abuses by making the insured cost-conscious."[55]

At a time when the public, and labor unions in particular, demanded more comprehensive health benefits, deductibles and other forms of cost-sharing served as a reminder that health care cost money, and that health insurance was not an entitlement to "free care." Blue Shield executive Charles Hayden favored cost sharing because if the insured "has to pay for it out of his own pocket, it becomes a matter of, 'how can I best spend this money and get the most out of it?' If he is spending somebody else's money, he does not give a damn."[56] A General Electric benefits manager insisted that deductibles were essential because without them health insurance represented "the means for destroying personal responsibility—and with it the weakening of competitive enterprise." Cost sharing, he argued, forced employees to take responsibility for budgeting medical costs, even when they had insurance.[57]

The growth of insurance policies with deductibles was astronomical. Between 1951 and 1961, the number of people covered by major medical increased from 108,000 to 34 million.[58] Although some employers offered major medical as a supplement to basic Blue Cross policies—providing near-comprehensive coverage to employees with both plans—major medical increasingly encroached on the Blues' market share throughout the 1950s.[59] Labor unions pressured employers to choose Blue Cross or prepaid group medicine instead, but employers were enamored of major medical's initially lower premiums and cost-sharing features.[60] In the mid-1950s, for the first time Blue Cross and Blue Shield began to discuss adding deductibles and copayments (another type of consumer cost-sharing) to their health coverage as an alternative to increasing premiums. By 1966, some 39 million people had group supplemental major medical insurance, usually through their workplace. They had an average deductible of $100 and copayments averaging 20%, with a maximum benefit of $10,000. Increasing numbers of Blue Cross subscribers faced deductibles as well.[61]

What did consumers think about cost sharing? Several 1950s surveys of public attitudes toward health insurance included questions about major medical, deductibles, and copayments. A Michigan State Medical Society survey found that "almost a majority" of respondents approved of deductibles "when it is predicated upon a lowering of monthly premium costs."[62] When a Blue Cross survey mentioned deductibles as a hypothetical, some consumers seemed comfortable with the idea. "It's for the protection of the insurance company as well as the patient," said one woman. "A small bill of $25 anyone can pay nowadays," said another. One individual stated that a deductible would allow companies to "eliminate a lot of small claims and give you better coverage."[63]

Twenty-four percent of the respondents in the Blue Cross survey were already in a deductible plan and found it "satisfactory." Half were either "willing" (41 percent) or "glad" (9 percent) to consider such a plan. Most respondents' comments about deductibles were "mixed"; "in all, about a fourth of the responses were quite negative," and "the cores of resistance are most firmly entrenched in the younger members and lower class groups." Not "anyone" could pay a deductible without feeling financial pain; when asked about a hypothetical deductible of $50, one man replied, "There are so many times when $50 seems like a fortune to me and I don't think I am much different from the average person." A woman criticized deductibles because "most of the things that happen come in this small bracket and at the time it hurts to pay it. No, I do not like this. . . . I do not even carry it on my car."[64]

Family size played a crucial role in how the public perceived deductibles, since group insurance that covered dependents generally required a separate deductible for each member of the family. In other words, a $50 annual deductible for a family of six was actually a deductible of $300. Respondents critical of the deductible felt "that the primary financial drain of illness[es] is the frequency and periodicity with which they occur, especially in large or growing families." For example, one 34-year-old mother said of a deductible plan, "I don't think I would want it because it would take a pretty serious illness to get any benefit out of it. I am after the small things. With young children [I am] more after the minor things."[65]

In assessing the impact of deductibles, the Blue Cross survey's mostly upbeat account of health insurance turned surprisingly harsh. "Health insurance is seen as being . . . helpful in the realm of the 'rare' surgical procedures," the survey's anonymous authors concluded, "but of practically no value in the small illnesses which arise quite consistently in most families." And, in a comment that foreshadowed contentious debates to come: "To many of these individuals a deductible plan is in essence depriving them of health coverage."[66]

A Columbia University survey conducted two years later echoed many of these findings. In interviews with male members of General Electric's major medical insurance plan, which was widely admired, 66 percent of respondents were at least somewhat dissatisfied. When asked how their health coverage could be improved,

> the deductible was the principal target of their complaints. More than 230 men [out of 751] expressed dissatisfaction with the deductible, in contrast, for instance, to 37 who were critical of the coinsurance provisions. . . . It was the men with large families who were most likely to be critical of the per-person deductible (41 per cent of the men with 4 or more dependents mentioned the deductible, as opposed to 17 percent of the single men). We have seen that the Plan did not cover as high a proportion of the expenses incurred by large families.[67]

A study of federal employees with major medical insurance found that "the changes they most wanted were to have the individual deductibles abolished, reduced, or changed into family deductibles"—in other words, to have a single deductible for the entire family.[68] Another national study of three insured groups, led by the respected health researcher Odin Anderson, reported that "the majority, although not an overwhelming one, wanted either insurance that covered small expenses . . . or both small and heavy expenses." Like other studies, this one concluded that "the larger the family, the more likely is the desire for insurance which covers small expenses."[69]

Both the Blue Cross and Columbia survey respondents found copayments to be more acceptable than deductibles. However, once again large families, and people with chronic conditions that required frequent doctor's visits, felt that copayments could create barriers to needed medical care. "Family budgets can be severely hit by repeated $5 and $10 office and home doctor visits," a guide for consumers noted.[70] "I think people in the country would be healthier, more inclined to see a doctor," said one respondent in the Columbia survey, "if they didn't have to pay $5 or $10 each time." For members of California's Kaiser Permanente health plan, Kaiser's small copayment of one dollar was among the plan's most popular features. "A person hesitates when he has to pay $5 for a visit," said one Kaiser member in the Columbia study, "but not $1 a visit." Another member recalled, "My son got sick a long time ago, and I hesitated to go because I didn't have $5 for the doctor. And he got pneumonia." But after her family joined Kaiser, "when the children get sick we don't hesitate."[71]

Although proponents of deductible plans touted their lower premiums, some people were willing, even eager, to trade lower premiums for better coverage. In 1960, the Federal Employees' Health Plan offered members a choice between several "low option" and "high option" benefits, the latter giving greater coverage with little or no deductible. Four out of five chose the low-deductible, high-coverage plans, "even though the additional amount was paid entirely out of their own salaries." Only 7 percent chose the cheapest plan. Sixty-seven percent of the lowest-income federal employees chose the high-option plans as well.[72]

Whether the public wanted it or not, the Blues increasingly added cost-sharing to their health plans throughout the 1950s. At a 1954 conference of the Cooperative Association of America, a speaker complained that Blue Cross was "introducing deductible and so-called 'co-insurance' features which only discourage people from going for medical care early when they need it. . . . Blue Cross is running a national campaign to narrow and reduce the services in the interests of keeping premiums down, when the need is for more comprehensive coverage."[73] Labor unions objected to deductible plans, criticizing them as setting up additional "economic barriers to hospital care" for workers. A $300 deductible in a major medical insurance plan represented more than a month's income for a substantial number of American workers.[74] "Major medical is misnamed," concluded an American Federation of Labor pamphlet. "It should be called 'minor medical' because it will pay for only a minor part of a family's medical costs."[75]

Both coverage limitations and cost-sharing practices worked against the goal of preventive health care. Critics of the Blues and of commercial insurers pointed out how lack of comprehensive coverage kept people away from the doctor until it was too late to stop small problems from becoming serious ones. Although it seems that no studies were done on health outcomes for people in different types of insurance plans during this period, some anecdotal evidence pointed to a lack of preventive care for those with Blue Cross or commercial coverage. A 1962 consumer guide cited the case of a group of workers who had only Blue Cross hospitalization coverage. When their union switched coverage and the workers joined the Group Health prepayment plan, their new doctors found that many of the employees' children had not received basic immunizations, including polio shots.[76]

Like "comprehensive coverage," "preventive care" became a term disliked by private insurance leaders because of its associations with

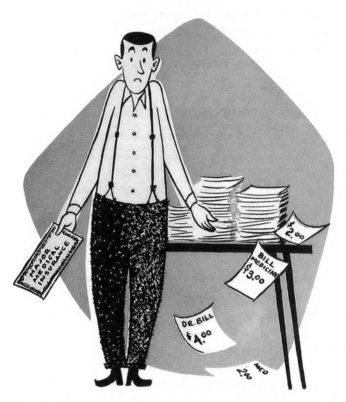

FIGURE 7. "Major Medical Should Really Be Called 'Minor Medical'": An AFL-CIO cartoon shows the impact of deductibles and copayments on an insured worker as his medical bills keep coming. *Catastrophic Illness Insurance: A Barrier on the Road to Health* (AFL-CIO Publication no. 51, May 1957). Michael M. Davis Collection, New York Academy of Medicine. Reprinted with permission of the George Meany Archive.

group practice and prepayment. At the private HIF meetings in 1954 delegates discussed a policy statement that would have put the insurance industry on record as being "concern[ed]" with "curative services only. In other words, we are not concerned with preventive services." This made some of the Blue Cross officials in attendance nervous. "I think it would be a great mistake to let it be known that we aren't concerned with" prevention, said one, and another expressed incredulity that HIF leaders had actually agreed to put forth a proposal for "the avoidance of preventive care." Some delegates defended the position, saying it was intended only to reaffirm the basic principle of "the insurance mechanism."[77]

Insurers at the meeting also wished to avoid coverage for long-term care, home health services, or chronic conditions. Charles Hayden of Blue Shield and the AMA, never reluctant to use colorful language, felt that the insurance industry must "draw a distinction between maintenance and medical care. I'm not interested in setting up a Blue Cross or Blue Shield Plan or any other kind of plan, because grandma has to be lifted on the pot twice a day. I'm not interested in that, because I don't think that's a medical problem."[78]

Despite this and many other derisive comments about coverage for preventive and long-term care, in the end meeting participants agreed to strike out the phrase "curative services only" from HIF's document. Although insurers did not want to come out in public as opposing prevention, they were aware that the policies of their industry tended to discourage preventive care, and that public and physician demands for more of such care called into question the basic principles of private insurance.

Most of the health insurance in force during the 1950s actually did the opposite of encouraging prevention: it drove people to use, and over-use, hospital services. Blue Cross especially, which covered care in the hospital but not the doctor's office, was beloved by the hospitals (who had, after all, invented the program) because its subscribers kept hospital beds filled. Heavy use of services contributed to both the rising cost of hospital care, and climbing costs for Blue Cross coverage.

Affordability was one of the initial goals of the Blue Cross model. However, by the early 1950s, plans were already having trouble keeping costs down. Concerns about rising expenses led the Blues to pioneer the study of hospital utilization trends. What they found was troubling. Michigan Blue Cross studied its membership in 1954 and reported that "Blue Cross members misused their hospital stay in nearly 36 percent of the cases," including "unnecessary admissions and overlong stays." Analysts believed that most of the misuse was deliberate—some on the part of the patients, but primarily on the part of physicians who understood that their patients would be covered for hospital care only. At a Pennsylvania state hearing on Blue Cross rate hikes in 1957, a highly respected physician, when asked if he had ever hospitalized patients because he knew they had Blue Cross, answered, "Of course. . . . Doesn't everybody?"[79]

Even necessary hospital care costs were rising as hospital capacity expanded because of Hill-Burton, and new medical technologies and surgical techniques were developed. Along with the rest of the economy, the cost of hospital supplies and wages rose throughout the 1950s. As a result, the average cost per patient-day doubled between 1946 and 1955.[80] Blue Cross responded by repeatedly increasing its premiums.

Throughout the decade, rate hikes for health coverage affected employers, workers, and unions. In 1955, Cleveland AFL and CIO leaders protested rising Blue Cross premiums, voicing concern "not only for their members, but for retired workers, widows and other fixed income groups, who may have serious difficulty or find it impossible to meet the increased cost."[81] When the New York chapter of Blue Cross asked for a 40 percent rate hike in 1957, labor leaders denounced the request, claiming that "commercial thinking and standards have begun to creep in to Blue Cross policy making."[82]

Commercial insurance also became more expensive. The rise of major medical resulted from the public's demand for comprehensiveness, but due to the deductible these plans made coverage even less comprehensive, and definitely made it more costly. Major medical contributed to the inflation of health care costs by allowing providers to charge what they wished, and also by favoring hospital use while discouraging preventive care.[83]

As this chapter has shown, leaders of the private insurance industry were fully aware of the limitations of private insurance coverage, and agonized over their implications even as they defended them. Blue Cross leaders and insurance executives worried that too much discussion of uninsured low-income people and senior citizens would imply that "voluntary health insurance can't do the job" and would lead to the dangerous conclusion that "any area of unmet demand will leave a vacuum for government to fill."[84] They were right, at least in part: the failure of the private insurance industry to meet the health coverage needs of America's senior citizens would be a crucial factor in the passage of Medicare.

Supporters of a private health insurance system would lose the battle against government insurance for the aged, but they still won the war. Medicare would embody many of the features of voluntary insurance, such as exclusion and cost sharing. Private health insurers after World War II created a system and a set of ideas that shaped the public plans that followed, not just by leaving so many uncovered, but by defending the principle that health insurance, by its very nature, was *not* intended to provide everyone with health care or economic security. In what political scientist Deborah Stone describes as a "struggle for the soul of health insurance," employers and private insurers insisted on rationing coverage via experience rating, limitations, cost sharing, and exclusions, and pushed back against public demands for economic security and comprehensive care.[85]

Abe Oseroff, administrator of Montefiore Hospital in Pittsburgh and founder of Pittsburgh Blue Cross, attended one of the Health Information Foundation's private meetings in 1954. He was quiet for most of the discussion, but after hearing the delegates agree on the need to resist comprehensive coverage and to expand disincentives for consumers to use medical care, he finally spoke. Oseroff expressed dismay at the direction the meeting had taken. "I was under the impression in the Blue Cross field . . . that we were attempting to cooperate . . . in the development of a health program that would bring to all the people the health services as they were needed," he said. "Now, the emphasis this afternoon has been upon the development of an insurance formula which would provide protection to the insurer, rather than to the insured."[86] Oseroff might have been speaking for the millions of Americans with private insurance whose incomes remained vulnerable to the costs of sickness, as well as the millions left out altogether.

PART III

*New Entitlements and
New Movements, 1965–80*

CHAPTER SIX

Entitlements but Not Rights: Medicare and Medicaid

"The doctors claimed that the fight was over government control of medicine. That wasn't it at all. The fight was over whether decent medical care is a basic right—like the right to food, shelter, clothing, and education. The people and Congress decided that it was."[1]

— Senator Clinton P. Anderson

Senator Anderson's enthusiasm was understandable in the heady days after Medicare's victory in July 1965. He was co-sponsor of the bill, and the battle against the AMA and Republican opponents in Congress had been hard fought. But did Medicare really bring health care into the realm of "basic rights"? Anderson may have forgotten temporarily that the United States did not define food, clothing, and shelter as official social rights. Medicare and Medicaid created massive and enduring federal and federal/state insurance systems to cover many medical costs for the elderly and the poor, but they did not confer a universal right to health care. And, like all other elements of US health system growth, Medicare and Medicaid created and enforced certain kinds of exclusion and denial even as they expanded access. For example, Medicare rationed coverage by age, and Medicaid by income, gender, and parental status.

In the 1950s, following the defeat of Truman's national health insurance proposal, reformers narrowed their ambitions by announcing a new plan targeted to the elderly only. Insurance for seniors would be seen as less threatening by the American Medical Association and the insurance industry, because it would cover those least likely to have private insurance. Also, it could be grafted on to the Social Security system, so no new administrative structure would be needed. Building on Social Security meant the program would be financed by payroll taxes, reinforcing the idea that recipients would earn their new benefits, rather than receive government handouts. The public viewed the elderly as an especially deserving group, in great need of medical care. In order to avoid confrontation with the medical profession, and to reflect the private Blue Cross model, reformers initially limited the proposed senior coverage to hospital care only, not even including doctor bills in the hospital.[2]

Health insurance for the elderly was the brainchild of officials in the Truman administration. The idea was next adopted by the AFL-CIO, whose member unions were involved in bargaining with employers for health benefits for retirees, but feared that the expense of such benefits would erode wages and protection for younger workers. Labor leaders found a sponsor in Rep. Aime Forand (D-RI), who first introduced a plan for health insurance tied to Social Security in Congress in 1957. President Eisenhower did not support the bill and conservative Southern Democrats blocked it in committee, but the hearings brought national attention to the idea of public medical insurance for the elderly.[3]

Between 1959 and 1961, a special Senate subcommittee to study the problems of citizens over age 65 held hearings in cities around the nation. The hearings gave older Americans a chance to air their hopes and fears about health care. In Boston, 40 senior citizens lined up to speak to the Congressmen. Some complained of the indignities of charity medical care, and described their experience at neighborhood clinics as "being herded along like animals." At the Florida hearing, a citizens' group urged Congress to "increase financial assistance to the aged so they could live out their lives in health."[4]

The Forand bill was reintroduced in 1960, this time under the sponsorship of Senators Clinton Anderson and John F. Kennedy. Kennedy believed that health insurance for the elderly, now named Medicare, could be a winning issue for Democrats and made it a major topic in his 1960 presidential election campaign. Kennedy's running mate Lyndon Johnson noticed that "medical care for the elderly repeatedly got the biggest applause" during stump speeches.[5]

The proposal's growing popularity spurred the AMA to action. The doctors' organization proposed an alternative program called Kerr-Mills, sponsored by Oklahoma Senator Robert Kerr and Arkansas Representative Wilbur Mills, both conservative Democrats, which offered matching grants to the states for assistance to the very poor elderly only. (As seen in chapter 1, the AMA had insisted on restricting federal help to the poorest of the poor since the 1930s.) Kerr-Mills passed in Congress in 1960. Opponents of more comprehensive programs believed this would end the movement for medical insurance for the aged, but Kerr-Mills, administered by the states, reached only a small minority of those in need because of its strict eligibility requirements.[6] At the same time that Kerr-Mills rationed coverage by both age and income, evidence was growing that a majority of elderly people, not just the very poor, needed assistance with medical bills.

The Problem of Insuring the Elderly

In 1900, there were only three million people over age 65 in the United States. By 1958, there were over 15 million, nearly 9 percent of the population. Older Americans had more health problems and spent 50 percent more on medical care than those under 65, and in some categories—hospital care and prescription drugs—they spent at least twice as much.[7] Although Social Security had greatly improved economic conditions for this part of the population, more elderly people than young people still lived in poverty, and Social Security payments were too small to cover high medical expenses. Existing state and local assistance programs, as well as the new federal Kerr-Mills program, were extremely limited and did not come close to meeting the health security needs of the elderly.

Private health insurance also fell short when it came to covering senior citizens. The insurance industry categorized people over age 65 as "substandard risks," because on average they were sicker and required more medical care than younger groups. Some Blue Cross/Blue Shield plans tried to assure continued coverage after 65 with higher premiums, but for commercial insurers, exclusion of the elderly and cancellation of policies at age 65 were "the rule rather than the exception."[8] A 1964 Senate subcommittee concluded that "private health insurance is unable to provide the large majority of our 18 million older Americans with adequate hospital protection at reasonable premium cost."[9]

Senior citizens' letters to members of Congress in support of Medicare complained of their problems with private health insurance, including expensive premiums, limited coverage, sudden cancellation, and inability to get coverage at all. "Our Social Security check is small[;] the Blue Cross is high," wrote an elderly Oklahoma woman to Rep. Carl Albert. Another senior worried, "I know that my (private insurance) policies would not be sufficient to cover the cost of hospital care, should I require it. The charges are just too great. And doctor's fees too enormous. What about elder citizens who do have real ailments, but are unable to procure health and hospitalization insurance? Something needs to be done." A 67-year-old Alabama woman and her 71-year-old husband had paid over $200.00 a year for Blue Cross/Blue Shield insurance for 11 years when their policy was suddenly cancelled. "I therefore feel very strongly that we need Medicare under such circumstances," she wrote to her senator, Lister Hill. "We think it is simply outrageous for Insurance Compan[ie]s to get so much money over the years and then let people out in such a manner."[10] Mrs. Joseph Tomisek of Chicago wrote to the *Tribune* about the high costs of doctors' visits, and "no x-rays, electrocardiograms, or blood tests included either"; she thought the Medicare plan "would be of inestimable value."[11] (In the end, those screening tests would not be covered under Medicare either.)

As industry executives had predicted (and feared) a decade earlier, the inability and unwillingness of private insurers to extend coverage to the elderly had led inexorably to calls for government intervention. Seniors' discontent with private insurance pushed many of them to support the Medicare proposals being discussed in Washington. And this time, the supporters of health care reform managed to organize a campaign powerful enough to take on the AMA.

The Battle over Medicare

In his February 9, 1961, message to Congress, President John F. Kennedy announced his support for a medical insurance program for the aged attached to Social Security. Medicare became a pillar of his domestic agenda. And unlike Roosevelt and Truman, Kennedy took the fight to the public.

Kennedy relied upon the support of organized labor and senior citizens in his fight against the AMA. In 1961, the AFL-CIO, with the encouragement of the Democratic National Committee, created the National Council of Senior Citizens (NCSC) out of its retiree membership, who were already well organized and easily reached via union newspapers. In 1962, the NCSC sponsored a letter-writing and postcard campaign to deluge Congress on behalf of Medicare. They also sent mass mailings to seniors around the country asking for their support.[12]

In May 1962, the NCSC pulled together the most visible public event the health reform movement had ever witnessed. President Kennedy accepted the group's invitation to address a Medicare rally at Madison Square Garden in New York, where he appeared before a cheering crowd of 20,000 senior citizens. In his speech the President insisted that Medicare did not represent socialized medicine or a threat to doctors' independence, reminding the audience that similar arguments had been made against Social Security in 1935. The crowd grew hushed as Kennedy spoke of his own father's devastating stroke. Joe Kennedy could pay his own hospital bills, the President admitted, but "what happens to him and to others when they put their life savings in, in a short time?"[13] Major television and radio networks broadcast the speech nationwide and to simultaneous rallies being held around the country by local branches of the NCSC.[14] Such a noisy public display of support for national health reform was unprecedented.

But the AMA had already put its public relations machine in high gear, and was employing "every propaganda tactic it had learned from the bitter battles of the Truman era," writes Ted Marmor.[15] The message was the same but the media were new, including radio, records, and television. In 1961, the AMA launched "Operation Coffee Cup," recruiting Hollywood movie star Ronald Reagan to record a speech opposing Medicare. The LP record was then mailed to AMA "ladies' auxiliaries" around the country, made up of doctors' wives. The ladies were to gather around the record player for coffee, listening to Reagan declaim that Medicare "was simply an excuse to bring about . . . socialized medicine" and that it represented the beginning of the end of freedom in America. Then, they were instructed to write their congressmen.[16] The AMA also produced anti-Medicare posters, literature, and petitions for physicians to display in their waiting rooms. The elderly were not really bad off, insisted the AMA, and did not require government insurance. Medicare threatened American traditions of voluntarism and freedom; it would "substitute decision-making by a small elite corps of federal administrators for the independent decisions of millions of consumers of medical services."[17]

Not all patients reacted as the AMA hoped to the waiting-room propaganda. "When I go to a doctor, it is for medical and surgical help, not political advice on matters which he seems to have a personal or selfish interest in," an Oklahoma constituent complained to his Congressman. A 65-year-old man visited his doctor and noticed "he had a petition asking all his patients to sign up against this [Medicare] program. . . . I told him no, I would not sign it." This citizen was angered enough that he demanded to make a speech before Congress in support of Medicare.[18]

Traditional tactics of physicians' opposition began to backfire.

When the AMA commissioned a study that found a majority of senior citizens had sufficient private health coverage, the media rushed to discredit it. Reporting that the doctors had only surveyed an affluent, all-white sample of elderly people, the *Chicago Defender* newspaper concluded that "this kind of opposition [to Medicare] in the long run will hurt the prestige of the American Medical Association."[19] United Auto Workers leader Walter Reuther's description of the AMA's propaganda campaign was pungent: "If they put it in bags, it would help your lawn grow better."[20]

Arguments that Medicare was un-American gained little traction. President Kennedy insisted, "This program is not socialized medicine. . . . It is a program of prepayment for health costs with absolute freedom of choice guaranteed. Every person will choose his own doctor and hospital."[21] The AMA lost one of its longtime allies in 1962 when the American Hospital Association reversed its traditional opposition and passed a resolution in support of Medicare, in exchange for promises that Blue Cross would play a role in administering the new program.[22]

This time around, the AMA was not winning hearts and minds. By 1962, polls showed 69 percent of the public in favor of Medicare.[23] The mobilization of senior citizens on behalf of the plan continued after Kennedy's tragic assassination. "Hundreds of energetic, elderly persons crowded into City Hall" at 1964 Medicare hearings in New York, reported the *New York Times*, whose reporter was surprised by the seniors' active participation; she noted that "the elderly persons had climbed two long flights of stairs" to get to the all-day hearing.[24]

The new President, Lyndon B. Johnson, vowed to carry on what Kennedy had started. He immediately took up the banner of Medicare and campaigned vigorously on the issue during his 1964 election campaign. Johnson's strong support for Medicare was inspired by Kennedy's legacy, and also by the labor and civil rights movements. In the spring of 1964, on a visit to Appalachia, Johnson witnessed coal miners protesting the loss of their company health benefits. This experience helped to convince the president to push urgently for Medicare.[25] Johnson, who supported the fight against racial discrimination far more vigorously than Kennedy, also saw Medicare as part of his overall civil rights agenda. In a phone call to Martin Luther King Jr. as the civil rights leader was preparing to march in Selma, Alabama, LBJ mentioned Medicare alongside voting rights as legislation that would benefit African Americans.[26]

Civil rights activists had understandably been less interested in medical care for the aged than they were in the urgent fight against racism and segregation. Baseball star and civil rights advocate Jackie Robinson wrote in a 1962 newspaper column that he wished JFK would fight as hard for civil rights legislation as he was fighting for Medicare, "to wipe out the deadly virus of racial prejudice."[27]

Still, some civil rights organizations had thrown their support behind Medicare early on. In 1962, one Chicago group, the African American Heritage Association, called for a national "all-out effort" of blacks on behalf of Medicare. The National Medical Association, the organization of African American doctors, voted to back Medicare that same year, in defiance not only of the AMA but also of its own leadership. Members waged a "bitter floor fight" at the NMA's 1962 annual meeting; the supporters of Medicare, led by Dr. Montague Cobb, won the vote by 106 to 71.[28] Cobb, a tireless advocate of racial justice, insisted that medical rights and civil rights were inextricably connected. "It is noteworthy," he said, "that in a roll call of the recent Senate vote . . . the senators who opposed medical care for the elderly through Social Security were almost to a man those who traditionally oppose civil rights legislation."[29]

Although Martin Luther King Jr. would not make a major public statement on health care until 1968 (see chapter 7), he strongly argued for a connection between voting rights and social legislation such as Medicare: black Americans, King wrote in the *New York Times* the day before passage of the 1965 Voting Rights Act, needed "the full power of the ballot" so that they could elect legislators to support "the Medicare, housing, schools and jobs required by men of any color."[30]

In 1965, health insurance for the elderly had the full, vocal support of the President, backed by the labor movement, civil rights leaders, and senior citizens. With LBJ's landslide election and a Democratic majority in Congress, Medicare seemed poised for victory. The AMA quickly proposed a new voluntary program that would cover doctors' bills for the elderly as an alternative, which was co-sponsored by Congressional Republicans.

But the doctors were outmaneuvered by LBJ and his new ally, powerful Ways and Means Chairman Wilbur Mills. Following pressure from the President to support his bill, Mills dramatically expanded the Medicare proposal by adding two new programs: a voluntary system to cover doctors' bills—virtually identical to the AMA's alternative plan—that would become known as Medicare Part B; and Medicaid,

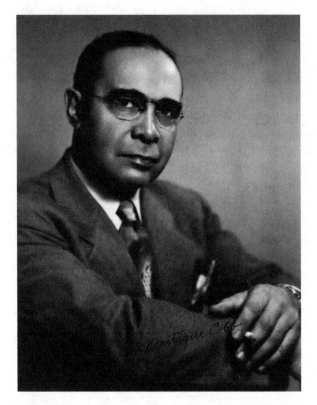

FIGURE 8. W. Montague Cobb, President of the National Medical Association, a leading advocate of racial equality in health care and Lyndon Johnson's ally in the fight for Medicare. National Library of Medicine.

health insurance for public assistance recipients, an expansion of Mills' own Kerr-Mills program. The resulting "three-layer cake" (Medicare Part A, Medicare Part B, and Medicaid) helped deflate the AMA's and Republican opposition and win Congressional support for the package.[31] The bill was approved by the House 313 to 115 in April 1965, and by the Senate 68 to 21 in July. Johnson used his powers of persuasion to break the Southern Democrat voting bloc, convincing several powerful senators to vote in favor. Half of Congressional Republicans also supported Medicare.[32]

Johnson's celebratory speech did not mention rights, but he did invoke FDR's "freedom from fear." Medicare, the President declared, meant that "a great burden will be lifted from the shoulders of all Americans. Older citizens will no longer have to fear that illness will wipe out their savings, eat up their income, and destroy lifelong hope of dignity and independence. For every family with older members it will mean relief from the often-crushing responsibilities of care." LBJ emphasized that Medicare recognized society's obligation to the elderly, and the deservingness of senior citizens: "For the Nation it will bring the necessary satisfaction of having fulfilled the obligations of justice to those who have given a lifetime of service and labor to their country."[33] On July 30, 1965, Johnson flew to Independence, Missouri, so that he could sign the Medicare bill with Harry Truman at his side. "You have made me a very, very happy man," said the former President, finally savoring a victory against the AMA.[34]

Johnson succeeded where Truman failed because he commanded congressional majorities and brilliantly persuaded members of the opposition, but also because he was backed by organized popular support. Civil rights activists, "energetic elderly persons," and organized labor provided the public pressure needed for both JFK and LBJ to act and to succeed as health reform leaders. After Medicare won, Johnson credited these activists for their help. He invited both the director

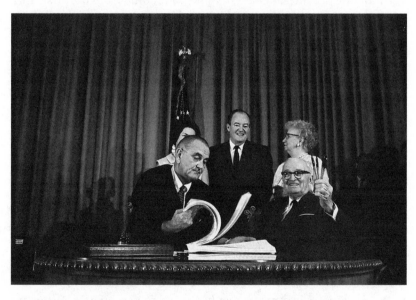

FIGURE 9. Lyndon B. Johnson signs the Medicare Bill with former president Harry Truman looking on triumphantly, Independence, Missouri, July 30, 1965. Behind them are Lady Bird Johnson, Vice President Hubert Humphrey, and Bess Truman. Harry S. Truman Library, Independence, Missouri.

of the National Council of Senior Citizens, Lawrence Oxley, and the head of the National Medical Association, Dr. Montague Cobb, to witness the Medicare signing ceremony alongside Harry Truman. Cobb in turn praised Johnson for his continued commitment to "ending racial discrimination from American life." It was clear that the civil rights leader and the president each felt that Medicare's victory would not have been possible without the other.[35]

Medicare also helped the civil rights movement get closer to one of its goals: the racial desegregation of Southern hospitals.

Medicare and Civil Rights

Shortly after the bill's passage, the Johnson administration turned Medicare into a highly effective tool for racial desegregation. The 1963 Supreme Court ruling *Simkins v. Cone* had declared the "separate but equal" provision of Hill-Burton unconstitutional, and Title VI of the 1964 Civil Rights Act expressly forbade racial discrimination in federally funded institutions. However, a majority of Southern hospitals remained segregated at the time of Medicare's passage. In Medicare, the federal government had a new and powerful weapon: the threat of withholding potentially huge amounts of funding from hospitals that refused to desegregate.

The Office of Equal Health Opportunity (OEHO) in the US Public Health Service worked with the Social Security Administration to enforce federal civil rights laws in Southern hospitals that wanted to receive Medicare funds. Hospitals had to prove that they were compliant before being certified for Medicare. Most Southern hospitals complied quickly, as least on paper, in order to receive the federal dollars, and by October 1966 the vast majority had been certified. Significant inroads were made against official segregation in this brief period. Sociologist Jill Quadagno describes the shakeup at several Southern hospitals: "Many hospitals admitted their first black patients, made room assignments without regard to race, removed barriers in waiting rooms, operating rooms, and cafeterias, and offered staff privileges to black physicians for the first time."[36]

But some hospitals resisted. Health policy historian David Barton Smith describes the turmoil in Mobile, Alabama, where a white hospital, the Mobile Infirmary, openly refused to desegregate. When investigators arrived from Washington to confirm that a group of white physicians were behind the resistance, the local newspaper launched a furious campaign against federal interference, and Governor George

Wallace called OEHO's refusal to certify the infirmary "heartless" and "immoral." The house of the local civil rights leader in the compliance campaign was firebombed, and a white female physician who had provided federal investigators with information was found shot to death. Eventually, the Mobile Infirmary did begin admitting some black patients and received its compliance certificate in July 1967. Federal officials dropped their investigation of white doctors' admitting practices in Mobile, which Smith calls "tantamount to capitulation."[37]

Paper compliance with civil rights regulations did not necessarily mean real progress toward racial equality in health care. Medicare-certified hospitals found many ways to avoid true desegregation. Some hospitals employed a strategy of converting their accommodations to all private rooms so that black and white patients would not have to share—even using Medicare funds to do this. Compliance could be won by showing the admission of black patients and proving the desegregation of waiting rooms; but hospitals could continue to refuse privileges to black doctors, so that they could not admit their own patients or practice at the hospital. In Atlanta, half of the members of the black Atlanta Medical Association applied for admitting privileges at dozens of hospitals that had been declared "compliant"; none were fully admitted, and two were given temporary privileges only.[38] In addition, Medicare Part B, insurance for physician services, was specifically exempted from Title VI of the Civil Rights Act, so white doctors could still exercise discriminatory hospital admitting privileges, as they did in Mobile.[39] "We are intelligent enough to know that because a hospital put on paper an affirmative response to compliance, this is not assurance that justice will be done," declared the Atlanta physicians. "Changes are not 'automatic'—they are 'systematic.'"[40] The battle against racial discrimination in hospitals would continue with Medicare as a major new weapon. But informal types of segregation, including economic segregation, would prove even hardier enemies than official Jim Crow.

The High Cost of Medicare

In the mad dash to political compromise, Medicare's framers deliberately kept mechanisms for cost control out. Any regulation of physicians' fees or hospital costs might be seen as government interference in the practice of medicine, which the legislation expressly forbid. An Alabama resident wrote Lister Hill, "If prices charged for public utilities can be regulated, it does not seem beyond reason to control prices in the more urgent field of human life and health."[41] Such pleas were ignored by Congress.

The hospital payment provisions of Part A were drafted in secret negotiations between the American Hospital Association, Blue Cross, and the Social Security Administration. The terms that emerged from those meetings made clear why the hospital industry threw its enthusiastic support behind Medicare. Hospitals could charge Medicare "retrospectively" (after services were delivered) for what it deemed "reasonable costs"—to be determined entirely by the hospitals. In addition to reimbursement for reasonable costs, hospitals also received a 2 percent bonus, with no upper limit, to cover administration, supplies, drugs, depreciation on buildings and equipment, and even public relations. The federal government paid an extra 7.5 percent to for-profit hospitals and nursing homes, to go straight to their bottom line.[42]

Physicians' fees under Part B were equally unregulated. Payment was fee for service based on "prevailing," "reasonable" charges—their "reasonableness" again determined by the physicians themselves, with no oversight by the government or anyone else.

Leaders in Washington did worry that the lack of cost controls in Medicare might lead to "growing pressure toward high prices." A month before Medicare's launch, LBJ asked doctors and hospitals to "exercise intelligent self-restraint" to "prevent unreasonable costs for health services."[43] But doctors, hearing of the "prevailing charges" rule, began raising their fees even before Part B's implementation. The first year of the program, physicians' charges shot up dramatically. "Doctors' Fees Up as Much as 300% under Medicare," the *New York Times* announced.[44]

Some of the increase was due simply to the new reality that many doctors who served the poor elderly were being compensated, by Medicare, for the first time for patients who had previously been unable to pay—a longtime goal of health reform. "I'm not raising fees, I'm eliminating a discount," explained one New York MD.[45] But many doctors were also charging far more than they had before Medicare. At a 1967 hearing on health costs, a Minnesota surgeon told Senators that "we doctors, like our patients, act as if the Government's money is no money. If the patient isn't going to have to pay us for our services out of his own pocket then he doesn't care how much we charge—and neither do we." As a result, Medicare patients were being "overhospitalized and overtreated" and "the medical profession consequently is being overcompensated for its services."[46]

In 1968 President Johnson again pleaded, "I appeal to the entire medical profession in this country to exercise restraint in their fees and their charges." But his calls went unheeded. Medicare's reimbursement mechanism and preservation of fee-for-service payment created a strong incentive for doctors to charge more, and eventually contributed to the US medical profession becoming the highest paid in the world. Hospital costs also grew dramatically. In the decade following Medicare's passage, the average cost per patient per day more than doubled, and hospitals' total assets rose from $16.4 billion to $47.3 billion. Alongside the growing costs of medical care in general (due to new technologies and treatments, higher labor costs, and overall inflation), Medicare payments to doctors and hospitals helped drive the rise in national health expenditures from $198 per capita in 1965 to $336 by 1970.[47]

Medicare's Benefits and Limits

In the first years of the program, Americans were less concerned about Medicare's costs and more about its benefits to the nation's seniors. Many saw the program as a major step forward in the nation's quest for better health and security. Medicare meant that seniors could use doctors and hospitals without fear of financial disaster. It was also a benefit earned through work and tax paying, that applied to the poor and middle-class elderly alike. When former president Harry Truman, himself a senior citizen, was issued the first Medicare card in 1966, he announced, "For many it is a step from charity, to security with dignity."[48]

Medicare allowed many seniors access to quality medical care for the first time. Desire F. Metzemakers of Lawrence, Massachusetts, who previously had not been able to afford the surgery he needed, felt "personally indebted" to President Johnson after receiving "exceptionally good care in the Lawrence General Hospital, all of which was assumed by the program that [the President] fought for and insisted on passage in the Congress of the United States." An Atlanta couple whose hospital bills were covered by Medicare expressed appreciation that "the fact that this Federal Program has been of such great financial assistance helps them face the future with a feeling of greater comfort."[49]

"I woke up the other night and knew I had to write to you and say thank-you Mr. Johnson from the bottom of my heart," a woman wrote the President from California. Her father was dying of cancer at a small hospital, and even though the family was low-income, "if he was a millionaire and had a lot of pull he could never receive any better care anywhere in the world. . . . We could never have made it without 'Medicare'!"

"My husband (77) had a cerebral stroke and was in the hospital 5 weeks," wrote another California woman to the President. "He just passed away and I don't know what I would have done without Medicare. We had a little savings but it would not have been a drop in the bucket toward hospital costs. Thank you again and may God bless you for this wonderful aid."[50]

Johnson must have been gratified by this outpouring of appreciation for the new benefits of Medicare. But the program also had its limits. Especially, it fell short of fully protecting recipients against health insecurity. Because Medicare was based on the principles of the private insurance industry, beneficiaries found themselves experiencing many of the same limitations and cost sharing that burdened people who had private insurance. Although it is mostly famous and appreciated (and reviled) for its generosity, Medicare also rationed in various ways, including deductibles, caps, limits on hospital stays, and exclusion of some types of care.

Medicare Part A coverage was a carbon copy of Blue Cross and many private insurance hospitalization plans. It covered hospital costs but not the charges of practitioners. In other words, Part A paid for the hospital room but not the physician, the operating room but not the surgeon, the anesthesia but not the anesthetist (unless practitioners were hospital employees). And the plan paid these costs only after a $40 deductible and 20 percent copayment. After ninety hospital days, Medicare no longer paid anything. There was no limitation on the overall amount of out-of-pocket costs beneficiaries had to pay. Enrollment in Part B, insurance for doctors' fees, was voluntary and not automatic. Unlike Part A, which was funded by payroll taxes, Part B required premium payments, initially $3 a month. Both Part A deductibles and Part B premiums increased in 1970, to $53 and $4 respectively, and continued to rise every decade since then.[51]

Deductibles, copayments, and premiums prevented some seniors from seeking care and coverage. A 1971 study found that Medicare Part B enrolled proportionately fewer lower-income and nonwhite seniors, and "whites make greater use of the benefits . . . than do nonwhites." The report suggested that the extra costs of Medicare "might have discouraged lower income people from securing health care because they couldn't afford the (now) $50 deductible nor the 20 percent coinsurance."[52] Flat-rate copayments and deductibles disproportionately affected poorer seniors, just as they did in private insurance. An Alabama senior reported, "I'm 74 years old, a widow, my social security income is $210 a month and I have no other income. I've been hospitalized 3 times in the last 3 months and I owe doctor and hospital bills over and above Medicare that I just cannot pay."[53]

Medicare's coverage limitations raised immediate concerns. Because of the potential expense, the plan offered no coverage for prescription drugs outside of the hospital or for long-term care in nursing homes, both an increasingly important part of seniors' health care. Just five days after Medicare became law, Illinois Senator Paul Douglas held a press conference to urge that coverage be extended to prescription drugs.[54] His and other calls for a Medicare drug benefit were denied for the next four decades, until the creation of Medicare Part D in 2003. Long-term care also was not included due to concerns about its potential expense.[55]

Medicare's limitations proved beneficial to the private insurance industry, which immediately began offering "Medigap" plans to cover the Medicare copayment and additional services. In this way, Medicare created an entirely new market for supplemental private health insurance. As early as March 1966, Blue Cross announced its new "Medicare Booster Plan." "Our approach has been to develop a structure of benefits that take over where Medicare leaves off," the company explained.[56] "Persons age 65 and over have been faced with a growing problem in financing those portions of their hospital and medical bills which are not covered by the federal Medicare program," noted the Health Insurance Association of America. By the mid-1970s, around 12.6 million Medicare recipients had purchased some form of supplemental insurance. These policies covered expenditures Medicare did not, such as the copayments that begin on the sixty-first day of a hospital stay, some doctors' bills above a deductible, out-of-hospital prescription drugs, medical appliances, and equipment. Medigap policies were offered by reputable insurers, including Blue Cross / Blue Shield, but the industry admitted that some companies in this market subjected seniors to "high pressure sales tactics, fraudulent representation, false or misleading advertising, overinsurance, replacement of already adequate policies, inadequate coverage at excessive rates, intentional inadequate disclosure or misstatement of coverage."[57]

In the mid-1970s, the costs and limitations of Medicare were major concerns reflected in letters written by older Americans to the National Council of Senior Citizens and members of Congress. The NCSC received a flood of such mail during its vigorous campaign in support of Senator Edward Kennedy's national health insurance proposals. A decade after Medicare's passage, costs had increased but the benefit limitations remained the same. As the price of drugs and supplemental insurance policies continued to rise, some seniors found Medicare unable to bring them health or economic security.

The lack of prescription drug coverage proved to be a major problem for people with chronic conditions. An elderly business owner whose wife was crippled by a stroke made slightly too much money to qualify for Medicaid, but "Medicare does not pay for any of our medicines." He invoked his ancestors' sacrifices in slavery in his plea for help with drug costs: "We were brought over here in chains and help[ed] build this country . . . hoping you will help people to understand that can help us." A retired union member from Colorado wrote, "I have Blue Cross, Blue Shield and Medicare but . . . I have to pay for the full price for my medicine. . . . They are taking everything Senior citizens have almost." A nurse practitioner in North Carolina reported that "some people feel that it is useless to come see a doctor if they then cannot afford the medication that he will prescribe."[58]

Medicare conferred a right to (partial) health coverage for seniors, but it did not confer a right to care. Although the vast majority of physicians accepted Medicare, doctors remained free to refuse Medicare patients, or to charge patients more than Medicare would reimburse them. "It is so hard to find a Dr. that works with Medicare, BC and BS," wrote the Colorado pensioner. "I went to one Dr. here, and Medicare paid him 123 and he had charged me 154. Now we have to make up the difference to pay him off." An Oregon man wrote, "It is getting harder and harder to find a Medical Doctor that will even accept my Medicare card anymore simply because it takes too much effort and it also takes to long for the Doctor to be paid for his services." He concluded with a claim to health care rights: "Frankly sirs this is simply one hell of a way to treat the old people that worked a lifetime and paid the Social Security Taxes along with doing a little dying bleeding and paying taxes to support our beloved country. . . . Decent Medical treatment should be a 'right' and not a privilege as it is all practiced to-day in America."[59]

Lack of coverage for long-term care forced a 72-year-old man to return to work, "16 to 18 hours a day to help pay for my wife's care in a Convalescent hospital. . . . For the past nine months I have paid an average of $700 a month for her care, and couldn't get help from Medicare because the care was considered purely custodial." Again invoking the sacrifices made throughout a long lifetime, he asked, "What can be done for the old folks who have built this great country to what it is[?]"[60] A Texas woman wrote to President Johnson, "The nursing homes and hospitals rates have increased since Medicare went into effect. I thought Medicare was to help the elderly but it hasn't been any good for those confined to nursing home."[61]

Medicare's premiums, copayments, and deductibles took a bite out of already strained budgets. "We have been advised by Medicare that starting July 1st our premium is again going up. Entrance in a hospital went up $20," wrote R. Hirsh in 1977, complaining of the lack of reward for long sacrifice: "We OLD PEOPLE in our 70s-80s and yes in our 90s helped get our beloved country to the status it is in by working for 25c an hour after the 1929 depression. . . . Our Medicare goes up one dollar each year, my Blue Cross premium better than doubled. . . . I guess we are the forgotten citizen instead of the senior."[62]

One frequent complaint in the seniors' letters was not directed at Medicare's cost or coverage; instead, it was directed at the program's unavailability to anyone under 65. Despite Medicare's many problems and limitations, it offered a form of very desirable coverage and security that remained out of reach for the majority of Americans. Medicare's rationing by age created a new set of rights claims, as a citizen's sixty-fifth birthday triggered a right to coverage that was denied to younger people who might be equally or even more in need of aid. Several people wrote to the NCSC asking if there was any form of help for those under age 65. (In 1962, Congress partly addressed this problem by allowing severely disabled people under 65 to apply for Medicare.)[63]

Citizens' complaints about Medicare reflected the limitations in the program's ability to protect seniors from the full cost of sickness, as well as objections to rationing by age. But overall public opinion on Medicare was, and continues to be, extremely positive. It is among the nation's most popular and fiercely defended social programs.

Medicare offers a kind of security to seniors that is unavailable anywhere else in the health care system. Eligibility is automatic. It protects not just seniors but their families from the burden of paying for a significant portion of the health costs of the elderly. The vast majority of doctors and hospitals participate, allowing seniors greater choice than most private health insurance plans. Its low administrative costs have made Medicare a model for broader national health insurance proposals. Despite its large share of the federal budget, politicians have not (yet) dared to attempt cutting Medicare benefits. Perhaps most important, Medicare is social insurance earned by a lifetime of work and tax paying (and sacrifice, as the letter writers above assert). As the Medical Committee for Human Rights proclaimed in 1967, "Already, the elderly have been granted a new dignity in the doctor's office and in the hospital. Those over 65 have finally been freed from the yoke of episodic charity and its concomitant indignities, and have become *paying patients*."[64] Medicare did not establish a right to health care, but it did confer an honorable entitlement on the nation's seniors.

For Medicaid, the third layer of the three-layer cake whipped up in 1965, the story was very different.

Medicaid: A Separate and Unequal System for the Poor

During the fight over Medicare, the AMA had proposed as an alternative a program of health coverage for poor seniors. Such a program, Kerr-Mills, already existed in limited form. Originating in a 1950 federal program that helped pay the medical bills of welfare recipients, Kerr-Mills, cosponsored by Medicare architect Wilbur Mills, had been adopted by 28 states by 1965.[65] In the midst of the Medicare battle, Mills grafted a version of the AMA's proposal—expanded to include the non-elderly poor—onto the Medicare bill. He named it Medicaid.

Medicaid (Title XIX of the Social Security Act) offered federal grants to encourage states to provide medical assistance for certain categories of low-income people. States could choose whether or not to participate in Medicaid, with the federal government paying from 50 to 83 percent of the state program's costs. By making participation optional on the part of states, Medicaid clearly avoided establishing a right to this assistance.

Medicaid required participating states to make medical assistance programs available to all recipients of "categorical" federal welfare programs (Aid to Families with Dependent Children and federal aid to the blind, disabled, and needy elderly). But additional eligibility requirements and program budgets were entirely up to the states. By 1970, all but two states (Alaska and Arizona) had joined Medicaid (Arizona would be the last holdout, until well into the 1980s).

While states had great leeway regarding whom they would cover, they could not choose to offer less than the minimum levels of medical benefits set by the federal government. Extending what Kerr-Mills had established, in some states Medicaid provided far more comprehensive coverage than Medicare, including inpatient and outpatient hospital services, laboratory and x-ray costs, nursing home care, and doctors' bills. Federal matching funds were provided for states that wanted to provide even more coverage, including prescription drugs. But the program's payments to hospitals and doctors were far less generous then Medicare's.

The differences between Medicare and Medicaid were striking. The split between the two programs exacerbated and made permanent the placement of the poor and the middle class into two separate tiers of the health care system. Medicare, as noted, was to be an honorable entitlement earned via payroll contributions, Medicaid a stigmatized public assistance or "welfare" program. While Medicare rationed on the basis of age, Medicaid would ration on the basis of income, gender, parenthood, and welfare status. The long-held notion that the poor and the middle class and affluent deserved different types of coverage and care became the law of the land.

"Means Test Medicine"

Medicaid enshrined in federal law an age-old method of rationing: the "means test," or income requirements. The program disqualified individuals or families with too many "means" because they were presumed capable of paying on their own. The means test had long been criticized as a humiliating invasion of privacy. Postwar European welfare states repudiated this form of rationing, preferring benefits conferred as a right of citizenship. But the means test remained a staple of state, local, and federal welfare programs in the United States (as it does today).

On the national level, means-tested health programs had been proposed earlier as alternatives to universal, compulsory health insurance. In 1947 Republican Senator Robert Taft, a bitter opponent of Truman, proposed a means-tested program for the poor only. The ideological component of the means test, and the justification of a two-tier medical system based on income, were evident in Taft's rhetoric. He said that hard-working Americans should pay for their own medical care, and those that could not should "have to take it [medical care] the way the State says to take it."[66] Truman supporters lambasted the means test and Taft's plan in a pamphlet: "What do they stand for: Taft: *Charity medical care*! . . . This means charity care after you apply for charity and pass a 'means test'—a snooping investigation into your family's and your relatives' income." Truman's national insurance proposal, on the other hand, would mean "Medical care *as a right and not as charity*."[67]

The means test had a practical component: it was one way of rationing scarce resources. According to a 1952 public health report, "inadequate funds" for welfare and health services "mean that eligibility requirements must be more stringent to reduce the number of persons served."[68] The means test was also a way to ensure that only the truly needy received aid; one doctor announced in 1961 that "we [physicians] view the means test as a device for weeding out free-loaders and social parasites."[69]

The means test became a central feature of the 1960 Kerr-Mills legislation. Applicants for Kerr-Mills benefits had to submit to detailed investigations of their assets. Twelve states had "family responsibility" provisions requiring not just the applicants but also their family members to submit to the means test. According to a Senate report, "A number of elderly persons in Buffalo, when informed of this provision reportedly told the welfare commissioner, 'Please kill my application. . . . I don't want my son questioned.'" The report concluded with a harsh assessment of Kerr-Mills: "In 'means test medicine,' far too much emphasis is placed upon the means test and not enough upon the medicine."[70]

Seniors increasingly saw the means test as a personal affront. One citizen wrote pointedly to Congress that "I have noticed over the years that the US Government has taken very good care of General Eisenhower, furnishing him with the very best of medical and hospital care at the tax payers expense. . . . And I don't believe that there is anything mentioned about a pauper's oath as our senior citizens are forced to take under the Kerr-Mills Bill."[71] In New York, one large labor union (the International Ladies' Garment Workers' Union) "became so angry at the harshness of the means-test administration . . . that it advised its members not to use Kerr-Mills."[72] The backlash against means testing increased support for Medicare among senior citizens. The Senate report quoted earlier pointed out that, in contrast to Kerr-Mills, "a social security–financed program would not spend millions in investigating income and assets of applicants and their relatives."[73]

Despite the strong criticism of the means test by both citizens and members of Congress, the 1965 Medicaid legislation left the practice intact. Medicaid was basically an extension of Kerr-Mills to the very poor under age 65.[74] Unlike Medicare Part A, eligibility for Medicaid was far from automatic; means testing would be required.

In all the fuss over Medicare, Medicaid went virtually unnoticed until the summer of 1966. Then newspapers began to pick up on the story of "the Sleeper Provision of the Medicare Act," whose "Cost May Dwarf That of Care for the Aged" (*Chicago Tribune*).[75] While some states were slow to adopt Medicaid and others created the most miserly programs possible, larger, wealthier states like New York quickly took advantage of Medicaid's "medically needy" (medically indigent) provisions to expand coverage to many more people. Medicaid costs in these states began to grow far beyond what policy makers had envisioned.[76] By 1968, President Johnson was already forced to ask for program cuts.

Spiraling costs, as well as negative publicity generated by unscrupulous physicians accused of profiting from "Medicaid mills," became the major Medicaid stories of the late 1960s and '70s. The positive side of the story, that Medicaid was beginning to improve the overall health of the poor, went mostly unnoticed.[77] Also hidden from public view were the stories of the people who began using the new form of coverage.

Experiencing Medicaid

When the federal Department of Health, Education, and Welfare held hearings across the country in 1968 and 1969 to gauge the public response to Medicaid, dozens of poor women came forward to describe their experiences and also to offer powerful criticism of the program. The participation of these women at the hearings received virtually no notice in the press and no specific response from government, but their testimony offers a glimpse into recipients' experiences with the early Medicaid program, and with the two- tier medical system in general.

Poor women at the hearings showed a surprisingly uniform response to Medicaid. Many expressed gratitude for the existence of the new program. The words of Mrs. Bessie Goodwin of Bedford Stuyvesant in Brooklyn, who identified herself as a "Medicaid card holder," were typical, and stirring. "My statement today is based upon what Medicaid has personally meant to me and members of my community," Mrs. Goodwin stated. "For the first time in my life I am able to get medical care like other Americans for myself and the members of my family. Since Medicaid, I do not have to wait until someone falls seriously ill before we rush to see the doctor, which was usually in the emergency room of the nearest hospital."[78]

But welfare recipients at these hearings also testified that Medicaid exacerbated the indignity of being poor and continued to put up barriers to obtaining medical care. Several women and their minister described conditions at Grady Hospital, the city hospital in Atlanta, which was the only place in town that would accept Medicaid cards. As a result, overcrowding became horrendous. Emergency room waits ranged from eight to ten hours. Many Medicaid recipients lived far from the hospital and did not have transportation to get there. They were denied certain drugs, glasses, and other items they needed. After the women's stories, the Reverend Austin Ford asked the hearing, "Why should not these people be as free to go to any hospital as to go to Grady?"[79] He raised an issue central to the critique of welfare medicine: that in a system and culture that worshipped free choice of physician or hospital, the poor were denied that choice.

Even in the hospitals and clinics that did accept Medicaid, welfare patients were treated separately and differently from others. Lucy Priggs of Washington, DC, who was diabetic, described waiting for two hours at DC General Hospital to get syringe needles while dozens of private-pay patients got to go ahead of her and received their needles.[80] Many women also spoke of the stigma of the separate line that Medicaid clients had to stand in; as Odell Young of Columbus, Ohio, described it, "when I went in the [University Hospital] clinic you are sick to start with and here stands a line of paid customers here (indicating); here is the welfare customers here. . . . What I would like to talk about," she continued, "is the poor people having a little more human dignity. We poor people that are on welfare everywhere we go we stand in line. We are marked by people [for] holding a card. 'You are welfare. You go to the clinics. That is what you do.'"[81]

One of the biggest problems facing poor women seeking health care was a shortage of doctors willing to accept Medicaid. Mrs. Young of Columbus told of a doctor she knew who "has got a big sign up on his door, 'Welfare Clients Monday and Wednesday Only.' Tuesday, Thursday and Friday you can die . . ."[82] A welfare rights activist in Washington, DC, testified that she called dozens of doctors on a list of those accepting Medicaid, and only a few of them actually agreed to make an appointment with a new Medicaid client. Several other women at the Washington hearing also testified that doctors who claimed to take

Medicaid either limited the number of Medicaid patients or refused them altogether.[83]

Especially moving testimony came from a migrant farm worker at the San Francisco hearing. She spoke of the importance of Medicaid to herself and her family after she was badly burned in a fire: "I don't know what I'd do without Medi-Cal. . . . I had no money, no insurance, when I received the Medi-card, I was losing the arm, it cost $1,200. So you see, I didn't lose my arm, so I'm proud of the Medi-card. . . . So I say, everybody needs it." But she went on to tell the audience that about three months earlier, her ten-year-old boy, who was born with severe birth defects, suddenly "got trouble with [his] bladder, and he [could] not make water. And we were so afraid, and we took him [in] the morning, about 9:30, we took him to five doctors in Morgan Hill, and nobody wanted to take him. He was all night and all those hours not making water, and he was all swollen. He would just holler and holler. And we went to these five doctors, and they don't want to see him. I say, 'I've [got] the Medicard'; they say 'No.'"[84]

While a shortage of doctors plagued Medicaid recipients, another aspect of the program that received notice at the hearings was the strict eligibility requirements that excluded a great proportion of the nation's poor and virtually all of the working poor. A Mrs. Flanagan of Baltimore, spoke of her oldest girl, who had her left lung taken out at age two. Local welfare programs helped pay her annual medical bills of several hundred dollars a year until Mrs. Flanagan went back to work. "So, since I went to work they cut me off from medical assistance. . . . I have a boy, he is five. He had a fractured skull in May. So I still owe for his hospital bill and I have taken him back for these stitches to be removed and they said, 'Mrs. Flanagan, how much money do you have? To remove the stitches will be $10.' So I said I only had $6. So they refused to take the stitches out. So I brought my child back and removed the stitches myself from his ear." Mrs. Flanagan made too much money to qualify for Medicaid, even though she could not afford $10 for her son's stitches to be removed. This was one of the most frequent comments of people testifying at the hearings: concern that the working poor and lower middle class were the hardest hit by medical bills but were not eligible for any aid whatsoever. Panelists recognized the problem, and one HEW representative at the Washington hearing actually asked Mrs. Flanagan whether she had considered leaving her job and her husband to qualify for welfare and Medicaid. She replied proudly, "No. My family has never been broken up."[85]

Medicaid recipients and poor women told their stories of the impact of poverty medicine on their own lives. At the same time, several of them offered a broader, more systematic critique of Medicaid and American health care itself. One theme identified state rather than federal control of poverty medicine as the source of many of its inequities. A San Francisco welfare activist declared that "the Federal Government should take more responsibility for the Medicaid program and not leave it up to the States to set up their own eligibility requirements. Many States exploit and abuse low-income people. . . . This happened in California when Governor Reagan tried to cut-back on the Medi-Cal program. The Federal Government should provide for equal standards of medical care in all States."[86]

The problem with Medicaid, insisted Etta Horn, a DC activist, was that it was a welfare program rather than a health care program. Any program that served only the poor was stigmatized as inferior. "Hospitals and doctors know that all Medicaid patients are poor and many of us are black, and will therefore often discriminate against us by refusing us service," Horn said. "Experience has taught us that we will only get good service when there are also middle-class people participating in the same program. We therefore advocate that the Federal government begin now to move toward a National Health Insurance that will guarantee that all Americans will be able to pay for hospitalization and chronic illness."[87]

The speakers at the Medicaid hearings took their own experiences as poor women seeking health care for themselves and their families and turned them into an indictment of welfare medicine itself. They took to task the two pillars of the US welfare state—states' rights and categorical eligibility, or non-universalism—that kept programs scattered and fragmented and set the interests of the poor and the middle class against each other. Like Medicare for seniors, the Medicaid program created new avenues for poor people to express their critiques of the health care system and to formulate claims for a right to health care—claims that would become more vocal and explicit in the 1970s.

The testimony at the HEW hearings pointed to one major way in which Medicaid was not a right to health care: the ability of physicians to refuse Medicaid patients. Doctors' unwillingness to accept Medicaid became a perennial problem with the program. Although a few physicians made a great deal of money from Medicaid, most private general practitioners chafed at Medicaid's lower fee payments and the ever-present bureaucratic delays in reimbursement. The program's inferior status in the US health system and its lack of a powerful political constituency made it vulnerable to budget cuts, keeping physician reimbursement low. Medicaid's budget problems, inefficient state bureaucracies, and the continuing refusal to encroach on physician autonomy combined to lead many doctors to drastically limit their Medicaid caseloads or to refuse Medicaid patients altogether.

In a 1976 survey of Floyd County, Indiana, only two of twenty-one physicians would accept Medicaid. In some towns and rural areas, no doctors at all accepted Medicaid, and patients had to be taken to the nearest city.[88] But as the hearings testimony above showed, it was nearly as hard to find a doctor to take Medicaid in the city as it was in the country. In 1978, all the physicians in Huntsville, Alabama, stopped taking new Medicaid patients. Many already had accepted Medicaid and could "all relate personal horror stories about six- or eight-months delays in payments, mountains of paperwork and low reimbursement rates."[89] So many doctors were refusing Medicaid recipients that patients had begun using emergency rooms "just to be able to see a physician for minor services."[90] A clear example of the inefficiency of US-style rationing, Medicaid's stinginess in one area (doctor reimbursement) ended up costing the system more money in another area (emergency rooms).

In a 1974 article titled "Sorry, No More Medicaid Patients for Me," a California family practitioner explained why he was closing his office to recipients of Medi-Cal, the state Medicaid program. He believed that Medi-Cal encouraged frivolous visits (moral hazard), giving the example of a regular patient who, once he joined the program, suddenly began coming to his office "every time he had a scratch or runny nose." Even worse, the state delayed paying about one-third of his Medi-Cal claims, and the doctor was spending increasing amounts of time fighting reimbursement denials. Finally, the rate of payment was so low that he would need to drastically increase his patient volume to make a decent living. A small-town doctor in Alabama with a high Medicaid case load echoed these objections, saying that his reimbursement rates were so poor that he was no longer breaking even and his practice was losing money.[91]

Difficulty finding a doctor who accepted Medicaid would continue to be a major obstacle for the poor. In the 1970s, poverty advocates and civil rights groups would begin to protest Medicaid refusal via lawsuits, protests, and other means (see chapter 7).

Medicare and Medicaid created entitlements to different types of coverage for large groups of people, rationing by age and income, but they did not create an obligation on the part of providers to provide care for those covered. The programs expanded access to care for millions and greatly improved the health status of elderly and poor Americans. But, whether honorable entitlement or stigmatized welfare assistance, neither Medicare nor Medicaid made health care a right.

The correspondence and testimonies of those who were the primary beneficiaries of these programs, however, suggest the emergence and expression of rights consciousness among many Americans. These voices may not have constituted a single movement, but they articulated a sustained critique of the US health care system's failure to recognize what they regarded to be one of the most basic of human rights. Soon, organized movements would begin to include health care rights among their demands.

CHAPTER SEVEN

The Rise of Health Care Activism

When we think of the social and political upheavals of the 1960s, health care does not readily come to mind. Yet nearly all of the activist groups of that era confronted the American health care system. No coordinated, large-scale movement emerged to specifically address medical inequality; instead, each social movement approached health care in its own way. African Americans, Latinos, women's liberation activists, and middle-class consumers were among the groups that challenged discrimination and unjust rationing in health care, and all of these movements formulated a conception of the right to health care. But they faced great and, in the end, insurmountable obstacles in bridging the distance between racial and economic discrimination, between civil rights and human rights, and between individual and social rights.

Health Care Civil Rights Activism after Desegregation

Official hospital desegregation occurred far more smoothly than school desegregation. As seen in chapter 6, apart from a few cases there was no movement of "massive resistance" to bar blacks from hospitals or from white wards. Hospitals had a compelling financial incentive to desegregate in order to receive Medicare dollars from the federal government.

But the formal desegregation of hospitals did not lead to the end of racial discrimination in hospital care. In 1966, Dr. Leonidas Berry told members of the National Medical Association, "There are widespread reports of many hospitals north and south which were given government approval for Medicare participation where racial discrimination and defiance of title VI [of the Civil Rights Act] continue to exist."[1] Some hospitals in both the South and the North continued to practice *de facto* racial separation by keeping charity and welfare patients separate from "pay" patients, and even, as mentioned previously, by converting all their patient rooms from semiprivate to private.[2] Throughout the country, hospitals continued to turn away or transfer patients who could not pay, disproportionately affecting low-income African Americans. As a result, many hospitals remained predominantly white or predominantly black.

During his Chicago protest campaign in the spring of 1966, Martin Luther King Jr. focused on housing segregation, but he also spoke out against inequalities in health care. King decried the high infant mortality rate in Chicago's black neighborhoods, and denounced the federal government's inaction in responding to complaints of hospital discrimination, telling his supporters, "We must move beyond sending complaints to Washington and act directly." King's speech in Chicago included his most famous pronouncement on health care: "Of all forms of discrimination and inequalities, injustice in health is the most shocking and inhuman. . . . It is more degrading than slums, because slums are a psychological death while inequality in health means a physical death."[3]

As civil rights militancy grew in the mid-1960s, the National Medical Association, the organization of black physicians, adopted a more aggressive and rights-based approach to racial discrimination in health. At its 1967 convention, NMA President Lionel Swan thundered, "I want to give notice that the National Medical Association . . . will continue to fight with all its resources against all health institutions and facilities that discriminate against Negro physicians and their patients. Let the racists know that as long as they continue this nefarious practice, they will have no peace." Berry wrote in the NMA's journal of "the new concept of 'medical rights' which is smoldering in the hearts and minds of many."[4]

Using increasingly militant language, activists defined health care discrimination as part of the US "system" of oppression that kept the poor and minorities in perpetual second-class status. They talked not only of racial but also of economic injustice, and of how the two were connected. The Chicago chapter of the Medical Committee for Human Rights (MCHR) condemned the "system of health care that pours a thousand poor people daily in the emergency rooms at County. . . . We must do away with the patterns of racial and economic discrimination which are inimical to medical ethics." The MCHR then joined its civil rights advocacy with a demand for universal health care rights: "These barriers deny the right to health care which should be inherent in our affluent, scientifically advanced community."[5]

Activist groups denounced high infant mortality and hospital refusals not as unintentional byproducts of health care injustice, but as criminal neglect and even deliberate attempts to reduce the black population. In 1967, a Chicago neighborhood group announced a study showing that the infant mortality rate in Cook County was significantly higher than in surrounding white suburbs and concluded, "we use the term 'genocide' to pinpoint the reason."[6] The following year, when Chicago Mayor Richard J. Daley suddenly called for punishing hospitals for emergency refusal after a white infant died, the *Chicago Defender* asked why its reporting of "hundreds" of black deaths due to rejection by white hospitals had been ignored. The paper quoted a civil rights activist's statement that "black people are being systematically exterminated" by emergency refusal and inadequate access to health care.[7] African Americans' distrust of the US medical system, which was rooted in a long history of discrimination and medical experimentation without consent, only worsened in 1972 when reports of the Tuskegee Study emerged. The media broadcast shocking revelations that the US Public Health Service had studied poor black sharecroppers suffering from syphilis for four decades, withholding treatment from them even when effective antibiotics became available.

Rights groups charged that hospitals and nursing homes continued to defy the Civil Rights Act. In 1972, the Leadership Council on Civil Rights complained that the federal office charged with investigating compliance had failed to act "even where clear, overt discrimination exists," and had taken no action against 200 hospitals that were noncompliant or had not responded to requests to demonstrate compliance.[8] Democratic Representative Don Edwards of California issued a press release announcing that in 1973 "there still exists in this country a dual system of health care for non-whites which has been allowed to continue despite enactment of Civil Rights laws" and compared the situation to *de facto* school segregation. "The signs barring admittance to non-whites which once hung above the doors of many of our hospitals have been taken down," Edwards said, "but segregation remains."[9]

The Campaign to Enforce Hill-Burton's Obligations to the Poor

Supreme Court–mandated desegregation, the Civil Rights Act, and Medicare were proving insufficient to truly dismantle hospital discrimination. Starting in the early 1970s, activists looked to a new legal strategy: the reinvigoration of the Hill-Burton Act's uncompensated care and community service requirements. As discussed in chapter 4,

hospitals receiving federal funds had been required since 1946 to provide a "reasonable level" of care to the poor, but this had never been
officially enforced. A campaign by welfare rights activists to more fully
enforce Hill-Burton compliance powerfully challenged hospitals' ability to refuse patients on the basis of income.

The Hill-Burton cases were made possible by a new alliance of poor
people—particularly African American women—with federally funded
legal aid attorneys.[10] As part of President Lyndon B. Johnson's War on
Poverty, the Office of Economic Opportunity opened legal aid offices
around the country to give poor Americans access to attorneys. Legal
aid lawyers in the South worked with local antipoverty groups to bring
lawsuits against Hill-Burton hospitals that were turning away poor
patients and patients on Medicaid.[11]

The most important case was *Cook v. Ochsner Foundation Hospital*,
brought in 1970 against ten New Orleans hospitals receiving a total of
$18 million in Hill-Burton funds. *Cook*'s plaintiffs, all of whom were
African American Medicaid recipients, included Rosezella Cook, who
was denied treatment for heart disease at Methodist Hospital because
of her inability to pay the $35 emergency room fee; Sallie Lee, with ar-
thritis and hypertension, who was turned away from Ochsner Hospital
for the same reason; and Monica Hunter, who sought care for severe
abdominal and head pain, and was turned away first from Methodist
and then from Hotel de Dieu Hospital, both of which refused Medicaid patients.[12] The women brought the suit "on their own behalf, on
the behalf of their minor children and on behalf of all others similarly
situated." The Louisiana district court agreed that the hospitals' policy
of "sparingly admitting or refusing Medicaid patients clearly discriminated against a very substantial segment of the public and violated the
'community service' obligation under the [Hill-Burton] Act."[13]

Cook v. Ochsner and several other class action lawsuits brought by
poor people and their advocates finally pushed the federal government
to pay attention to the uncompensated care requirements. HEW initially proposed that Hill-Burton facilities devote 5 percent of their
operating costs to free care, but this was scaled back to 3 percent after "a landslide of protests" by hospitals.[14] In 1975, Congress enacted
an amendment to the Hill-Burton program that required hospitals to
comply with the uncompensated care requirement for 20 years after
receipt of federal funds, and to enforce the "community service" obligations "in perpetuity." These obligations required hospitals to offer service to members of the community regardless of race, creed, national

origin, or Medicare / Medicaid status. Many of the new regulations, particularly the ban on Medicaid discrimination, represented clear victories for the welfare rights movement, but their implementation would not be simple. Advocates for the poor continued to complain of "widespread facility noncompliance and ineffective enforcement" of hospitals' obligations.[15] While some hospitals tried diligently to provide their fair share (and sometimes more) of uncompensated care, the updated Hill-Burton requirements did not prevent rampant refusal and "dumping" of uninsured and Medicaid patients from becoming a major crisis in the 1980s (see chapter 8).

The distinguished poverty lawyer Sylvia A. Law later said of the Hill-Burton campaign, and of poor people's health activism in general, "Programs for the poor lead to poor programs."[16] Since it would benefit only the very poorest Americans, Hill-Burton enforcement lacked a broad-based constituency of support (unlike Medicare, which benefited the middle class also). The Hill-Burton enforcement cases were only a partial victory. Welfare rights activists continued their fight to make health care more accessible to the poor—not only through lawsuits, but also through demanding representation and rights in the hospital system.

"Welfare Mothers" Create the Patients' Bill of Rights

The National Welfare Rights Organization, which brought together welfare recipients to demand the full benefits to which they were entitled and sought to bring greater political power to the poor, was active from 1966 through 1973. At its peak in 1969, the organization had approximately 22,000 dues-paying members, but thousands more participated in its actions throughout the country.[17]

After four years focusing solely on welfare issues, the NWRO formed a Health Rights Committee early in 1970. As its name indicated, the Committee insisted that health care be treated as a right: "Just as all people have *welfare rights*, we believe they also have *health rights*. . . . NWRO maintains that quality health care, both in prevention and treatment, is a basic right and should be provided for all people on the basis of need rather than the basis of income."[18]

In order to implement these ideals, the NWRO sent the American Medical Association a list of suggestions for updating the physicians' Code of Ethics. The activists demanded that the AMA declare it unethical for physicians to refuse service to Medicaid patients; to deny service on the basis of race, religion, ethnicity, or national origin; to allow experimentation on poor patients that they would not allow on their own private patients; and to deny poor patients the rights of privacy and dignity. Finally, the NWRO demanded that "the AMA reverse its opposition to National Compulsory Health Insurance."[19] They received no response.

The NWRO got more attention from its attempts to shake up the hospital organizations. The Health Rights Committee won a victory in the spring of 1970 when it managed to get a group of welfare mothers invited to a meeting of the Joint Commission on Accreditation of Healthcare Organizations (JCAHO), the national agency overseeing hospital accreditation, in Chicago. The commissioners greeted the NWRO members with "grim face[s]," but after the meeting the JCAHO agreed to create a consumer advisory board and, for the first time in its history, to add antidiscrimination language to its list of hospital standards.[20]

The Health Rights Committee next targeted the formidable American Hospital Association. Members traveled to Houston to picket the AHA's 1970 convention and confront delegates. TV cameras showed welfare mothers marching in front of the convention center with signs reading "Condition Tax Exemption on Health Care to the Poor—Don't Fight It, AHA!"[21] To avoid further disruption of the proceedings, AHA leaders agreed to give Mrs. Geraldine Smith, financial secretary of NWRO, an opportunity to speak.

In her speech to the assembled delegates, Geraldine Smith launched an attack on the AHA from the perspective of poor mothers on welfare. "The American Hospital Association is hypocritical, selfish, parochial, and patronizing," she declared. It "hides behind a screen of concern for the disadvantaged," while perpetuating "a dual system of health care" and "preaching freedom of choice." Smith then presented the AHA with a list of demands, including more outpatient clinics; 51 percent community membership on hospital boards; formal patient grievance mechanisms; open medical staff privileges; making admissions and collections policies available to the public; opening JCAHO survey reports to the community; including unaffiliated physicians on utilization review and evaluation and audit committees; transferring patients only on medical indications; translation services for non–English-speaking patients; and "keeping patients informed." Other demands addressed the right of access for low-income people, including equal treatment for ward patients and the demand that hospitals "not refuse Medicaid,

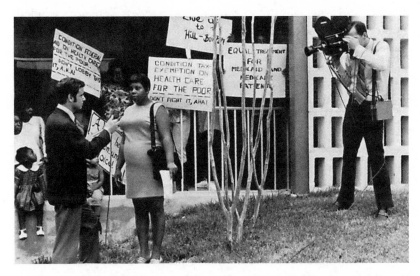

FIGURE 10. Geraldine Smith of the National Welfare Rights Organization is interviewed by a television crew following her impromptu speech at the 1970 American Hospital Association Convention in Houston, Texas. Reprinted by permission, from *Hospitals* (October 1970). Copyright 1970 by Health Forum Inc.

Medicare or medically indigent" patients. But Smith's focus was on rights that would benefit all patients, not just the poor.[22]

The AHA delegates responded to Geraldine Smith's blistering speech with silence—or "courteous attention," according to one report—and afterward "the house proceeded to conduct its business without further reference to the NWRO complaints."[23] Although the welfare mothers' presence did not alter the meeting's agenda, the AHA journal ran a piece on the protest and speech, including photographs. Shortly afterward, hoping to preempt the demands from below, the AHA drafted its own version of a Patients' Bill of Rights.

Pressure from welfare rights activists had forced the AHA into action, but the Bill of Rights approved by the hospital association's members in 1973 would bear little resemblance to Smith's demands. Its twelve provisions included rights like informed consent and medical privacy, which were important to middle-class and wealthy patients as well as the poor, and represented an important step forward for individual rights. However, the bill did not list any rights that might cost hospitals money or that would involve shifting control from hospitals and physicians to patients. Rights to consumer participation in governance and especially enforceable rights to access were not included. Point Seven of the AHA Patients' Bill of Rights did stipulate that "the patient has the right to expect that within its capacity a hospital must make reasonable response to the request of a patient for services."[24] The vagueness of this statement was both self-evident and deliberate. Columnist Joan Beck of the *Chicago Tribune* complained of the AHA's Bill of Rights, "None of this goes nearly far enough. . . . Terms aren't defined. Wording is vague. And no mechanism is provided for enforcement."[25]

Hospitals did not exactly rush to implement the new Bill of Rights. Many were slow to adopt it, some refused altogether, and the American Medical Association registered its displeasure with the entire concept.[26] But, as consumers became more demanding and rights talk permeated political debates, hospital attorney John F. Horty argued that it was probably in hospitals' best interests to adopt the AHA bill or aspects of it, since it guaranteed maximum flexibility for hospitals and was entirely voluntary and unenforceable. Horty warned hospitals to adopt such bills "or the courts will tell them what it means." They could pick and choose among the rights they would advertise to patients, Horty noted; "If the hospital feels that a Patient's Bill of Rights serves its purpose, it should carefully review the language and delete any portions of points or entire points which are not applicable to the institution." He especially cautioned against Point Seven, which threatened to guarantee care, and also a provision requiring continuity of care.[27]

Despite the built-in flexibility of the AHA's Bill of Rights, eighteen months after its announcement, only about one-third of the nation's 7,000 hospitals had adopted it in any form.[28] There was no national grassroots organization pressuring hospitals to accept the Bill of Rights or to put them into practice, because by the end of 1973, the NWRO was in tatters following the death of leader George Wiley and various internal divisions. Activists continued to work at the state level, but the organization no longer had a strong national presence.[29]

Hospitals resisted poor people's demands that would have led to wholesale restructuring of the health system. But, despite the limits of its victories, the Health Rights movement of the NWRO made a permanent mark on the US health system. Hospitals and health agencies still seek consumer participation—sometimes meaningful, sometimes token—in decision making. Many hospitals now post "Patients' Bill of Rights" and "Hill-Burton Uncompensated Care" notices in their waiting rooms, however watered down and difficult to enforce their provisions may be. The movement permanently injected rights language into the health care system, although it has not always been used in ways that poverty advocates would have intended (such as the managed care Patients' Bills of Rights proposed in the 1990s, which would have applied only to people with insurance). NWRO health activists also had some long-lasting successes on the state level. One example was a Medicaid children's health screening clinic in Clark County, Nevada, opened and operated entirely by the local welfare rights organization.[30] Welfare rights activists got as far as they did because of their boldness (disrupting the AHA convention and JCAHO meeting), their timing (they were able to work with lawyers funded by the Johnson Administration's poverty programs), and their creativity (targeting Hill-Burton and the hospital accreditation agency, two relatively obscure but crucial institutions). By refusing to separate civil rights from economic rights, welfare rights advocates questioned the very foundations of a health care system that rationed by race and by class.

The Campaign against Hospital Flight

Even after the Civil Rights Act, Medicare, the new Hill-Burton rulings, and Patients' Bills of Rights, some hospitals found other ways to minimize serving minorities and the poor. Growing costs throughout the 1970s forced hospitals, including community nonprofit hospitals, to place greater emphasis on their bottom lines. In addition, inner-city populations were dwindling and becoming heavily minority. In the absence of universal hospital insurance, one way to guarantee greater revenues and to serve growing populations was to relocate some or all hospital services and buildings from poor inner city areas to wealthy suburbs where patients could pay. As the phenomenon of "hospital flight" became increasingly common in the 1970s, it was challenged by civil rights organizations at both the local and national levels.

In Chicago, community activists forced the federal government to get involved when St. George Hospital in Englewood, a poor black neighborhood on the South Side, announced that it would close and use its recently awarded Hill-Burton funds to open a hospital in suburban, all-white Palos Heights, 30 miles away. Chicago physicians accused hospital leaders of "robbing the inner-city community of vitally needed health care resources" and demanded action from HEW, the federal Department of Health, Education and Welfare. After receiving a response the doctors described as "vague and elusive," Dr. Andrew Thomas, president of the Cook County Physicians' Association, suggested that black doctors take over the abandoned St. George facility and run their own hospital. Finally, HEW stepped in and mediated an agreement that led to the improvement and expansion of two affiliated hospitals on the South Side, the addition of minority representatives to their boards, and hospital affirmative action hiring programs for local residents.[31]

Other attempts to curb hospital flight ended in failure. Civil rights advocates brought federal lawsuits in 1977 and 1978 against hospitals in Wilmington, Delaware, and Gary, Indiana. In Wilmington, 800 hospital beds at the downtown Medical Center were replaced by a new facility in a suburb not served by public transportation. The plaintiffs, a neighborhood group, targeted HEW, claiming that suburban hospital expansion at the expense of inner-city residents was a violation of the Civil Rights Act. A district court ordered HEW to investigate Wilmington General Hospital, but this led only to a weak negotiated settlement—the hospital agreed to provide a shuttle bus between facilities—that angered the plaintiffs. In Gary, Methodist Hospital reduced services at its inner city location while opening a modern new suburban facility; 90% of patients at the suburban branch were white, while 80% at the "left-behind downtown facility" were black.[32] Plaintiffs filed similar lawsuits in New York City, San Antonio, and St. Louis, but none were successful or had a significant impact, either on the pace of hospital flight or on the federal government's willingness to force civil rights compliance on hospitals that fled the inner city.[33]

Community Health Centers

For many years, public health advocates had argued that community-based clinics could be more effective than high-tech hospital care in caring for everyday and long-term health needs.[34] In the 1960s, the federal government seemed to increasingly agree. Although continuing to subsidize hospitals via Hill-Burton and Medicare, the Johnson administration also funded a new program to establish neighborhood clinics throughout the country.[35] The Community Health Centers program was run by the Office of Economic Opportunity, the quintessential agency of Johnson's War on Poverty. The first federally funded clinic opened in 1965, and by 1970 there were over 100 such clinics in 44 states and the District of Columbia.

The Health Centers program embodied many of the aspirations of health care activists. Clinics were supposed to provide comprehensive services on the basis of need, not ability to pay; emphasize preventive care; and be run by members of the local community (embodying the War on Poverty principle of "maximum feasible participation" by the poor). Some clinics truly embodied these goals, especially the pioneering Tufts-Delta Health Center in Mound Bayou, Mississippi, led by physician-activist Jack Geiger, a cofounder of the Medical Committee for Civil Rights. This unique clinic practiced the ideal of community participation, hiring local women as nurses and offering training for area residents that would lead to jobs at the Center. The Delta Health Center also put into practice a broad conception of health care that went beyond medical services. For example, realizing that people of the Delta were not just sick but also malnourished, staff began distributing food as well as medicine, and sponsored a 500-acre cooperative farm run by local residents.[36]

In keeping with the era's spirit of grassroots activism, many neighborhood-based organizations and even radical groups like the Black Panther Party opened clinics in deprived areas. Alondra Nelson points out in her history of Black Panther health activism that the organization was influenced by United Nations and World Health Organization declarations of social rights. In 1971 the Panthers' national newspaper echoed the WHO's expansive definition of health and declared that it was "one of the most basic human rights of all human beings." Following a directive from leader Bobby Seale in 1970, local Panther chapters opened health centers in major cities throughout the country. More than 150 doctors, nurses, and medical students volunteered at the Panthers' busy Chicago clinic, named the "People's Free Medical Care Center."[37]

Medical provision by activist groups sometimes led to opposition from local governments. Chicago Mayor Richard J. Daley tried to impose licensing requirements on all health facilities that were "not solely owned or operated by physicians" and used the requirements to attempt to shut down several clinics run by community groups, including the Panthers.[38] When the city's Board of Health tried to close a Black Panther clinic on the South Side because it lacked a license, hundreds came out in protest. Ronald "Doc" Satchel of the Black Panther Party argued that "clinics charging fees, and exploiting welfare clients with assembly line treatment aren't required to have a license." Protesters coming out in support of the clinics ranged from members of the militant youth group the Young Lords to neighborhood residents like

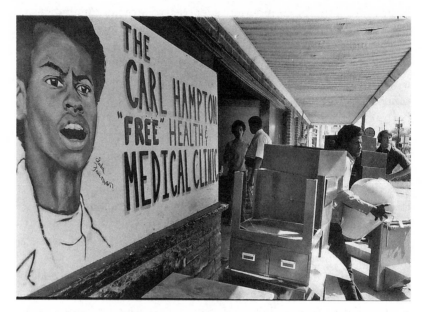

FIGURE 11. The Carl Hampton Clinic, run by the People's Party II, a Black Panther organization in Houston, Texas. Photo by Fred Bunch, *Houston Post*, May 15, 1971. Reprinted with permission of the *Houston Chronicle*.

Gladys Hunter, who told a reporter that the clinic "represents something poor black people have never had before." The *Chicago Defender* noted that "The Panther medical clinic would not exist if city medical facilities for the poor were adequate."[39] The city's attempt to shut down the clinics was later overruled by a judge.[40]

Community health centers also met opposition from the still-conservative organized medical profession. In 1967 the new President of the American Medical Association, Milton O. Rouse, continued the long tradition of AMA disapproval of competition from clinics by declaring that government-sponsored health centers were "unnecessary and 'wasteful.'"[41] Community hospitals in Lee County, Arkansas, and Imperial Valley, California, faced pressure from local medical societies to refuse admitting privileges to physicians who worked for local Office of Economic Opportunity health centers. When a Chicago doctor arrived in Tucson, Arizona, to open an OEO health center, "We encountered some significant hostility, both in the medical school and in the medical community. . . . The concern there was mainly from a few doctors in the community in private practice who thought it was a 'comminist' [*sic*] enterprise, and they were afraid of competition from the health center."[42]

Latino Rights and Health Care

Health care had long been a concern of Latino organizations in the United States. Starting in the mid-1960s, the United Farm Workers' (UFW) campaign publicized the horrific health conditions of migrant workers on the nation's farms.[43] Toward the end of the decade, the Chicano (Mexican American) and Puerto Rican movements added a more radical and militant dimension to Latino health activism. These activists argued that the poor health status of Latinos was rooted in the fundamentally racist nature of the health care system. Like the Black Panthers, Latino militants did not demand more and better services from the existing system; they insisted that communities set up and control their own alternative health institutions, and pushed for a broader definition of health that included better nutrition, housing, education, and workplace conditions.

Latinos experienced health disparities and both official and informal discrimination. Segregation of health care institutions into "White" and "Mexican" prevailed throughout the Southwest and California well into the 1960s. Even in the absence of official segregation, the language barrier and patients' immigrant or migrant status created severe obstacles to obtaining health care. Most health facilities lacked Spanish-speaking personnel and translators. At some locations, Spanish speakers were simply refused services. One clinic physician in California refused to help a patient with translation because "Mexicans should learn English." Some health workers openly showed resentment of Spanish-speaking clients, described by some patients as "*Me hacen mala cara*" (they give me a dirty look).[44]

Chicano activists argued that community self-determination was essential to better health for minority groups. A medical student writing in the *American Journal of Public Health* in 1970 reported enthusiastically that "the health practices and health status of the Mexican American people could be radically improved through the Chicano movement."[45] In Los Angeles and San Diego counties, local Chicano groups set up drug prevention and rehabilitation programs, free clinics, and birth control and health information centers. The Brown Berets, a militant Chicano youth organization, opened health clinics throughout California and in Chicago.[46]

Chicano and Puerto Rican movement clinics embodied the principle of community participation. At the UFW's Rodrigo Terrones Memorial Clinic in Delano, California, "the farm workers have complete say over how it's run and what services should be made available."[47] The Bobby García Memorial Clinic in Albuquerque, New Mexico, founded by Las Gorras Negras (the Black Berets, another militant youth organization), accepted "*no* government money." The clinic was staffed three nights a week by volunteer doctors, and one of the Black Berets, a young man named Marvin García, was "taking a course in Lab Sciences at the University of N. M. so that he can serve the Clínica as an assistant lab technician." An article in the Black Berets' newspaper proudly reported the ways in which this clinic was different from what the community was accustomed to. The waiting room was painted in warm colors and decorated with Chicano murals, "not portraits of rich gringo doctors." Patients were followed up after their visits, and even offered transportation home or to the hospital. Most important, care "is completely FREE." The García Clinic "stands as an example of what health care should be but almost never is, under the US system: a human right, not a privilege," the article concluded.[48]

In New York City in 1970, members of the Puerto Rican Young Lords organization commandeered an x-ray van belonging to the Tuberculosis Association. They hung a banner on the "liberated" vehicle reading "Free Health Care for All," and renamed it the Ramón Betances Health Truck, after the nineteenth-century Puerto Rican independence leader. The technicians on board were sufficiently impressed that they volunteered to stay and help offer free chest x-rays to neighborhood residents. A mother of six observing the scene approved, saying that "anything that benefits the people is right."[49] The free x-rays were part of the Young Lords' emphasis on preventive health care in the community. Another of their New York City campaigns involved group members going door-to-door with free urine tests to detect lead poisoning. In Albuquerque, the Black Berets went even further by forming a Chicano People's Health Corps, whose members would be trained to give full physical exams. According to the Berets, "The main goal is to create a system of preventive medicine."[50]

At the national level, more mainstream Latino health care activism focused on two of the major culprits behind health disparities: a lack of Latino medical professionals, and a lack of translation services for Spanish-speaking patients. The National Chicano Health Organization, formed "to insure first class health care for the Chicano community," announced that less than 1 percent of medical students in the country were Hispanic.[51] "Off hand, I would venture the guess that there are not more than a hundred Chicano MDs in the Southwest and California," reported one activist in 1970. "It is, I believe, due in large part to the discriminatory and racist character and practices of medical schools that such a drastic shortage of Chicano physicians and dentists and psychiatrists is the condition."[52] In Dallas, where 10 percent of the population was Mexican American, less than 1 percent of maternal/child health staff were Spanish speaking; the Leadership Conference on Civil Rights argued that this situation was to blame for the extremely low rates of prenatal care for Mexican American women in the city.[53]

The Women's Movement and Access to Health Care

The feminist health movement of the 1960s and '70s is remembered more for its demands for reproductive rights and its powerful critique of the sexism of the medical profession than for advocating universal access to health care. Yet women's health activists did draw connections between the nature of US rationing and the health system's treatment of women. In 1971, the first edition of the now-classic bestseller *Our Bodies, Ourselves* argued that profit-driven medicine had led to an epidemic of unnecessary surgeries on women, especially hysterectomies (removal of the uterus), at the same time that women without access to primary care died of preventable cervical and uterine cancers. The authors declared: "We believe that health care is a human right and that society should provide free health care. . . . Health care for everyone is possible only outside of the profit system."[54]

The women's movement directly challenged the system by opening independent feminist health clinics. Most were dedicated to providing reproductive services such as birth control and abortions, but some also offered full preventive and primary care services. About 50 feminist clinics had been established in the United States by 1976. Whatever services they offered, says historian Sandra Morgen, the clinics all embodied the "concept of control by women": self-help, the subversion of medical hierarchy, and free, low-cost, or sliding-scale care.[55] Like community clinics and dispensaries before them, some feminist clinics inspired opposition from the local medical profession. In Chico, California, doctors refused to work at the feminist health center because local hospitals would blacklist them if they did; the clinic had to import physicians from San Francisco.[56] But other physicians dedicated their careers (and in later decades, would even risk their lives) to providing reproductive services to women.[57]

Some members of the women's movement and Latino/Black Power movements argued for an approach to women's health rights that would encompass the right to be free from forced sterilization as well as to limit fertility. Groups that focused exclusively on the needs of poor women developed an even broader definition of women's health. Health workers at the Delta Health Center, in one of the most economically deprived regions in the country, "argued that women's reproductive health could only be understood within a broad context of health care," writes historian Jennifer Nelson, a context that included access to primary care, decent housing, and sufficient food.[58]

Organizations of working class women focused particularly on issues such as maternity insurance and affordable child care. Women at the Rank and File Action Conference held in Chicago in 1970 endorsed a "Declaration of Rights of Women Workers" that included health care as a right. Although these activists were probably not aware of labor activist Florence Greenberg's speech at the 1938 National Health Conference, they were carrying on her legacy by calling for health to be added to the list of "inalienable rights" of working people.[59] The Coalition of Labor Union Women in the 1970s strongly criticized discrimination against women in health insurance, including higher premiums and limited or nonexistent maternity coverage.[60] The women's movement achieved an important victory with the Pregnancy Discrimination Act of 1978, which requires employers to treat pregnancy the same as any covered disability. However, insurance companies in the individual market continued to exclude maternity and to charge higher premiums to women (the 2010 Affordable Care Act intends to ban this practice).

Alongside the demands of civil rights and feminist activists for greater health rights, several organizations devoted themselves specifically to transforming the US health system. The first was the Medical Committee for Human Rights, the interracial group of physicians founded in 1963 (formerly the Medical Committee for Civil Rights). Initially, the MCHR had been a mainstream civil rights organization focused on preventing the exclusion of black doctors from hospital practice (see chapter 4); its members joined the 1963 March on Washington and provided medical care to protesters injured in civil rights marches. By the late '60s, the organization became more militant; its physician members treated protesters clubbed in anti–Vietnam War protests, cosponsored clinics with the Black Panthers, and agitated for community control of urban hospitals.[61]

Medical students joined the uprising against traditional medical authority when students from around the country met in Chicago in 1965 and founded the Student Health Organization (SHO). Medical student activists published newspapers, demanded representation in medical school governance, and attacked the AMA's conservatism. Local branches ran Summer Health Projects that enlisted medical students to provide health services in poor areas. New York City activists formed the Health Policy Advisory Center (Health/PAC), "an irreverent, anti-establishment think tank" that targeted the rapidly growing for-profit health system—hospitals and drug and insurance companies—which the New England Journal of Medicine editor Arnold Relman had dubbed the "medical industrial complex." Health/PAC's 1970 report, entitled The American Health Empire, called for a "democratic restructuring" of the health system that would put patients before profits.[62]

Did the wave of health care social activism in the 1960s and '70s succeed in transforming the American health system? The civil rights, Black Power, Latino rights, and feminist movements all advanced powerful critiques of the injustices of American health care and beliefs in equal access, universalism, and prevention. Yet the health care system in the 1970s remained inequitable, rationed on the basis of factors other than medical need, and focused on hospitals and technology. The social movements did succeed in bringing about some important changes: the erosion of unquestioned physician authority, the notion of individual empowerment through medical self-knowledge, and the beginning of the breakdown of racial and gender barriers in medical schools and eventually the medical profession.[63] Student activists, for example, succeeded in convincing over 100 medical schools to adopt affirmative action recruitment procedures by 1974.[64] But these changes did not fundamentally transform the health care system or the distribution of power and resources within it. Aspirations for a right to health care remained unfulfilled.

Activist organizations, especially by the early 1970s, fragmented into different identity or interest groups (African Americans, welfare mothers, women, Latinos, etc.) and often focused on single issues (e.g., abortion rights, the creation of ethnic studies programs at universities) rather than joining in a broad-scale movement aimed at changing deep-seated inequalities. This is a familiar critique of 1970s social activism, but it has specific implications when it comes to health care movements. Because the health care system itself was so fragmented, activists with limited resources could target only specific aspects of it—reproductive rights, Medicaid, hospitals—rather than the system as a whole. In addition, the traditional separation of civil and political rights from social and economic rights foiled activist goals. Demands for civil rights (hospital desegregation) and political rights (consumer representation in hospitals) proved more winnable than economic rights or rights to access (free care, Medicaid acceptance, an end to hospital flight), which were almost entirely repudiated. Although this era did leave behind a few programs that directly addressed health-care inequalities—particularly the remaining community health centers—rationing persisted and the right to health care remained elusive. However, rights rhetoric would reappear in a different and perhaps more lasting form as a new American consumer movement began to question the power of the health care industry.

The Consumer Movement and Health Activism

Health activists in the late 1960s and early 1970s increasingly used the word "consumer" to refer to the users or potential users of health care. A consumer had a more active role than the passive "patient." Health consumers, by gaining knowledge about health care and the health system, became "empowered" to make informed choices. Although consumerism has often been a conservative force in American life, at this time it took on an anti-establishment, anti-corporate edge.[65] In general, however, the 1970s consumer movement put less emphasis on a basic right of access to health care for all, and emphasized the rights of middle-class consumers / patients to be protected from unsafe drugs and other health care industry abuses. In other words, it promoted regulation of the health system rather than fundamental change.

The Health Research Group, formed in 1971 as part of crusading consumer rights leader Ralph Nader's organization Public Citizen, became the most visible arm of the consumer movement in health care. The Health Research Group immediately upset the medical profession by publishing a "consumer directory" of physicians in Maryland that included their office hours, fees, and willingness to make house calls. Nader argued that health consumers needed such information for the same reason they needed comparisons of "autos and drugs"—to be able to choose the highest quality and the best value.[66] The language of consumer empowerment in medical care soon permeated popular culture, as books telling readers how to "talk back to your doctor" flooded the market. Public Citizen rankled the drug industry by publishing a guide to prescription medications titled *Pills That Don't Work* (the guide has been in continual publication since 1980 and is now titled *Worst Pills, Best Pills*).[67]

Along with drug companies and the medical profession, the private health insurance industry became a target of the growing consumer movement. Health insurance policies were derided for soaring premiums and deductibles, coverage limitations, and hidden exclusions, and insurance companies increasingly came under fire for fraudulent practices. Consumer advocates and journalists published books with titles such as *The Health Insurance Racket and How to Beat It*, *Your Health Insurance: A Story of Failure*, and *Blue Cross: What Went Wrong*, advising consumers to beware of the "small print" in insurance contracts where the deductibles and exclusions might be hidden.[68] Television news programs began highlighting the burden on consumers of inadequate health coverage. In 1970 journalist Daniel Schorr hosted a CBS special with the provocative title "Don't Get Sick in America" that described health insurance as a "shrinking security blanket." Schorr reported that even middle-class Americans with health insurance "were 'shocked' at the amount of money they had to pay for hospital care" beyond their coverage, leading to "on-going worry." A 1972 NBC program titled "What Price Health?" featured families wiped out by medical bills even though they were insured. Presenter Edwin Newman intoned, "Question: What good is health insurance if it doesn't cover your needs?"[69]

Health insurance scandals attracted nationwide attention, especially when insurance companies were accused of defrauding senior citizens. This was the case with Colonial Penn insurance company, whose leader Leonard Davis had created the American Association of Retired Persons to sell his Medigap insurance plan. Colonial Penn was sued by consumers in 1978 for consistently paying out less than half of its income in benefits to policyholders.[70]

In Washington, advocates of national health reform began using consumer complaints about private insurance as powerful evidence for their cause. Senator Edward Kennedy held numerous hearings on health care in the early 1970s that featured testimony from Americans "whose insurance ran out, excluded certain services or diseases, or required deductibles and partial payments by the policyholder which ran up to thousands of dollars before they were through. In some cases the family was bankrupted, in others long-accumulated savings were wiped out, and in many others debts were incurred which required regular payments that mortgaged a family's future."[71] The Kennedy hearings emboldened many individuals to take their health insurance problems public. They wrote hundreds of letters to Senator Kennedy, many mentioning hardships brought about by cost sharing and limited coverage. The Baldwins of Woodland, California, complained, "We pay around $480.00 a year for insurance and still when we get sick we have to pay half of it out of our own pockets." They had spent nearly all of their $10,000 in savings on Mrs. Baldwin's tumor operation. They pleaded, "For god sakes please get us some good insurance we don't want it for nothing we want to pay for it." A woman wrote that after her sister was hospitalized, "the insurance company only paid $180 out of $2500. . . . I don't think they should be allowed to charge so much, they're so hardened, it's your money or your life."[72]

A few state governments responded to consumer activists' demands to take action against unfair health insurance practices. Michigan, Pennsylvania, and North Carolina launched investigations into insurance discrimination based on race or gender.[73] In several states, insurance commissioners (and rival commercial insurance companies) challenged the tax-exempt status of Blue Cross / Blue Shield plans, which they argued behaved more like a for-profit company than a public service.[74] Consumer advocates found an influential government ally in Herbert Denenberg, the popular insurance commissioner of Pennsylvania, who became known nationwide as a "hell-raising" critic of the industry. In 1972, *Time* magazine reported that Denenberg had "ordered all the 1,157 insurance companies that do business in Pennsylvania to appoint ombudsmen to hear consumer complaints. . . . Complaints are pouring in to Denenberg's office at an annual rate of 50,000, up from 25,000 in 1971." Denenberg forced private health insurers to negotiate with hospitals for better prices, and repeatedly refused Blue Cross requests for rate hikes.[75]

The new consumer activism, following a decade of social movements questioning the basic foundations of American institutions, seemed to be pointing toward a sea change in the United States' approach to health care justice. In August 1971, an article on the front page of the *New York Times* announced, "Subtly but unmistakably, Americans from all strata of society and all economic classes are swinging over to the idea that good health care, like a good education, ought to be a fundamental right of citizenship." Public support for some form of national health insurance program was running 2 to 1.[76] The *Times* and many other commentators, as well as President Nixon and congressional leaders, believed that some form of national health insurance would be adopted soon. But then, so had Harry Truman in 1946.

From Rights to Cost Control

In 1971, President Richard Nixon announced that American health care was undergoing a "massive crisis" and declared that a national health plan was the "highest priority" of his administration. Unlike later Republican presidents, Nixon saw no contradiction between his basic conservative philosophy and bold government action on domestic issues.[77] Nixon's national health proposal, announced that same year, included two concepts that would prove extraordinarily powerful and long-lasting. Both would also reaffirm rationing at the expense of rights. The first was the "employer mandate," which would require employers to provide health insurance for their workers. The employer mandate later became a pillar of the Clinton health plan. The other was a concept that most Americans had never heard of in 1971: the "health maintenance organization," or HMO, a form of prepaid group practice insurance. HMOs (discussed in greater detail in chapter 9) embodied ideals of efficiency and cost reduction, and also provided a bold new model that appealed to Nixon's desire to be seen as an innovator.[78]

The American Medical Association had already proposed an alternative bill, named "Medicredit," that offered tax credits for the middle class to purchase private health insurance and a Medicaid-like plan for the poor. Senator Edward Kennedy had put forth a sweeping proposal for national, compulsory health insurance that would cover everyone. Soon the American Hospital Association, the insurance industry, and dozens of others chimed in with their own plans. At one point in 1971, there were 22 competing health care bills before Congress.[79]

The battle over the many different proposals highlighted the basic principles of rights and rationing at stake in the creation of a national insurance system in the United States. Kennedy's plan emphasized universalism and equal coverage. He denounced the income-based methods of rationing health care: "We ought to have one set of standard . . . benefits for all Americans. And it ought to be a quality set of benefits for all Americans. Not one set for the poor, one set for the middle income and another for those that are employed and those that are unemployed."[80] Labor unions and the Committee for National Health Insurance, a labor-led coalition of consumers, workers, and seniors, passionately supported Kennedy's original proposal because it repudiated means testing and cost sharing, both of which had negatively affected working people. The AFL-CIO slammed Nixon's plan for including cost sharing because it "would further expand the already wide gap in health between the poor and the more affluent."[81]

Both the Nixon and the AMA proposals included copayments and means testing, not just to save money, but as a matter of principle: health care was not a universal right and the government had no obligation to ensure equitable coverage. Senator Clifford Hansen of Wyoming, cosponsor of the AMA's "Medicredit" bill that had garnered the support of over 100 Senators and Congressmen, argued on national television, "I don't say it is a constitutional right, simply because we've been born in America, never to live in poverty, never to need any doctor, or never to have to serve in the military. I think along with the great privileges of citizenship go some personal responsibilities. And so specifically I would say that I don't think it's a person's right to the best possible medical care."[82]

Both Nixon's proposal and the AMA's would require employers to purchase coverage from private insurance companies, which infuriated supporters of universal coverage; United Auto Workers leader Leonard Woodcock thundered that the private insurance industry "has failed to deliver the health care or protection that legitimately has been expected of it." Renowned heart surgeon Michael DeBakey, a supporter of Kennedy's plan, said the Nixon proposal amounted to "subsidizing private health insurance companies."[83] The debates led nowhere. By 1974, Nixon had expanded his plan and Kennedy had modified his so that the two came closer to achieving a compromise, but labor leaders refused to budge. The Watergate scandal soon overshadowed national health insurance, and none of the bills ever made it to a vote.[84]

A consensus soon emerged that universal coverage would not be possible until health costs were brought under control. Democrat Jimmy Carter pledged a national insurance plan during his 1976 presidential campaign, a promise that won him the support of the powerful labor vote. But once in office he focused almost entirely on cost control, stating that "unrestrained health costs . . . restrict our ability to plan necessary improvements in our health care system." In 1975 US health

spending had reached $118.5 billion. A looming energy crisis and eco-
nomic troubles were becoming the nation's top concerns, and Carter
feared that "with current inflation, the cost of any national health insurance program . . . will double in just five years."[85] In an attempt to
slow medical inflation, Carter initially proposed a plan for hospital cost
containment, but it was quickly killed by the hospital lobby.[86]

After Carter's administration finally presented a proposal in 1978
that offered coverage for "catastrophic" health costs only, Ted Kennedy angered Carter by holding a press conference to denounce the bill
as too timid. The Massachusetts senator, who would soon announce
that he would run against Carter in 1980, insisted that the Democratic
midterm election platform must again include a plan "that will provide
decent health care across the country . . . for all Americans as a matter
of right and not of privilege."[87] With Carter facing a national tax revolt
(California's anti-tax Proposition 13 passed in June 1978) and drastically declining popularity, the president's plan received little interest
in Congress.

Medical expenses continued spiraling upward. By 1978 health care
was costing the United States $206 billion, or 9.1 percent of the gross
national product. There was widespread agreement with Carter's original position that health care reform was simply impossible because
the "costs will be staggering."[88] *New York Times* columnist Tom Wicker
argued the opposite: rather than putting the cart before the horse, "a
[national] insurance program, which could fix doctors' and hospitals'
fee schedules, would be the best way to stop health costs from rising
further."[89] But few commentators noted this argument. The media
and professional journals' discussions of cost inflation focused on
expensive technology, the costs of malpractice, increasing numbers
of aged ("the Graying of America"), and the inflationary aspects of
Medicare. Some analyses pointed to increased coverage itself as the
cause of rising expenditures. Medicare's "generous" coverage was forcing private insurers to follow suit. Too much insurance and coverage
by third parties meant that people were not aware of the true costs
of their medical care. Yet millions remained without coverage and
their access to health care was increasingly threatened by the system's
extraordinarily high costs; as the administrator of the federal Health
Resources Administration put it, "the effects of the burgeoning cost
of health care can be measured in unnecessary human suffering rather
than in dollars."[90]

The focus on cost control would lead to a new era in US health care history. Health care activists' vision of equality and universal coverage, which had been shared at least in part by Presidents Franklin D. Roosevelt, Truman, Kennedy, and Johnson, came to seem like a relic of a past era. All presidents since Carter, no matter their political persuasion, have placed cost control at the center of their reform efforts. And, as economist Rashi Fein has noted, because of the growing complexity and cost of the system, health reform became the realm of experts using a highly technical language, producing increasingly detailed reports that spoke to other experts rather than the public.[91] The struggle to connect health care reform to civil rights and social justice continued at the grassroots, but no longer seemed relevant in Washington.

Yet the more the presidents, the politicians, the press, and the public fretted about health costs, the faster those costs rose. By the 1980s, the United States had a health care system that embodied the worst of two worlds: extremely high and rapidly rising costs, combined with growing inequality and millions of people without coverage.

PART IV

Rights vs. Markets, 1981–2008

CHAPTER EIGHT

Emergency Rooms and Epidemics

In the 1980s, the United States experienced two national medical emergencies. The first was a nationwide increase in "patient dumping" by emergency rooms, as cuts in government medical assistance led private hospitals to reject uninsured, unprofitable patients, even if they were severely injured or dying. Second was a terrifying new infectious disease, AIDS, that struck down young people in the prime of life. Both crises led to revived rights demands, federal laws establishing new health rights, and new types of rationing. Activists demanded an end to discrimination based on health condition, and a universal right to health care. But the official rights to access created in the 1980s— the right to emergency room care and the right to federal funding for AIDS care and treatment—applied only to one part of the health care system and only one (albeit devastating) medical condition. They were responses to crises, not a coordinated plan to expand access to health care. These temporary fixes aided many Americans, but did nothing to stem the longer-term crisis of rising costs and growing numbers of people without health insurance, and may even have exacerbated them. In 1992 Bill Clinton was elected President on a promise to guarantee health care to all. But the failure of his administration's ambitious proposals forced a return to the consensus that fundamental health reform in the United States was impossible.

In the summer of 1981 the *Chicago Tribune* described a harrowing scene at Cook County, the city's massive public hospital. Very sick patients "could be seen lying on the floor at County's battle-scarred emergency room." Cook County normally took care of 90 to 125 indigent patients transferred from private hospitals each month, but after new Medicaid cuts the number had jumped to 365 in July and 560 in August. "Officials at County don't call this 'transferring,'" reported the *Tribune*. "They call it 'dumping,' a deliberate attempt to get rid of Medicaid patients." Patients who were "dumped" at County included a 60-year-old woman with severe pain, vomiting, and bowel obstruction who had to be operated on immediately for advanced cancer, and a woman with obvious symptoms of meningitis who was transferred to County for a CAT scan—even though the transferring hospital was well aware that County had no CAT scan equipment.[1]

"Dumping" was not confined to Chicago; transfers of indigent and Medicaid patients from private to public hospitals were increasing nationwide.[2] The increase happened suddenly. In 1981, the new President, Ronald Reagan, pushed for cuts to public medical care and other social programs. Congress slashed the federal contribution to Medicaid and allowed states to implement further cuts and reduce the number of people who were eligible. In response, some states drastically restricted Medicaid payment to hospitals. In Illinois and elsewhere, accepting Medicaid patients meant a hospital would lose more money than ever, and private hospitals began transferring such patients to protect their bottom lines. To add to an already compounded problem, the economic recession of the early 1980s had led to high unemployment and soaring poverty rates—the number of people in poverty increased by 13.4 percent between 1980 and 1982[3]—so more individuals became uninsured, ratcheting up the pressure on hospitals to provide care for which they would not be paid.

The emergency room dumping crisis was a particularly stark example of the transformation in health care brought about by Ronald Reagan's election to the presidency. Reagan, one of the most explicitly ideological presidents of the twentieth century, sought to end the growth of government embodied in the New Deal and Great Society in favor of spending cuts, privatization, deregulation, and faith in free markets. As a paid actor less than twenty years earlier, in his "Operation Coffee Cup" recording for the AMA, Reagan had denounced Medicare as "a short step to all the rest of socialism."[4] As president, his administration's health care goals were to cut Medicare and Medicaid spending, end the tax break for employer health insurance, and encourage private savings to replace the public's reliance on government entitlement programs.[5] "We cannot allow health costs to keep climbing," said Richard Schweiker, Reagan's Secretary of Health and Human Services. Instead of increased government regulation, "We intend to loose the forces of the market." The administration would support cost sharing for "less use of medical services by patients" and "convince people how to take control of their own health" through responsible personal behavior. The Reagan administration, according to one official, "attempts to make health care more like a business and less like a national free lunch."[6] The cuts to Medicaid, although not as drastic as Reagan wanted, were among the first actions taken by the Republican-dominated Congress in 1981.

Patient dumping was nothing new, as discussed in chapter 4. The journal of the American Hospital Association admitted that "it is a time-honored way of handling the problem" of patients who would lose the hospital money, even if this included the dumping of patients with life-threatening conditions.[7] Back in 1968, the director of admissions at Cook County Hospital claimed that 25.2 percent of the patients arriving at County were "transferred under unsafe conditions; for example, in shock, overmedicated, obtunded (dull or deadened). Patients were moved with unsplinted fractures, obstructed airways, and insufficient supplies of intravenous fluid which ran out before arrival at Cook County Hospital."[8] Another, even more common event was the transfer of nonemergency or stabilized patients to public or other "safety net" hospitals. In many communities, this was standard practice. "We've always been dumped on," said H. Robert Gregg, MD, president of Children's Hospital in Detroit. "All children's hospitals are dumped on. That's part of our business."[9]

Following the Medicaid cuts, some states capped the number of hospital days they would pay for Medicaid patients, resulting in a search for care that crossed state lines: "Patients from New Hampshire and West Virginia are coming to Boston hospitals for care because of severe restrictions in days of care allowed . . . in their own states," reported the journal *Hospitals*. On the West Coast, some hospitals issued bus schedules to their indigent patients, along with "'direction cards' and maps of how to get to the public or university hospital in town." Private hospitals and clinics in New York City gave uninsured patients "a referral slip with the name of the nearest municipal hospital."[10] Private, for-profit hospitals, which were growing in number in the 1980s, routinely rejected and transferred indigent patients. David A. Jones, the chairman of the for-profit Humana hospital chain, said that "in cities where there is a tax-supported hospital charged with caring for the indigent, Humana's hospitals have no qualms about transferring uninsured patients."[11]

Medicaid patients were never popular with private hospitals, but the 1981 cuts deepened their pariah status. Draconian cuts (in Illinois, Medicaid reimbursement for a hospital day dropped from $600 to

$450, and for a clinic visit from $150 to $50) led private hospitals to "panic" and transfer Medicaid patients at even greater rates. "We only take in Medicaid patients if their lives are threatened and we transfer them as soon as possible,'" said a spokesman for the private Michael Reese Medical Center in Chicago.[12]

The increase in rejections was not confined to Chicago. In 1982, both Children's Hospital in Denver and Beth Israel Medical Center in New York City publicly "announced that they will no longer provide non-emergency care to uninsured patients." Transfers of patients to DC General Hospital in Washington increased 374 percent between 1981 and 1984. In Texas, Dallas County's Parkland Memorial Hospital was spending "about $10 million annually on transferred indigent patients. The hospital has filed seven suits to obtain partial reimbursement from other counties," reported the journal of the American Bar Association, which also noted that the phenomenon was not confined to low-income patients: "Many middle-class but underinsured people are also being shunted from one hospital to another."[13]

For the first time, the popular media and mainstream medical and hospital journals began to identify dumping as a national problem. The *New England Journal of Medicine* and the *American Journal of Public Health* both published major studies on the dumping crisis. In 1982, *Hospitals*, the journal of the American Hospital Association, took its own readership to task with a two-part investigative report entitled "The 'Dumping' Dilemma: The Poor Are Always with Some of Us."[14]

Newspapers around the country reported shocking stories of dumping. *Miami Herald* readers learned about Ethel Dennis, a 76-year-old widow and former domestic worker who became very sick with tuberculosis and high blood pressure and was turned away by a neighborhood hospital because she had no insurance or Medicare card. In the parking lot, she went into convulsions. "A nurse came out of the First Aid room and gave the sick woman an injection," the newspaper reported. "Then, incredibly, she went back inside, leaving her patient lying on the ground, untreated." Four hours after she first asked for help, a private ambulance brought Ethel Dennis to Jackson Memorial, Miami's public hospital, where she died. In California, newspapers reported the case of 33-year-old Anna Grant of Contra Costa County, who went into labor but was turned away from a private hospital even though her unborn child showed signs of distress. "She was sent by ambulance to a county hospital, where the baby died."[15]

In 1982, the *Chicago Tribune* interviewed Louis Jackson, who had been transferred from a private hospital to Cook County Hospital while suffering from a severe bacterial infection. "I was too sick to know what was going on," Jackson said. Doctors at the private hospital stabilized his blood pressure "but I remember one of them saying, 'He can't pay' and another, 'Let's get him out of here.' The next thing I know, I was here (at Cook County)." He was still in shock during the transfer. Another patient shipped to Cook County, David Mann, was told by a private hospital that all its beds were full, even as he sat watching other patients being admitted. He ended up spending six weeks at County recovering from a severe heart infection. "I was dumped," Mann said, because of being on Medicaid.[16]

In 1985, the crisis reached the ears of Congress. Several sensational incidents of dumping by Brookside Hospital in Oakland, California, caught the attention of Alameda County's Democratic Congressman, Fortney "Pete" Stark. The story of Eugene Barnes, a 32-year-old uninsured African American man who was stabbed in the head and died after being refused treatment at Brookside, not only appeared on local TV stations and in newspapers, but also was reported by CBS anchorman Dan Rather on the national news on January 31, 1985.[17] Stark was infuriated at the number of dumping cases, or "ping-pong patients," in his district. "It is simply not acceptable to kick desperately ill people from one hospital to another because they can't foot the bill," he later said.[18]

Stark succeeded in adding an amendment to the Consolidated Omnibus Budget Reconciliation Act (COBRA) in 1986, creating the Emergency Medical Treatment and Active Labor Act, or EMTALA. EMTALA stated that, in any hospital receiving Medicare funds (thus virtually all US hospitals),

> If any individual comes to the emergency department and a request is made on the individual's behalf for examination or treatment for a medical condition, the hospital must provide for an appropriate medical screening examination within the capability of the hospital's emergency department . . . to determine whether or not an emergency medical condition . . . exists.

The requirement also applied to hospitals' treatment of women in labor. Hospitals found in violation could be fined $25,000 and have their Medicare status revoked.[19]

Because it was an amendment to the budget act, EMTALA was enacted swiftly, without public comment or a congressional hearing.[20] It is somewhat surprising that such a far-reaching law, and such a radical departure from hospitals' "no duty" tradition, received so little public notice. It may be that Stark wanted it that way; omnibus budget bills were a tried and true technique of sneaking legislation past scrutiny (EMTALA also became known in the hospital world as COBRA, which only added to the confusion).

Stark was able to quickly achieve his main goal—Brookside Hospital in his district became the target of one of the first EMTALA investigations. It received a warning from HCFA (the federal Health Care Finance Administration) and agreed to clean up its act in 1987.[21]

Overall, though, EMTALA had very little effect for the first few years of its existence, in part because it was so little known by the public or the hospitals. It took authorities years to develop official regulations to accompany the law—the final federal regulations were not published until 1994. Few hospitals were investigated and even fewer punished. Although understaffing at HCFA may have contributed, Democrats argued that the Reagan administration deliberately neglected EMTALA enforcement. Rep. Ted Weiss likened it to the White House's approach to its funding of the Contra rebels in Nicaragua: "If we don't like the law, we won't enforce it."[22]

Criticism of EMTALA came from both hospital leaders and the medical profession. Understandably, they complained about the problem of the uninsured being dumped on their doorstep. "We do not defend inappropriate transfers," said an American Hospital Association official, "but they should be recognized as signs that the delivery system is under stress." The focus on dumping would only "divert . . . attention from the more important issue at hand: adequate funding so that access to care can be assured for the indigent."[23] "It is not reasonable to ask community hospitals to risk financial ruin for the sake of a deficient social policy," wrote a doctor in the *Journal of the American Medical Association*. "The responsibility for the medically indigent and uninsured must be shared by everyone, not unilaterally imposed on a selected segment of our economy."[24] Creating access to just one type of care was the kind of irrational US-style rationing that led to higher costs overall.

Pete Stark, the Congressman responsible for EMTALA, did not see the law as a panacea. *New England Journal of Medicine* editor Arnold Relman pointed out that EMTALA "doesn't get to the heart of the matter. Without more support for indigent care, hospitals caring for uninsured emergency patients will be put at a serious economic disadvantage."[25] Stark agreed, pledging to propose federal indigent care reimbursement to hospitals to accompany EMTALA enforcement. He convened a hearing on federal support for safety net hospitals in March 1987, but it was fruitless.[26] Tacking on an "unfunded mandate" like EMTALA to a budget bill was one thing; allocating federal dollars to support hospital care for the uninsured was another, and next to unthinkable at a time when the Reagan administration's main goal was to *cut* Medicare reimbursements to hospitals. With this form of irrational rationing, Congress hoped to end the newspaper stories of people dying in parking lots, while avoiding any new or rearranged federal spending commitments.

Cost Containment and Cost Shifting

When Reagan took office, the US government was spending $73.4 billion, or 11 percent of the federal budget, on health care (in 1965 it had been only $5 billion).[27] The cost of Medicare and Medicaid had risen from $26 billion in 1976 to $56 billion in 1981.[28] Of this money, $36.8 billion was going to Medicare, whose policy of allowing doctors and hospitals to charge as much as they wished had led to large cost increases. In 1983, Reagan officials created a new hospital payment system for Medicare known as DRGs (Diagnostic Related Groups). Instead of paying what the hospital charged on a fee-for-service basis, the government would now pay a flat rate for each diagnosis. The new system was intended to give hospitals incentives to keep costs down. "If a hospital can treat a patient for less than this flat price, it makes money," noted a health industry official. "If it can't, it eats the loss."[29] DRGs transformed Medicare payments from retrospective (after the fact) to prospective (before the fact), and thus became known as "prospective payment."

Medicare cost containment encouraged hospitals to discharge patients more quickly and to avoid overtreatment. The average length of a hospital stay in 1983 was 10 days; by 1995, it had fallen to 7.1 days.[30] Soon, fears arose that patients were being discharged "sicker" as well as "quicker" and that undertreatment might replace overtreatment. DRGs might have been a factor in the dumping crisis, as hospitals scrambled to avoid patients with expensive conditions.[31]

The Reagan administration also attempted to lower doctors' fees in Medicare through the introduction of fee schedules. Although Medicare spending continued to grow, more than doubling between 1980 and 1990, the new cost control methods managed to keep the rate of

Medicare's price increases below that of private health insurance.[32] But in the long term, the new payment system did not help reduce overall national health expenditures, in part because many hospitals and doctors, in a practice known as "cost shifting," simply started charging more to privately insured patients.[33] Cost shifting is an example of the high cost of US-style rationing—placing limits on one area of the health system increases costs in another area.

At the same time that Republicans were attempting to control Medicare's spending, the newly Democratic Congress passed the largest Medicare expansion in history to that date, the Catastrophic Coverage Act of 1988. This Act attempted to address one of the major limitations of Medicare, its cutoffs of hospital stays over 60 days, by stipulating that Medicare would pay all hospital and doctor costs when they rose above $2,000 a year per recipient. The Act also added prescription drug and nursing home benefits to Medicare. Because all these new benefits would be so expensive, the Democrats decided to fund the law by a premium hike on most Medicare recipients, rather than an additional payroll tax on all workers. What was perceived as a new tax on seniors proved hugely unpopular, despite the Act's new benefits, and the next Congress repealed it in 1990.[34] The lesson many lawmakers took from the debacle was that in health politics, cost mattered more than coverage.

AIDS, Rationing, and Rights

The AIDS epidemic made its first terrifying appearance in the United States in 1981. Those stricken with the immunity-destroying virus faced not only debility and death, but also the severe stigma of a disease associated with the most marginalized groups in society—gays, drug users, the poor. However, more than any other group of disease sufferers in history, those with AIDS found a collective voice and fought back against discrimination, neglect, and violations of their rights. AIDS activists demanded, and won, dramatic changes in drug development and medical research, speeding discoveries in testing and treatment. They led public education and prevention campaigns and created formal and informal networks of support for sufferers. The AIDS movement also fought against health care rationing based on HIV status, and by 1990 began to call for a universal right to health care. Although they won limited rights to access for people with AIDS, activists were not able to dislodge the deep-seated inequities of the US health system.

AIDS led to new types of health care denial and revived old ones.

The attachment of stigma to sexually transmitted disease, and separation or refusal of patients with contagious disease, had been common throughout history.[35] Although eventually the virus was found to be spread only by direct transmittal of bodily fluids, fear of contagion was pervasive. Early in the epidemic, many health care workers refused to treat AIDS patients out of fear for their own safety. Surveys found that between one-third and one-half of primary care physicians refused to accept patients with AIDS.[36] Even when it became established that health care workers could protect themselves with simple precautions, refusal remained widespread. In San Diego in 1987, "as in most other cities, a handful of doctors handle nearly all the AIDS cases, and they are becoming overwhelmed by the increasing numbers of dying patients."[37] The epidemic created a new category of emergency room transfer or refusal: the dumping of people suspected of being infected with the AIDS virus.[38] Nevertheless, many health care providers insisted that AIDS patients had a right to care and they acted on that belief. As one example of their dedication, physicians and nurses led in the establishment of the famous AIDS ward at San Francisco General Hospital.[39]

AIDS created a new category for insurance rejections. Fearing that the disease would be catastrophically expensive, private insurers began refusing or dropping customers with AIDS or HIV (the virus and a test to detect it were discovered in 1984). Because the majority of early AIDS cases were concentrated in the white, middle-class gay community, a high proportion of HIV patients in the United States had private insurance at the time of diagnosis. But as the disease progressed, these same patients lost their coverage, either through job loss or from being dropped by their insurer, or both. They were then forced to spend all their resources on medical care until they became eligible for Medicaid. By 1993, Medicaid, which covered 11 percent of all US health spending, covered 25 percent of AIDS-related costs.[40]

This was the case for Wilson Roberts, whose story was featured in the *New York Times* with the sidebar "AIDS killed him, but our health care system tortured him." Roberts lost his engineering job and his health insurance after he became sick with the virus. He was refused hospital care after losing his private insurance, and spent his life savings on medical care before becoming eligible for Medicaid. Roberts died on his thirty-fourth birthday.[41] People with AIDS who lost their private insurance faced not only discrimination based on their condition, but also the barriers to care associated with being uninsured or on Medicaid. "I will be dead in three years, and the health insurance system will speed my death," said Stan Long of Los Angeles, whose insurer had cancelled his policy along with those of thousands of subscribers with HIV or AIDS.[42]

Insurance companies also found ways to reduce or eliminate benefits for AIDS for insured people. Many imposed an "AIDS cap" on group policies, lowering the maximum benefit for AIDS care only.[43] Some companies created a category of AIDS coverage that applied only to those sickened by "involuntary infection," excluding people who acquired the virus through sexual contact or through drug use. Furious at the implication that such infections were somehow "voluntary," one AIDS activist wrote to an insurance company official, "no one sets out to acquire this disease, all people with AIDS are innocent."[44] Some insurers even excluded from individual coverage members of occupations stereotypically associated with gay men. A California insurer included "beauty and hair salon employees . . . decorators and interior designers" on its list of "ineligible occupations."[45]

Health care access and coverage did not receive much attention from the AIDS movement for the first few years of the epidemic, when activists faced an emergency situation and had to deal with the government's neglect of the disease and the search for prevention and treatment. By 1990, however, a confrontation with the health care system became unavoidable. The epidemic's advance and the disease's long incubation period meant that tens of thousands of individuals were coming down with full-blown AIDS, pushing the health care system to a crisis point. By 1991, AIDS became the leading cause of death for men and women in the United States aged 25 to 44. Also, the grim reality was that AIDS patients before 1990 simply didn't live long enough to require much medical care; AIDS groups had focused on home and custodial care for sufferers, rather than access to the mainstream health system. By 1990, some treatments for AIDS were indeed being discovered, which brought the question of access to the forefront. People with AIDS and their supporters had to fight for access and care within "the most inequitable system of medical care among advanced democratic societies," in the words of AIDS researcher and advocate Ronald Bayer.[46]

ACT UP (AIDS Coalition to Unleash Power), the militant and highly effective AIDS advocacy organization, was founded in 1987 and initially focused on demanding quicker drug approval and access to new treatments for AIDS sufferers.[47] Then, in the early 1990s, both the

New York and San Francisco branches of ACT UP established committees devoted entirely to insurance and access issues for people with HIV/AIDS. These groups used strong rights language in their demands. "People with life threatening diseases, especially people with AIDS, face illegal discrimination, absurd premium increases and sudden policy cancellation. *They need protection*," a San Francisco activist wrote to the California health insurance commissioner in 1990. "Health care is a right and health insurance is a necessity, not a luxury." The Golden Gate Insurance Committee demanded that the state provide insurance data, including redlining practices and denials, "an end to disease-specific spending caps," price controls on premiums, mandated coverage of home care, preventive care, and experimental treatments, and an expanded statewide high-risk pool "and other forms of guaranteed access."[48]

ACT UP used in-your-face tactics to bring attention to discriminatory insurance practices. In 1990, activists staged a "phone zap" (flooding the switchboard with phone calls) against a company that had eliminated AIDS benefits unless the policyholder could prove "involuntary infection." The company, Galaxy Carpet Mills, relented and rescinded the rule. In May 1991, about 100 ACT UP members marched from the headquarters of the Health Insurance Association of America in Washington, DC, to the White House, carrying black coffins draped with the names of insurance companies accused of discrimination against people with AIDS.[49]

ACT UP also demanded a national commitment to funding for AIDS care and treatment. Demonstrators targeted President George H. W. Bush, including marching on his vacation home in Kennebunkport, Maine, for federal neglect of the epidemic. Alongside the more mainstream tactics of advocacy organizations across the country, ACT UP's militancy helped win a historic commitment from Congress to fund not just education, but access to care and treatment for the disease's victims. Thanks to bipartisan sponsorship by Senators Ted Kennedy (Democrat) and Orrin Hatch (Republican), Congress passed the Comprehensive AIDS Care Emergency Act in 1990 (later named the Ryan White CARE Act, after the Indiana teenager and AIDS activist who died that year after contracting the disease through a blood transfusion). The Act provided $880 million for the medical care and support of people with AIDS. Despite attempts by conservatives in Congress to cut funding or block reauthorization, the CARE Act thrived, and today assists half a million people annually. After Medicare and Medicaid,

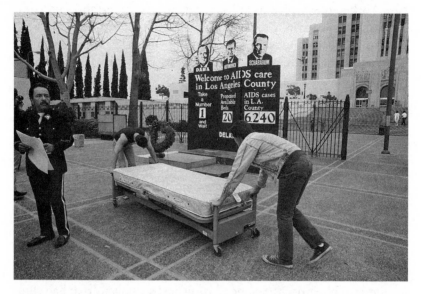

FIGURE 12. Rationing by health condition: ACT UP members protest a shortage of AIDS care facilities in San Francisco hospitals. Photo by Sara Krulwich, *New York Times*, February 8, 1989, A1. Reprinted with permission.

it is the third largest source of public financing for HIV/AIDS care in the United States.[50]

The allocation of significant federal resources to patient care and treatment—not just prevention, education, and research—was a huge victory for the AIDS activist movement's campaign for access. But again, like all the health care expansions in the United States, the CARE Act raised the question of why only certain categories of sick people deserved coverage and support. Some ACT UP activists noted that the arguments in Congress against the CARE Act (some conservatives tried to block reauthorization or cut funding) "have the same theme: they don't want to take money away from other people who also need it. National health care should circumvent this debate by guaranteeing treatment and medical care to every American whatever the need." Arguing that ACT UP should throw its support behind universal insurance, activists concluded, "National health care is just morally right. That our country has gone so long without it is a scandal."[51] Early in the 1990s, ACT UP created its own "Healthcare Campaign" and began joining national demonstrations in support of universal health insurance. In a "Medical Insurance Bill of Rights for People with HIV Disease," ACT UP declared that "health care is a right for all people."[52] Fighting for the health care rights of people with AIDS led activists to claim a right to health care for all.

People outside the AIDS activist community also acknowledged that the epidemic "has heightened America's awareness of the need for reform."[53] "AIDS highlights all the flaws in American health care," stated the president of New York City's Health and Hospitals Corporation, "the lack of preventive medicine, primary physician care, long-term facilities, home care, universal insurance, and drug treatment."[54] As AIDS in the late 1980s began to increase most rapidly in minority inner-city communities, the disease converged with existing epidemics of homelessness, poverty, racism, the emergency room crisis, and the closure of public hospitals. Health officials in New York City warned that a shortage of facilities would lead to widespread denials of care and bring the system to the brink of collapse.[55]

The Ryan White CARE Act helped avert such a disaster with its infusion of federal dollars to city hospitals.[56] Rather than providing broad funding for uncompensated care or the uninsured (as Congressman Stark had wanted following EMTALA), Congress instead allocated new dollars on the basis of disease category, because of both the devastating, emergency nature of the epidemic and the brilliantly effective activism of the AIDS/HIV movement.

Even in the era of Reagan and George H. W. Bush, Congress passed significant new coverage expansions (the CARE Act) and even new legislation (EMTALA) that created the first official right to access. But there was no fundamental change in a system that provided health care for some, not all. The CARE Act and EMTALA practiced rationing by applying only to specific groups of people (AIDS sufferers) or specific categories of care and facilities (emergency care). They were stopgap measures to avert the collapse of the system—to prevent Americans from actually dying in the street—rather than steps toward universal access. At the same time that these (literally) reactionary measures expanded coverage and rights for some, protection for others continued to contract—namely, the employer health benefits that covered a majority of the US population under age 65.

The Rise of the Uninsured and Bill Clinton's Attempt at Reform

In 1990, the popular magazine *Consumer Reports* published a major two-part report on health insurance. Alongside the usual advice about the

best/worst plans for consumers, the magazine introduced a series titled "Crisis," featuring stories and photos of individual patients, each
of whom was dealing with a calamity caused by inadequate coverage.
"Crisis: Delayed care" described a newly hired Nevada casino worker
who put off visiting a dermatologist because of his health insurance's
one-year waiting period, and died from a malignant melanoma. In "Crisis: Benefits end, costs don't," an attorney paralyzed in a bike accident
ran out of benefits after the first $250,000 and began paying for home
care out of his own pocket. "Crisis: Unaffordable premiums" described
a TV repair shop owner who struggled to provide benefits for himself
and his employees after his insurance premiums doubled following an
illness. "Crisis: Locked in" told the story of a woman who could not
change jobs after being diagnosed with glaucoma because her preexisting condition would exclude her from coverage anywhere else.[57]

These and other "horror stories" appearing throughout the media
emphasized a new point: the nation's health crisis had reached the
middle class. The heartrending tales were not about the poor, Medicaid recipients, AIDS patients, or any of the other marginalized groups
who had long suffered on health care's fringe; they were about "mainstream" Americans who thought they were protected if they worked
hard and played by the rules. They quickly learned that this was not so,
and they were shocked at their own powerlessness when they became
caught up in the health system's inequities and red tape, or lost their
insurance altogether.

The percentage of Americans covered by private health insurance
peaked in 1982. Then, the promise that private coverage would meet
the nation's health insurance needs began to crumble in earnest. Corporate downsizing, two recessions, increased global competition, and
the decline of manufacturing all contributed to US employers' inability
or unwillingness to continue offering benefits. The percentage of employees of medium and large businesses who received coverage from
their employer fell from 96 percent in 1983 to 82 percent in 1993.[58] By
1992, 37.1 million Americans had no health insurance, up from 29 million in 1979. There were 51.3 million who were uninsured for at least
part of the year. Eighty-four percent of the uninsured were workers or
dependents of workers. "Most uninsured Americans are middle class
working families," a health policy expert told the Senate Finance Committee in 1994.[59]

Employers dropped health care benefits as they became increasingly
unaffordable with the rising cost of medical care. For some businesses,

health care had become their greatest expenditure. In an example that made headlines, Lee Iacocca, the new chairman of Chrysler auto company, "was amazed to discover that Blue Cross / Blue Shield was Chrysler's largest supplier" and that health costs for workers accounted for $700 of the sticker price of each car the company produced.[60]

Iacocca's anger at the high cost of health care was matched by that of the American consumer. Employees were being forced to shoulder more of the costs of their coverage. In 1983, slightly more than half (54%) of full-time employees in medium and large firms contributed towards employer-provided health premiums for family coverage. Ten years later, over three-quarters (76%) of these employees paid health insurance premiums. The real average monthly contribution paid by employees for their health coverage more than doubled, from $45 in 1983 to $107 in 1993.[61] And, as the distressing "Crisis" stories in *Consumer Reports* illustrated, Americans were getting less while paying more.

In 1991, Pennsylvania Democratic Senate candidate Harris Wofford swept into office with an ad campaign announcing, "If criminals have the right to a lawyer, I think working Americans should have the right to a doctor. . . . I believe there is nothing more fundamental than the right to see a doctor when you're sick." Wofford, who had been a virtual unknown, became a "living symbol of the public's desire for change" in health care.[62] His victory launched health care reform as a major issue in the 1992 presidential election.

When Arkansas governor Bill Clinton accepted the Democratic nomination for the presidency, he announced his vision of "an America where health care is a right, not a privilege."[63] But the right to health care meant something different to Clinton than it had to LBJ, Truman, or FDR. Clinton insisted that he was not a traditional Democrat. The new health care system he wanted would cover everyone—the liberal goal of universal access—but it would also control costs and preserve the private health insurance market. Clinton rejected calls for a Canadian-style (or Medicare-style) centralized "single payer" system that would eliminate the private insurance middleman. Instead, he embraced a new philosophy of "managed competition" in which private insurers competed for the business of purchasers organized into "health alliances."

The slogans of Clinton's presidential campaign—"health care that's always there" and "health care that can never be taken away"—emphasized universalism and health security. Clinton was firmly committed to universal coverage, insisting that he would refuse to approve a plan that did not cover everyone in the country. These straightforward populist slogans contrasted with the actual bill that emerged from the negotiations of the Clinton Health Care Task Force, a group of over 600 experts chaired by First Lady Hillary Clinton. The Clinton Health Security Act, nearly 1,400 pages long, proposed a dauntingly complex system of managed competition: competing insurance companies organized into regional health alliances and overseen by a National Health Board. Under this system, everyone would be insured via an employer mandate, with subsidies for smaller employers and unemployed people.

By including a National Health Board to cap insurance costs and set "global budgets" for health care spending, the plan veered from the original idea of managed competition, which had emerged from a meeting of policy experts and health industry representatives known as the Jackson Hole Group in 1990. The concept envisioned a market-based system of private insurers that would control prices by virtue of competition. Adding government oversight to managed competition represented the "third way" that Clinton "so often seeks in truly polarized debates," noted the New York Times: "not pure Jackson Hole, not total regulation, but something that seeks to meet the progressive goals of making health insurance more affordable and more widely available without utterly dismantling the American system."[64]

Even strong supporters of health reform struggled to muster enthusiasm for the Clinton plan. Consumer advocates were dismayed at having been left out of the policy-making process. Speaking about the experts who advised Hillary Clinton in crafting the health proposal, the president of the Consumers Union complained that they were a "Who's Who of health special interests," dominated by hospital, pharmaceutical, and insurance executives. Organizations left out of the negotiations included the AMA, minority health care providers, and even senior citizens' organizations, including the National Council of Senior Citizens, which had played such a major role in the passage of Medicare.[65] Longtime single-payer advocates were outright opposed, claiming that the byzantine Clinton proposal offered "more bureaucracy, less consumer choice and a health system owned by a few insurance giants." Labor unions and the American Association of Retired Persons rebelled at the proposal's cuts to Medicare and Medicaid.[66]

The medical profession's reaction to the Clinton plan was mixed. By the 1990s, especially because of the rise of managed care, physicians were no longer the most powerful players in the health care industry. The increase in medical specialization meant that the AMA now represented only a small fraction of doctors in a divided and fragmented profession. Some physician groups, including the American Academy of Family Physicians and the American Academy of Pediatrics, endorsed the Clinton plan for its embrace of universal coverage. At the start of the debate, the AMA itself sought to break away from its past and work with, rather than against, the President toward reform, but in the end denounced the Clinton plan for its central spending controls.[67] Business organizations also opposed the plan because of the employer mandate.[68]

The strongest opposition of all came from the insurance companies. Even though universal coverage using managed competition would have brought them millions of new customers, insurers, like doctors earlier in the century, rejected any plan that would increase government regulation of their industry and loosen their control over the health care system. The Health Insurance Association of America, made up of smaller insurers, ran a $15 million advertising campaign against the Clinton plan, including the "Harry and Louise" ads (see below). Aetna, MetLife, CIGNA, Prudential, and Travelers, the insurance giants who had originally supported the idea of managed competition as members of the Jackson Hole Group, jumped ship when they heard about the proposed National Health Board to oversee spending by the health alliances.[69] As political scientist Jacob Hacker describes it, insurance companies "were not going to forfeit their central position in the medical sector without a fight."[70]

Public opinion, initially strongly in favor of reform, began to turn against the Clinton plan. The proposal was dauntingly complex and difficult to understand. Terms like "managed competition" and "global budgets" did nothing to capture hearts and minds. But the public did understand the term "rationing" and did not like it one bit. Opponents insisted that Clinton's plan would bring European- or Canadian-style rationing into American health care. "It all sounds to me like you're going to have some government setting prices," former president George H. W. Bush had admonished Clinton during a televised debate. The Health Leadership Council, a group led by CEOs of fifty major health insurance companies, drug and medical device manufacturers, and hospitals, ran advertisements around the country "raising the specter of health care rationing and warning of bureaucratic interference with patients' rights." The ads included a warning that "Washington bureaucrats" would "decide how much care can be given to you and your family."[71]

And with two middle-aged suburbanites named Harry and Louise, the Health Insurance Association of America created the most famous anti–health reform ad campaign of all time. The TV spots featured the couple fretting at their kitchen table about how the President's plan would interfere in their relationship with their doctor. They worried that health care reform would bring rationing: "you know, long waits for health care and some services not even available."[72] The widely accepted definition of rationing as a sinister, European or Canadian activity was crucial to opponents' strategy of focusing the public's fears on how health care reform would take something away from them. Because no one talked about how the current system already rationed, Clinton and his supporters could not emphasize the plan's goal of *ending* rationing by health coverage and ability to pay.

Postmortem analyses of the reform episode agree that the Clinton administration lacked a political strategy to match its complicated technical maneuverings. Unlike the famously skillful LBJ, who could wrap congressmen around his little finger, "the Clintons seemed unable to focus on and execute the politics of reform," as Blumenthal and Morone put it.[73] (Clinton also lacked the popular mandate LBJ enjoyed after his landslide victory, having received only 43 percent of the vote.) Like Harry Truman, Clinton had no plan to mobilize popular approval. It didn't help that both the opponents' advertising campaigns and the densely complex proposal itself sowed confusion rather than bringing clarity. Kennedy and Johnson had won support for Medicare in part because people understood it—it built on Social Security, which they were already familiar with. But Clinton had refused to consider a plan built on the already popular Medicare system. Kennedy and Johnson had also brought the cause directly to the people, with Madison Square Garden rallies and stump speeches. Clinton's plan became bogged down in committees of "experts" working behind closed doors. "Health care is a right, not a privilege" and "health care that's always there" were ideas around which ordinary people could mobilize. "Health alliances," "managed competition," and "National Health Board" not only failed to capture the public's imagination, but also made it much easier for opponents to attack the plan.

By the fall of 1994, Congress declared that the Clinton health reform proposal was dead. The campaign against it had frightened Americans by telling them that their rights would be taken away and their health care rationed. Scare tactics once again prevented a serious discussion of how rationing already occurred and how rights were being curtailed in the existing system. Instead, defeat led to the abandonment of national reform. Incremental, modest changes could still be discussed, but "universal coverage" became an untouchable subject in Washington. Inaction on the part of the White House and Congress meant that huge changes would take place in the health care system over the next decade with little or no federal oversight. Between 1994 and 2008, more and more Americans would lose their health insurance, pay more for their coverage, or face a new kind of rationing in the form of managed care. As the experience of exclusion and rationing spread to more of the population, the right to health care for all would rise again as an urgent demand.

CHAPTER NINE

At the Breaking Point

National health reform legislation failed in Washington in 1994 but succeeded in 2010. During the period in between, the number of uninsured Americans continued to grow. The Clinton administration won some incremental reforms, but the conservative president, George W. Bush, who followed in 2001 sought to replace government intervention with the free market. The United States experienced two major disasters, the terrorist attacks of 9/11 and Hurricane Katrina, which also became health crises involving survivors with chronic illnesses and no health insurance. But the biggest story in American health care became the hardships of people *with* health insurance. Managed care restrictions, higher out-of-pocket costs, exclusion of preexisting conditions, and many other aspects of private health insurance forced the middle class to experience health care denials and a lack of health security on a large scale. Americans' anger at insurance companies helped Barack Obama win the 2008 election on a promise of sweeping reform — and a claim that health care is a right.

Back in the late 1990s, however, survivors of the Clinton health care debacle had predicted that major health reform would not be possible in the United States any time soon. The media, politicians, and health policy analysts all agreed that any new changes proposed would have to be incremental, addressing only part of the nation's health insurance problems. Any moves toward more sweeping reform would no longer take place on the national level, but could continue quietly, in individual states. Certainly, there was to be no more discussion of a right to adequate health care for all.

Alongside this pessimistic retreat, two bipartisan reforms during the late Clinton administration did attempt to incrementally expand health coverage. The first was the Health Insurance Portability and Accountability Act of 1996, which created some modest restrictions on insurance companies' ability to reject applicants, but ended up doing little to actually improve health insurance portability[1] (the law became much better known for its patient privacy stipulations). A second incremental but important step was the creation of SCHIP, the State Children's Health Insurance Program, in 1998. SCHIP expanded Medicaid by allowing states to cover children from families with income up to 200 percent of the poverty level, and later also made it possible for some states to offer Medicaid to the uninsured parents of covered children. By 2006, SCHIP programs had reduced the number of uninsured children nationwide by 20 percent, although 8 million remained uninsured.[2]

Because of SCHIP's reliance on the federal / state Medicaid funding model, the program could not cover every eligible child, and eventually some states had to put children and families on waiting lists as state funds dwindled.[3] These waiting lists did not make headlines; they were business as usual in the American way of rationing. Even though it could not come close to meeting the need, SCHIP was the most important expansion of coverage since 1965. Like Medicaid, the program was means-tested, and it rationed on the basis of income and family status (when adults became eligible, only parents of SCHIP children could apply). Like Medicare, it rationed by age, but this time children rather than elders were the beneficiaries. Coverage for children only was politically palatable; few members of Congress were willing to argue against a Medicaid expansion for vulnerable kids, although President George W. Bush was less hesitant in refusing to expand SCHIP in the following decade.

But even as SCHIP covered more poor families and HIPAA allowed some portability of coverage, the number of Americans without health insurance continued to rise, from 39 million at the time of the Clinton reform defeat, to over 41 million by 1999.[4] Two central factors contributed to the increase: the continually growing cost of medical care, which forced employers to drop benefits or increase their cost to employees; and major economic shifts that led to greater job instability, unemployment, temporary and part-time work, and the decline of the manufacturing sector that had traditionally provided generous benefits to blue-collar workers in the United States.[5] The crisis was reaching beyond the poor, the unemployed, and the underemployed. It was increasingly evident a full-time job was no longer a path to health coverage. The authors of the 2006 book *Uninsured in America* argued that the health insurance crisis was creating a new "caste" of the working poor whose lack of coverage led to a downward spiral of chronic bad health, disability, and insecure employment.[6] The 1996 Clinton welfare reform law, which moved poor mothers off the welfare rolls and into paid work, left many former welfare recipients without health insurance as they lost their Medicaid eligibility.[7] Between 2000 and 2003, nearly four million people (including dependents of workers) lost their employer-provided health coverage.[8]

Early in the 2000s, there was new attention to the health consequences of uninsurance. In 2003, *USA Today* reported that the "myth" that "the uninsured get access to care when they really need it is fading as study after study documents its falsehood."[9] In a series of reports released between 2000 and 2004, the prestigious Institute of Medicine of the National Academy of Sciences (IOM) reported that the uninsured received about one-half the amount of health care compared to those with insurance. People without health coverage had fewer preventive screenings, received fewer effective treatments, and died of cancer and other major diseases at higher rates than the insured. The IOM's headline-grabbing conclusion was that 18,000 Americans died every year because they lacked health insurance.[10]

But the plight of the uninsured was only part of the turn-of-the-century health crisis. People *with* health coverage were experiencing a new kind of explicit rationing in the form of "managed care." It was not only uninsured Americans who were being denied care that they needed. More than ever before, the crisis spread to the middle class.

HMO Horrors: The Backlash against Managed Care

Managed care and its most common manifestation, the health maintenance organization (HMO), were survivors of the Clinton reform proposals. The concept dated back to the prepaid medical plans of lumber and railroad workers early in the twentieth century, and the medical cooperatives of midcentury. The term "managed care" had been coined around 1970 by Minnesota physician Paul Ellwood, who proposed that a system merging health care delivery and finance would allow for greater efficiency and encourage preventive and comprehensive care. While the Clinton plan's emphasis on managed care organizations, which were unfamiliar and threatening to much of the public, clearly played a role in its defeat,[11] the end of the Clinton reform did not mean the end of HMOs—just the opposite. By 1996, a *Wall Street Journal* reporter wrote that "faster than almost anyone expected, managed care has become the *de facto* national health policy of the United States."[12]

When Congress passed the HMO Act in 1973, there were between 30 and 40 managed care organizations in the United States, and 90 percent of them were nonprofit. The expansion of HMOs was encouraged in 1981 when the Reagan administration eliminated federal subsidies for the HMOs and instead promoted the plans as an opportunity for private investors to make money. Although some of the major HMOs, such as Kaiser Permanente, remained not-for-profit, managed care increasingly lost touch with its nonprofit roots. By the mid-1980s there were over 600 HMOs in the United States, 60 percent of which were for-profit. Plans began to merge and consolidate, until only a few national organizations dominated the industry, including Kaiser Permanente, Blue Cross/WellPoint (including many formerly nonprofit Blue Cross plans converted to for-profit), Humana, and UnitedHealth.[13]

HMOs were popular with employers because of their initial cost savings compared to traditional fee-for-service plans, and the number of Americans enrolled in HMOs peaked at 81.3 million in 1999.[14] But many HMO members did not like what they were getting. HMOs practiced a new kind of rationing, one that was much more obvious to the consumer. While fee-for-service medicine encouraged doctors to order more tests and treatments, managed care aimed for the opposite. Doctors were paid a set fee per patient (known as capitation), giving them a financial incentive to keep treatment costs low. HMO members were assigned to a primary physician whose role was that of a "gatekeeper" required to approve all treatments and referrals to specialists. Some managed care companies paid doctors bonuses tied to how much they kept costs down.[15] While a reduction in unnecessary tests, treatments, and specialist visits would undoubtedly benefit the whole system, consumers feared—and many began to experience— denials of needed care.

Managed care denials could take many different forms. In addition to the "gatekeeper" primary physician keeping a lid on referrals, HMOs had armies of staff to perform "utilization reviews" of treatments ordered by doctors, and could deny payment for treatments the HMO deemed unnecessary. Utilization review, as the most explicit form of rationing in managed care, received much negative attention in the media, especially when denial resulted in death or injury to the patient, as in the case of a California patient whose leg had to be amputated following the HMO's refusal to extend a doctor-ordered hospitalization.[16] Some HMOs issued blanket rules shortening hospital stays for common procedures, including childbirth, which led to a public and media outcry against "drive-through deliveries" and "drive-through mastectomies."[17]

Managed care greatly reduced the choice of physician or hospital because HMOs required their members to use only those providers designated "in network," who had contracted with the HMO. Patients who required care from out-of-network providers had to pay very high fees. During the Clinton reform debate, Americans had been "threatened with the specter of 'losing the right to choose our own doctor,'" wrote Long Island resident Lillian Polak to the *New York Times* in 1998. "Now, six years later, health maintenance organizations are choosing our doctors for us."[18] It was hard not to note the irony: the Clinton plan had been sunk by Harry and Louise's warnings that consumers would lose their power to choose; now that worst-case scenario had come true, but in the private rather than the public sector.

Even the right to emergency care was compromised for members of some HMOs. Utilization review meant that a patient could be denied coverage for an ER visit if the condition turned out to be non-emergent—for example, if chest pains feared to be a heart attack were diagnosed as a digestive problem. Some HMOs required "preauthorization" for emergency care, meaning that patients "find themselves having their treatment delayed while the hospital seeks authorization for payment [or] having treatment denied if the authorization is refused," according to a study by the consumer group Public Citizen. In-network rules meant that some emergency patients were "being shuffled from the hospital to another in a dangerously unstable condition because their HMO has a contract with the second hospital."[19]

Even as they sought to lower costs, many managed care organizations devoted a large percentage of their revenues to administration, overhead, and profits. Critics worried that for-profit companies had a built-in incentive to reduce patient care. The Association of American Medical Colleges reported in 1995 that for-profit HMOs were paying out an average of only 70 percent of their premium revenue for medical costs; "The remaining 30 percent went for administrative expenses — and profit." The numbers in Illinois were even worse, according to a study by the Illinois State Medical Society, which found many for-profit plans in the state allocating only 60 percent of their income to medical care. Nonprofit plans, on the other hand, spent a much higher percentage of premium income on care, such as Harvard Pilgrim Health Care (89 percent) and Kaiser Permanente (94 percent).[20]

Much criticism of HMOs came from the medical profession. Physicians, who had benefited from the fee-for-service arrangements under traditional health insurance, were dismayed by many aspects of managed care. In addition to eroding the cherished tenet of free choice of doctor, managed care threatened the doctor-patient relationship and physician autonomy. In a system in which treatment decisions were increasingly subject to second-guessing by HMO officials, "physicians have lost their voice," lamented one doctor.[21] As HMOs squeezed physician payments, the incomes of American doctors began to decrease for the first time since the Great Depression. Between 1993 and 1995, primary care physicians in California, a state where HMOs dominated the market, experienced a drop in earnings from $172,100.00 to $146,000.00 (still not a pittance, exactly).[22]

Managed care was indeed reducing some health costs, but concerns about lowered quality and denials of care began to dominate the debate. Opinion polls "showed that the insurance industry had become public enemy number one," according to sociologist Jill Quadagno. *Time* magazine's cover of April 14, 1997, blared, "THE BACKLASH AGAINST HMOS."[23]

Consumers became even more frustrated when they discovered that they were unable to sue HMOs in court for neglect or malpractice, because of an obscure but important federal law named ERISA that granted legal immunity to a large segment of employer-sponsored health plans.[24] The lack of legal redress for HMO members led to demands for a new Patients' Bill of Rights (also known, more accurately, as the Managed Care Consumer Bill of Rights). The bill, introduced in Congress 1997 and supported by President Clinton, would have allowed patients to sue their HMOs. "Too many managed-care firms and other insurance companies have decided that the shortest route to higher profits and a competitive edge is by denying patients the care they need and deserve," thundered Senator Ted Kennedy, not surprisingly a strong proponent of the legislation.[25]

Although a federal Patients' Bill of Rights never came to be, there was a rush in the states to pass legislation regulating HMOs. In response to denials of emergency care and refusals to reimburse, many states passed "prudent layperson" laws, mandating that health insurers pay for emergency room visits for conditions that a reasonable person would deem to be an emergency. The outcry against "drive-through deliveries" and "drive-through mastectomies" led to state laws requiring minimum hospital stays for childbirth and some other conditions. Other state laws mandated that female members of managed care plans be given direct access to an obstetrician and gynecologist without a referral from their primary care physician. In the absence of the power to sue, dozens of states created Independent Medical Review procedures for patients questioning denials of care by their HMOs. By 2001, all but three states had passed some form of legislation regulating managed care.[26]

The federal Patients' Bill of Rights died, but Congress did pass a "Newborns' and Mothers' Health Protection Act" in 1996, requiring health plans to cover a minimum hospital stay of 48 hours after a normal vaginal birth and 96 hours after a Caesarean delivery. Although this law was puzzling to health policy analysts and even some women's health activists who had long argued for shorter hospital stays and the de-medicalization of childbirth, it made sense as a symbolic blow in the backlash against managed care.[27]

Some experts felt that the backlash was getting out of hand. Managed care was actually beginning to slow medical costs; in 1996 medical spending rose only 2.5 percent, while total consumer prices rose 3.3 percent.[28] The health policy scholar David Mechanic argued that "inordinate" attention was being paid to managed care, at the expense of the much bigger problem of the uninsured. The consumer, media, and political "bashing" of HMOs, Mechanic argued, arose because managed care "makes patients acutely aware of rationing."[29] Bare-faced rationing, with middle-class patients as the rationed ones, was too much for the American public to stomach.

Other commentators noted that rationing by HMOs may have been more obvious, but in other ways managed care was a continuation of US health care business as usual. Earlier forms of health insurance that emphasized hospital care and paid doctors on a fee-for-service basis had encouraged too much medical care, while HMOs seemed to encourage too little. Both types of insurance were built around the needs and goals of the insurance company rather than the needs of the patient. *New Republic* writer Jonathan Cohn argued that both HMOs and traditional insurance failed to serve "people with the worst medical conditions. . . . In that sense, managed care hadn't so much altered the evolution of American health insurance as reinforced it."[30]

The backlash led to managed care plans loosening some restrictions. Many companies began offering preferred provider organizations (PPOs) that allowed greater access to "out of network" specialists. Then health costs began to rise again. While in 1996 employer health insurance premiums rose less than 1 percent, the lowest increase in history, by 1999 they were climbing by 5.3 percent and by 2003, 13.9 percent.[31] The managed care revolution's promise of cost control was fading. At the turn of the millennium, new conservative leadership decided to turn over rationing to the market.

George W. Bush and the Market

"I'm absolutely opposed to a national health care plan," presidential candidate George W. Bush told the audience during a televised debate in 2000. "I don't want the federal government making decisions for consumers or for providers."[32] Asked about the problem of the uninsured, Bush boasted that the state of Texas, when he was governor, "spent $4.7 billion a year . . . for uninsured people. And they get health care." Bush was referring to state reimbursement of hospitals that provided care for the uninsured in emergency rooms. "Now, it's not the most efficient way to get people health care," the soon-to-be President acknowledged.[33]

George W. Bush believed that emergency rooms were solving part of the nation's health care problems, and that the market would be able to take care of the rest. Reflecting the major emphasis in conservative thinking of the time, Bush contended that the American health care crisis stemmed from the way the insurance system shielded individuals from the true cost of health care. In an influential 1997 book, *Market-Driven Health Care*, Regina Herzlinger of the Harvard Business School argued against third-party payment and for a system that offered consumers what they wanted most, which she argued was "convenience and mastery." Conservative think tanks like the Cato Institute and the Heritage Foundation produced voluminous research and proposals arguing for an end to federal tax subsidies for employer-sponsored coverage and their replacement with individual health savings accounts that would allow consumers to purchase policies of their choice in the private market.[34]

Bush's position on health care represented a kind of conservatism different than Ronald Reagan's. Both Republican presidents emphasized cost control, but Reagan attempted this by imposing restrictions on federal payments to providers (see chapter 8), and Bush by placing the impetus for controlling costs on the consumer through mechanisms like higher health insurance deductibles. Bush also aggressively sought to deregulate private insurance and drug companies while at the same time redirecting federal Medicare and Medicaid payments toward them—a goal that was not always consistent with cost control.

Republican Health Care Reform:
The Medicare Modernization Act of 2003

However much conservatives reviled the growing costs of entitlement spending, Medicare was still a "third rail," a program incredibly popular with a large constituency (seniors) that voted in large numbers. Bush would not push cost controls in Medicare as Reagan had attempted; indeed, he would dramatically expand it—on his own terms—by giving private insurance and drug companies a greater role in the program. Some critics from the left charged that Bush's ultimate goal was to privatize Medicare altogether.[35] During his 2000 campaign Bush had seized on the popular goal of adding a prescription drug benefit to Medicare, and by 2003 he had succeeded, becoming the first and only Republican president to propose and win a major expansion of health coverage.

Medicare's lack of prescription drug insurance had been a major drawback of the program since its inception. Lyndon Johnson had balked at including drug coverage because of the cost. But as seniors increasingly depended on new, expensive drugs that could control chronic conditions like diabetes, high cholesterol, and high blood pressure, the lack of coverage for medications in Medicare became a huge problem. Democrats had proposed adding prescription drugs to Medicare as part of the catastrophic coverage proposal in the 1980s. Drug coverage was included in the failed Clinton health plan, and Bill Clinton first proposed a "Medicare Part D" for prescription drugs in 1999.[36]

But Republicans did not want to simply expand Medicare to allow the federal government to negotiate with drug companies and provide a standard drug benefit to seniors. Bush and his supporters instead sought a major role for private insurance companies in Medicare. Not only would this fit with an ideology in favor of private competition and opposed to more government, but it also guaranteed support for the new legislation from the powerful pharmaceutical industry, which would resist any attempts at price controls on their products.[37] Congress passed the $400 billion drug benefit in 2003. With its convoluted "donut hole" that covered prescriptions only above and below a certain amount, Medicare Part D again expanded benefits while creating new exclusions.

Another part of the 2003 Medicare Modernization Act, and the centerpiece of the Bush administration's market-based strategy, was the creation of health savings accounts (HSAS). HSAS allowed consumers to save up to $2,000 a year tax-free in an account to be used solely for health costs. Holders of the accounts were required to purchase or accept an employer's offer of health insurance with a high deductible. Bush made the case for HSAS by arguing that they would lead to lower costs. "Health-care costs are on the rise because the consumers are not involved in the decision-making process," Bush argued. "Most health-care costs are covered by third parties. And therefore, the actual user of health care is not the purchaser of health care. And there's no market forces involved with health care. It's one of the reasons I'm a strong believer in what they call health savings accounts."[38]

Despite Republican enthusiasm, health savings accounts did not catch on as quickly as supporters hoped. In early 2009, about eight million people were enrolled in HSA-eligible insurance plans. However, more than 40 percent of those people had never opened an account because, according to the *New York Times*, "if you're having trouble affording health insurance to begin with, it's going to be hard to scrape together extra money to put into an HSA."[39] HSAS did fit with the overall trend toward high-deductible insurance policies and the increase in overall out-of-pocket costs experienced by consumers in the early 2000s. Higher deductibles and more cost-sharing were supposed to bring down health costs overall, but like every other incremental health reform, they failed to do so. In addition, high-deductible health plans, as seen in chapter 5, discouraged preventive care and created greater economic burdens for families with children and individuals with chronic illnesses.[40]

In bringing market principles to health care, Republicans—and, increasingly, many Democrats—hoped to tame medical costs, break the connection between employment and health coverage, reduce the number of uninsured, and bring greater choice and autonomy to consumers. At the same time, the reforms they advocated involved significant government subsidies to private businesses. Medicare Part D channeled Medicare dollars to health plans and drug companies without price controls; Medicare Advantage plans, another approach favored by the Bush administration, paid private insurance companies 12 percent more in tax dollars than traditional Medicare; and health savings accounts generated significant fees for private banks (and tax breaks for more affluent account holders).[41] While seniors and families were supposed to put their own "skin in the game" by using more of their own money to buy health coverage, more of their tax dollars were being paid to private, for-profit companies. The use of the government to build up business was nothing new in the United States, but the Bush-era health reforms embodied a particularly strong contradiction between free-market rhetoric on the one hand, and federal subsidy to private entities on the other. And while politicians tinkered with donut holes and private Medicare plans, deep-seated problems in the American health system remained unaddressed.

Health Care in the Aftermath of Disasters: 9 / 11 and Katrina

Two devastating millennial disasters — the terrorist attacks of 9 / 11 and Hurricane Katrina — brought the inequities of American health care starkly into public view. Survivors of these catastrophes faced special difficulties obtaining access to health care because of job loss, displacement, and the destruction of health facilities. But the tragedies they experienced highlighted problems in US health care that were far from new: uninsurance, the linkage of health coverage and employment, no continuity or coordination of care, racial disparities in health, stringent requirements for Medicaid, and a shortage of primary care and safety net providers.

Government responded to the health care crises of 9 / 11 and Katrina in dramatically different ways. Congress agreed to expand Medicaid to temporarily cover survivors of 9 / 11, but refused to do the same for victims of Katrina. These contrasting responses added another chapter to the history of rationing and the denial of health care rights in the United States.[42]

Apart from the devastating loss of life on September 11, 2001, the immediate health concern following the terrorist attack on the World Trade Center in New York was the potential impact of the massive dust cloud on survivors and residents of lower Manhattan. But soon another long-term health problem emerged: the loss of health insurance by people who had worked in the Twin Towers and their families. A crisis of lost jobs quickly became a crisis of lost health coverage, for the families of the dead as well as for survivors and their families. The Federal Emergency Management Agency (FEMA) had no plans for the continuation of health coverage after a disaster.

In the stunning voluntary response to 9 / 11, many of the organizations and businesses offering aid recognized victims' need for health coverage as a priority. The investment banking firm Cantor Fitzgerald, which lost nearly 70 percent of its New York workforce in the attack, pledged to continue health coverage for victims' spouses and children for at least 12 months "at the company's cost." Labor unions, particularly service worker and public employee unions, also offered extended health benefits to survivors of the disaster and to the families of victims.[43]

Non-unionized tower employees and their families had a more difficult struggle. Many had no health coverage even before 9/11. Many were immigrants afraid to seek benefits. Smaller companies could not afford to come up with the types of payouts and services to victims that some of the World Trade Center's wealthier employers offered. The families of two security guards killed in the attack complained that the private security companies had never even contacted them with condolences for the loss of their loved ones, much less offered them help with finances or health care.[44] In addition to the efforts of the service unions, some private organizations were created to assist low-income survivors and victims' families, including Windows of Hope, which raised money to aid the families of WTC restaurant workers and "committed to fund five years of health insurance coverage for all of the families."[45]

Loss of health insurance also became a problem for the thousands of workers who lost their livelihoods in New York's temporary economic downturn following 9/11. Economists estimated that the city lost nearly 80,000 jobs, primarily in low-wage industries, as a direct consequence of the attacks.[46] New York City was already home to large numbers of people without health coverage; the added pressure of the newly uninsured threatened to overwhelm the city's indigent care system and its medical budgets. Government needed to expand health coverage, and quickly, argued the director of New York's Health and Hospitals Corporation, to ensure the "financial stability of the city's health care system." The best and quickest way to do this was through Medicaid.[47]

Although New York already had much experience with Medicaid expansion, the temporary program it created following 9/11 was unprecedented. Disaster Relief Medicaid dropped the "grueling" application process in favor of a simple, one-page form, and "those eligible g[o]t a Medicaid card the same day."[48] Normally, a program making it easier to get a government benefit would have faced an "avalanche of opposition" but, as the New York Times surmised, "The uninsured and their advocates have found far more universal support after Sept. 11, as

New Yorkers have faced all kinds of medical needs, including mental health services and continuing medical treatment that had been interrupted by the attacks." The national sympathy for New York's plight, particularly the sympathy emanating from Washington, enabled Governor George Pataki and Mayor Rudolph W. Giuliani to push through Disaster Relief Medicaid, a program that otherwise would have been unthinkable in the US political culture of hostility to welfare.[49]

Disaster Relief Medicaid eventually enrolled 400,000 people in the state, 250,000 of them in New York City. Many New Yorkers who enrolled in the program had lost their jobs because of 9/11, and most had no previous health coverage. Some had applied for Medicaid previously and been turned down because of income limits.[50]

Despite the specific linkage of Disaster Relief Medicaid with 9/11 and its aftermath, the program may have been most effective in relieving, if only partly, the longer-term crisis of chronic disease and uninsurance in the city. The program uncovered a "pent-up demand for health services" among New Yorkers. Participants eagerly sought mammograms, dental care, and preventive check-ups; many were able to fill prescriptions regularly for the first time.[51] Primary care physicians in New York reported that "patients with disaster-relief Medicaid have come in with complaints about everything from chronic abdominal pain to high blood pressure." A 42-year-old Bronx home health aide had always relied on emergency rooms to treat her asthma, and had never been able to afford medication. After joining Disaster Relief Medicaid, she obtained "her own prescriptions, bought reading glasses, and went to a dentist. 'I needed things but with no coverage, there was nothing I could do,'" she told a reporter.[52] A Hispanic woman, also asthmatic, told the *Washington Post* that "she had gone without treatment for long periods, buying medicine when she could afford it, at times borrowing inhalers from friends," but under the new program, "'Oh yes, I can go to the doctor!'"[53]

Disaster Relief Medicaid lasted only four months. A *Times* headline poignantly summed up the program's temporary nature: "The Doctor Will See You, for Now." Some recipients were absorbed into New York's expanded Medicaid system, but most ended up uninsured again.[54] New York politicians shifted their focus to the health needs of the rescue workers who had been exposed to hazardous dust following the disaster. A bill for special health coverage for rescue workers languished in Congress for nearly ten years, because of both the controversial nature of the rescue workers' diagnoses (it was difficult to prove direct linkages between the 9/11 dust cloud and the severe and often fatal lung and other disorders experienced by many rescue workers) and the program's high cost of $7.4 billion.

Following an ongoing public shaming on comedian Jon Stewart's *The Daily Show*, during which he called the failure to support the rescue workers' coverage "an outrageous abdication of our responsibility to those who were most heroic on 9/11," Republicans in Congress finally agreed to a more modest $4.3 billion bill at the end of 2010. If the United States had universal coverage, such targeted legislation would not even have been necessary, but this point went unnoticed in congressional debates focusing on the special deservingness of rescue workers. Proponents "argued that the nation had a moral obligation to provide medical assistance to rescue workers who spent days, weeks and even months at ground zero."[55] Huge popular support for the measure reflected this perception that rescue workers were especially deserving, and that lifetime health coverage was something to be earned by special sacrifice, rather than a right of citizenship—a form of rationing by moral worthiness. Republicans criticized the singling out of rescue workers, but on the grounds that the bill would drain the federal budget: "Every American recognizes the heroism of the 9/11 first responders," said Tom Coburn (R-OK). "But it is not compassionate to help one group while robbing future generations of opportunity."[56]

In 2005, a second major disaster exposed deep and continuing problems of uninsurance, illness, poverty, racism, and government neglect, for the whole world to see. Hurricane Katrina took its toll most swiftly on the elderly, the sick, the housebound, the wheelchair-bound, people confined to hospital and nursing home beds—those who found it difficult or impossible to escape. High rates of poverty in New Orleans and the Gulf Coast region meant that much of the population hit hardest by the hurricane suffered from chronic illness, but few had health insurance.

Before the hurricane, Louisiana had among the highest rates of uninsurance in the nation, with 26.4 percent of working adults lacking health coverage (only Texas was higher, with 30.7 percent).[57] Health disparities in the state were especially severe; the Louisiana Department of Health reported that 11.9 percent of African Americans in the state had diabetes, compared with 7.2 percent of whites, and that 15.8 percent of those who lived in households with income of less than $15,000 per year had the disease. Even higher rates of diabetes showed up among hurricane evacuees. An endocrinologist visiting a shelter in Lafayette, Louisiana, found that "500 of the 2,000 to 3,000 people housed there" had the disorder.[58] The *Washington Post* surveyed evacuees in Houston shortly after the hurricane and reported that half had no health insurance, and 40 percent had heart disease, diabetes, or high blood pressure, or were disabled. "When illness or injury strike, they were twice as likely to say they had sought care from hospitals such as the New Orleans Charity Hospital than from either a family doctor or health clinic."[59]

After Hurricane Katrina, it was chronic illness and poverty among evacuees, not the expected injuries that usually follow disasters, that challenged the medical resources of disaster agencies and volunteers. A physician at Houston's "Katrina Clinic" for evacuees explained, "We usually plan for a disaster involving explosions, trauma, wounds. We recognized this was not that kind of disaster. . . . We didn't need a (mobile) surgical hospital, we needed a big pharmacy. We needed a laboratory. We did not need an operating table, we needed an exam table." The *Houston Chronicle* reported, "As the crisis phase passed, people too poor for easy access to medical care for less-pressing problems in New Orleans sought it out in the Katrina Clinic. People who barely escaped New Orleans with their lives could now get attention for ingrown toenails." Physicians fitted people with eyeglasses, gave immunizations, and filled countless prescriptions.[60] *New York Times* columnist Nicholas Kristof spoke with a volunteer doctor who "discovered a previously undetected hole in a 4-year-old boy's heart. The mother said nobody had ever listened to the boy's chest before."[61] As Disaster Relief Medicaid in New York had led to a surge in previously neglected primary care, so did hurricane evacuation clinics expose the vast medical needs of an uninsured population.

But temporary help could do little to stem the outpouring of demand for medical care in the wake of Katrina. To the ranks of the uninsured were added hundreds of thousands of survivors who lost their health insurance when their workplaces and jobs were wiped out by the hurricane. Katrina's victims were, according to the *Chicago Tribune*, "one of the largest groups to lose medical coverage because of a single event in the nation's history"—it is difficult to think of a larger one.[62]

In the weeks following the hurricane, survivors were scattered throughout Louisiana, Texas, and most states in the union. Most were newly unemployed, many newly uninsured, and those enrolled in Medicaid faced the possibility of losing their benefits by leaving their home states. Thousands forced below the poverty line by Katrina turned to Medicaid for the first time. But in Louisiana, a majority found that they were not eligible for Medicaid because of the state's strict income cutoffs: applicants' incomes had to be below 20 percent of the official poverty level (20 percent of $16,000 for a family of three)—in some cases, as low as 13 percent. (This extraordinarily stringent standard helps explain the state's reliance on its Charity Hospital system to care for the poor.) As in most states, only certain categories of people were considered eligible for Medicaid, particularly single mothers with children; to qualify for Medicaid in Louisiana, the childless had to have an income of less than $174 a month.[63]

As a result of Louisiana's requirements, over half of the 6,000 state residents who applied for Medicaid in the weeks after the storm were turned down. Many of these individuals formerly had private health insurance, and some had been undergoing lifesaving treatments. Several newspapers reported the story of Emanuel Wilson, a 52-year-old school bus driver from New Orleans, who survived the hurricane but had to stop chemotherapy injections for intestinal cancer when he was turned down for Louisiana Medicaid.[64] Another New Orleans resident, Albert Bass, 47, formerly of the Lower Ninth Ward, was hospitalized for fever and liver problems right after the hurricane. His Medicaid application was denied, and "Now, tens of thousands of dollars in medical bills await a man with no income. . . . His asthma has worsened, but he has no money to pay for medications."[65]

On September 15, 2005, Senators Charles Grassley (R-IA) and Max Baucus (D-MT) introduced a bill, S. 1716, to create a temporary Medicaid program for Katrina survivors. The Emergency Health Care Relief Act of 2005 offered survivors in any state five months of Medicaid coverage, with greatly expanded eligibility—200 percent of poverty for children, pregnant women, and the disabled; 100 percent of poverty for all other adults—and simplified application procedures. And, unlike the state-federal cost sharing of traditional Medicaid, the full cost of the program would be paid by the federal government.[66]

The Grassley-Baucus bill received the enthusiastic support of health care providers and advocates for the poor. It was endorsed by the governors of the states most affected by the hurricane.[67] The plan was also expected to pass fairly easily because of its bipartisan sponsorship; Grassley was a major ally of the Bush administration. Congress could also look to the earlier success with Disaster Relief Medicaid as a

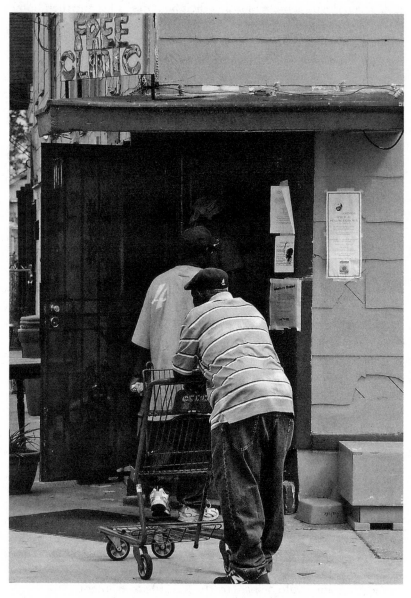

FIGURE 13. Nine months after Hurricane Katrina, New Orleans residents line up at "Common Ground," a free health clinic established by volunteer doctors, nurses, and pharmacists. Photo by Dana Yarak, March 2006.

model. As the Senate met on Monday, September 26, Grassley and Baucus "expected the bill to pass by a voice vote," according to the *Los Angeles Times*. But to their dismay, it was blocked by Republicans John E. Sununu of New Hampshire and John Ensign of Nevada. Sununu claimed he opposed the Medicaid extension because it would increase the already burgeoning national deficit.[68]

The next day, Secretary of Health and Human Services Michael Leavitt sent a letter to Senate leaders declaring the Bush administration's opposition to the Grassley-Baucus bill. He called the bill "inadvisable" and "a duplication of administration efforts." Leavitt argued that state-by-state waivers would allow hurricane survivors to receive Medicaid benefits without a massive new federal intervention. The Senate bill, on the other hand, "requires a new Medicaid entitlement for Katrina survivors, regardless of whether that will work best for those survivors or the states," Leavitt wrote.[69]

The bill's supporters reacted with fury. Sen. Blanche Lincoln (D-AR), whose state was dealing with thousands of evacuees from the Gulf states, attacked "the web of red tape that this administration is spinning over our ability to provide the basic needs of health care to people who have been devastated." "Could you please explain to us," Grassley and Baucus replied to HHS Secretary Leavitt, "why the Katrina evacuees do not deserve the same assistance provided the people of New York" after 9/11? Grassley, who chaired the Senate Finance Committee, even threatened to block the administration's proposed cuts to the overall Medicaid program if the White House failed to withdraw its opposition to the Katrina health bill.[70]

But the administration refused to budge, and the bill failed to garner any further momentum. Grassley gave up the fight, and went on to lead Senate efforts to enact major cuts to Medicaid in the 2007 federal budget. Katrina survivors were left without a health coverage plan that would even come close to the benefits temporarily offered New Yorkers after 9/11.[71]

The various government responses to 9/11 and Katrina were stopgap measures that only temporarily or inadequately sealed gaping holes in survivors' health security. They rationed health care with a new spin on the old category of deservingness, sending the message that 9/11 victims were more deserving than Katrina victims; that first responders were more deserving than average New Yorkers; that New York was more deserving than Louisiana. The programs' temporary or emergency natures were also a form of rationing: any new health care rights could not be allowed to last indefinitely. Such emergency measures could not and need not attempt to address long-term and continuing problems of chronic illness, health disparities by race and region, and unequal access to health care and health coverage.

Exploding Health Costs: Searching for the Cause and Cure

Solutions to the United States' long-term health crisis seemed elusive, even impossible. In a system that was already the most expensive in the world, how could it be feasible to cover more people? Echoing arguments of the Carter era, during the first decade of the new millennium a political and media consensus formed around the idea that no health care reform would be possible until—or unless—costs were brought under control. The rising cost of health care was "the worst long-term fiscal crisis facing the nation," wrote the *New York Times* in 2007, "and it demands a solution, but finding one will not be easy or palatable."[72]

Costs in both the public and private health systems were spiraling out of control. Many saw Medicare as the biggest problem, due to the aging population and government's legal obligation to fund entitlements. Bush's massive new Medicare Part D would only make the cost problem worse. Still, growth in the Medicare program averaged over several decades was only 4.4 percent per year, while private insurance costs were growing 7.4 percent per year.[73] According to the Congressional Budget Office, Medicare spending was not driving the rise in overall health expenditures, but the other way around: medical cost inflation forced the government to spend more on Medicare.[74]

While conservatives continued to blame entitlement spending as the central cause of high health expenditures, liberals and critics of the health care industry focused on private, profit-making medical care as the culprit. For-profit hospital chains, price-gouging "nonprofit" hospitals, voracious insurers, and "Big Pharma" were raking in trillions of health care dollars that they did not actually spend on health care. In a 2006 book and later a film titled *Money-Driven Medicine: The Real Reason Health Care Costs So Much*, financial journalist Maggie Mahar told "the story of how today's market-driven medical system gives Wall Street investors life and death control over our health care, turning medicine into a profit machine instead of a social service to meet human need." Marcia Angell, former editor in chief of the *New England Journal of Medicine*, published a 2004 book titled *The Truth about the Drug Companies* that named the pharmaceutical lobby and massive advertising campaigns by drug companies for medications of dubious benefit as the drivers of high drug costs.[75]

Conservatives took a different angle: they insisted that it was tort lawyers' quest for economic gain that led to huge, costly claims against doctors and hospitals, sent malpractice premiums sky-high, and forced physicians to practice defensive medicine or drove them out of the profession altogether. Medical malpractice reform, including placing caps on damages, became a top priority of the Bush administration; George W. Bush argued that reducing "frivolous lawsuits" was essential to bringing down the cost of health care. Critics of this approach pointed to research showing that malpractice awards to patients and their lawyers were actually not a significant driver of health spending. States that passed the kind of malpractice reform conservatives envisioned did not see a reduction in health costs. The real impact of malpractice on medical inflation, they contended, resulted from the massive number of serious medical mistakes that injured or killed patients each year. The Institute of Medicine's 1999 report that 100,000 patients a year died because of physician or hospital error—"more than die from automobile and workplace accidents combined"—received wide publicity. Few of these cases ever resulted in a malpractice suit.[76]

If high malpractice awards were not the main culprit in soaring health costs, perhaps the flood of patients who relied on high-tech, expensive emergency room care was to blame. ER "overuse" was resulting in billions of dollars in wasteful spending. Although emergency room visits had been rising since the 1970s and even earlier (see chapter 4), a major jump of 32 percent came between 1996 and 2006, from 90.3 million in 1996 to more than 119 million, according to the Centers for Disease Control and Prevention. Many analysts blamed the increase on the serious shortage of primary care providers, even for patients with insurance, forcing people to seek basic care in the ER.[77] Conservative commentators pointed to undocumented immigrants, whose estimated cost to the nation's emergency rooms was over a billion dollars, and even to the right to emergency care itself. University of Chicago legal scholar Richard Epstein argued that EMTALA's right to access had led to the epidemic of emergency room overuse.[78] As in the case of malpractice, conservatives saw rights (of patients, immigrants, ER health seekers) as drivers of the high cost of health care.

By the time of a revitalized health reform debate in 2008, a consensus had emerged in health policy circles around the major explanation for the country's astronomical medical costs. Put simply, the problem was too much medicine. In her widely praised 2007 book *Overtreated*, medical journalist Shannon Brownlee concluded that unnecessary care, including "too many tests and unnecessary treatments, too much surgery, [and] too many elective procedures" accounted for one-fifth to one-third of US health care costs. Overtreatment cost the health system twice: first the cost of the care itself, then the cost of the hospital injuries and medical mistakes that increased because of all the unnecessary care. Brownlee summarized decades of research by John Wennberg and colleagues at Dartmouth on medical overuse showing that physicians were driven to prescribe high-tech, unnecessary care mostly because they got "paid more for doing more," but also because of lack of evidence about the effectiveness of many procedures.[79] The idea that the problem of overtreatment could be fixed by "evidence-based medicine"—doctors and hospitals being given financial incentives to offer only those tests and procedures shown to be effective via clinical trials—became extremely influential in health policy circles and would make its mark on the Obama health reform law in 2010. But it was unclear whether evidence-based medicine would actually result in significant reductions in medical costs.

The Bankruptcy of the American Medical Consumer

Who was paying for all these high health costs? The answer was government, taxpayers, employers, and, increasingly, consumers themselves. If their employers still offered insurance, workers were paying more in premiums and cost sharing. Individuals and families in the private insurance market had to pay the most, because they did not benefit from the cost savings of pooled group insurance. In addition, aggressive insurance company practices led to many insured people finding out that they were not covered at all when they needed care. In a practice known as "rescission," insurers would "scour the medical records of policyholders who start filing expensive claims, looking for reasons to cancel their policies." Over a five-year period, the three largest insurance companies cancelled 20,000 policies via rescission.[80] This practice led to heartrending stories of patients who died after losing their insurance, and was condemned at congressional hearings in 2009. (It was banned in the 2010 Affordable Care Act.)

People who lost their insurance or were uninsured but needed hospital care also faced aggressive collections policies by hospitals. In a 2005 study that received major publicity, Harvard Law School's Elizabeth Warren reported that medical bills were the number one cause of personal bankruptcy in the United States. Many people filing for bankruptcy because of medical costs were insured—they had reached their coverage cap, they had massive deductibles and copayments, or their insurer simply refused to pay. Hospitals showed little sympathy; there were many well-publicized cases of prominent institutions, including Yale University Hospital, ruthlessly pursuing debtors, garnishing their wages and placing liens on their homes. These practices were reported throughout the mainstream media. The high-circulation women's magazine *Self* told the story of Joanne Jordan, a 27-year-old real estate agent with Hodgkin's lymphoma. "In May 2001, Jordan arrived home after a doctor's appointment, exhausted, to find a notice posted on her door by the county sheriff. Potomac Hospital's administrators had taken her to court and secured a lien on her house." A sidebar headline warned, "One accident, one diagnosis, and any woman can end up broke and even homeless."[81]

What had happened to the voluntary hospitals' charity role, codified under Hill-Burton? "Nonprofit hospitals, originally set up to serve the poor, have transformed themselves into profit machines," reported the *Wall Street Journal* in 2008. Because of mergers and the rising value of their investment portfolios, the income of the 50 largest nonprofit hospitals increased eight-fold between 2001 and 2006. Seventy-seven percent of US nonprofit hospitals were in the black, but instead of devoting the surplus to patient care, the *Journal* reported, they were using the money for fancy capital improvements. Northwestern Memorial Hospital in Chicago rebuilt its entire campus for more than $1 billion, and its CEO received a $16.4 million payout in 2006. At the same time, Northwestern spent less than 2 percent of its revenues on charity care. Hospitals aggressively sought well-heeled clientele—the University of Pittsburgh Medical Center spent $10 million on advertising in 2006.[82] Even as taxpayers continued to subsidize private hospitals to the tune of $32 billion dollars annually, the tradition of private control with minimal federal oversight allowed both profit and nonprofit hospitals in the 1990s and early 2000s to reap large revenues while increasing their charges to patients. Another venerable nonprofit institution, Blue Cross/Blue Shield, increasingly converted to for-profit insurance, much of it under the umbrella company WellPoint. Mergers and consolidation in the insurance industry and the loss of nonprofit alternatives led to greater market concentration and less competition, thus higher prices.[83]

Sicko and the Health Care Horror Story

In the 1990s and early 2000s, health care horror stories—anecdotes describing individuals' medical bankruptcies and denials of care—resonated throughout American culture. HMO abuses and denials of care, and evil insurance companies as villains, featured in the plots of the Hollywood movies *The Rainmaker* (based on a John Grisham novel) and *John Q.* (with Denzel Washington as a father battling the insurance company that denied his child a heart transplant).

Controversial filmmaker Michael Moore even made a feature-length documentary based around HMO horror stories. In 2006, Moore sent out a call on his website for descriptions of "what you've been through with your insurance company, or what it's been like to have no insurance at all, or how the hospitals and doctors wouldn't treat you (or if they did, how they sent you into poverty trying to pay their crazy bills) . . . if you have been abused in any way by this sick, greedy, grubby system and it has caused you or your loved ones great sorrow and pain, let me know."[84] The resulting film, *Sicko*, received a 15-minute standing ovation at the Cannes film festival and was released in the United States in June 2007. It was the second-highest grossing film of that weekend's releases and was nominated for an Academy Award for best documentary feature.[85] The film not only included stories of dying children turned away from hospitals or accident victims forced to choose which finger to be reattached, but also presented admiring portraits of health care in Britain, France, Canada, and Cuba. Conservative groups were infuriated, arguing that Moore ignored less appealing aspects of other countries' health care systems, particularly waiting-list rationing of elective procedures.[86]

The health care horror story played a major role in the 2008 presidential election. Democratic candidate Barack Obama became the first presidential candidate to share his own family's insurance story with the public. Obama's mother, Ann Dunham, had died of ovarian cancer at age 53. Repeatedly, Obama told audiences how his mother "ha[d] to spend the last months of her life in the hospital room arguing with insurance companies because they're saying that this may be a pre-existing condition and they don't have to pay her treatment." The telling and retelling would always lead to the conclusion, "there's something fundamentally wrong about that." Ending preexisting condition exclusions by insurance companies was a personal as well as a political fight for Obama.

The 2008 campaign was unusual also because it featured direct discussion of the right to health care. During the October 7, 2008, debate between Obama and Republican candidate John McCain, moderator Tom Brokaw asked, "Is health care in America a privilege, a right, or a responsibility?" McCain replied that health care is a responsibility, but Obama said, "Well, I think it should be a right for every American." Then he told the story of his mother's battle with insurance companies on her deathbed.[87]

Obama was, as we have seen, far from the first political leader to proclaim the right to health care. But by invoking his own mother's story as the source of that claim, Obama was the first to do what so many ordinary Americans had done in confronting the limitations and injustices of their health care system: to take from his own experience with rationing a belief that health care should be a right for all, not just for some.

EPILOGUE

Rights, Rationing, and Reform

On March 23, 2010, Congress passed the Patient Protection and Affordable Care Act (PPACA), the most comprehensive reform of the health system in US history. Health care reform was a top priority for President Obama, even as the country faced a collapsing economy and two continuing wars. "I am not the first president to take up this cause," Obama told Congress in his special address on health care in 2009, "but I am determined to be the last."[1] As the president noted, a victory on health care reform would be absolutely historic. Obama would succeed where Truman, Nixon, Carter, and Clinton had failed.

But even before the ink had dried, conservatives were calling for the Act's repeal. They declared the Affordable Care Act unconstitutional because of a provision known as the "individual mandate," which requires all Americans to buy health insurance by 2014 or face a fine. Members of the Tea Party movement marched on Washington declaring that the law was a government takeover of medical care. As of this writing (May 2012), the nation awaits a Supreme Court ruling on the Act's constitutionality.

Many Americans see this battle over health care as pure politics. Not a single Republican in Congress voted for the bill. The debate over the legislation in 2009–10 was bitterly partisan and included such infamous moments as Representative Joe Wilson yelling "You lie!" at the President during his speech to a joint session of Congress, and an uproar over Republican accusations that the law would establish "death panels" to deny care to the elderly. Amidst all the vitriol, central questions about what reform would really mean for the health care system and the people who used it were lost. Does the Act establish new health care rights for Americans? Does it continue or does it attempt to change the way health care is rationed in this country?

Neither rights nor rationing is explicitly addressed in the legislation. Both concepts played a part in the rhetorical debates around the bill, but do not appear in concrete form in its actual provisions. As the bill's title indicates, the central goals pursued by Obama and Democrats in Congress were patient protection, meaning the curbing of abuses by private insurance companies, and the affordability of insurance. Although the Act will greatly reduce the number of uninsured, universal coverage was not part of the final bill. The primary thrust of reform, then, is regulation and affordability in insurance markets, not rights and rationing. The only official right mentioned in the text of the law, apart from language ensuring that existing rights (such as those enforced by the Civil Rights Act) not be curtailed, is the "Preservation of the right to maintain existing coverage."[2] This was an important part of the political campaign leading up to the bill, because Obama was aware that insured Americans' fear of losing their current insurance was an important factor in the defeat of the Clinton proposal. Not surprisingly, the word "rationing" does not appear in the law at all. But, as in every aspect of American health care, issues of rights and US-style rationing are implied throughout the Act.

The PPACA bans some of the major insurance company practices that lead to bankruptcy or loss or denial of private insurance. The act forbids companies from placing caps on annual and lifetime coverage, which benefits the relatively small number of people who end up with very expensive, catastrophic health costs, but also increases security for everyone with insurance. In one of the most praised and eagerly anticipated features of the law, insurance companies will no longer be allowed to exclude people because they have a preexisting condition. The law also bans the practice of rescission, insurance companies canceling policies when a policyholder gets sick. Health plans will no longer be allowed to charge higher premiums to women than men. New plans must offer a variety of preventive services, such as cholesterol screenings, vaccinations, and birth control, without copayments.

Although the Act does not state it this way, each of these provisions seeks to put an end to insurance company rationing by health status and by gender. Such regulations could also be seen as conferring a right to coverage on individuals, no matter their health condition. When the first restrictions on insurance companies' ability to exclude came into effect in June 2010, the government announced them as a "New Patients' Bill of Rights." But some of these provisions will apply to only a small segment of the insurance market, the segment in which individuals will buy private coverage in the new exchanges. Due to pressure from religious conservatives, the law does allow discrimination by health condition by restricting coverage of one type of medical procedure: abortion. Finally, although the coverage expansions will significantly improve access to care, the PPACA does not declare health care to be a right.

The Affordable Care Act also sends a mixed message about the right to health security, or protection from high medical costs. Most of the plans available through the new state exchanges will still be high-deductible plans. The Act does put caps in place that will limit consumers' out-of-pocket spending on medical costs up to $6,000 annually for individuals and $12,000 for families.[3] These amounts are lower than those that the majority of people with high-deductible plans can pay now, but the costs can still lead to significant expenditures for individuals and families with chronic or severe health problems. As discussed in chapter 5 of this book, deductibles in health coverage can also discourage people from seeking needed health care. The majority of people who will move from being uninsured to having health coverage in 2014 might find that they have no choice other than a high-deductible plan.

"Affordable care" is a central goal of the Act. Very few people will be able to buy private, individual coverage on their own, even if the insurance exchanges do lead to price competition among health plans. To address this problem, the PPACA will provide extensive government subsidies to allow individuals with moderate incomes to buy coverage in new state exchanges. The law does not confer a right to health insurance, but it does confer a right to a subsidy to buy insurance, thereby going some way toward alleviating rationing by income. (The right to buy insurance at all in the exchanges is entirely denied to undocumented immigrants.)

Still, those subsidies will apply only to a specific, narrowly defined group of people, those who are not covered by employer insurance. Americans who already have group insurance through their employer will keep it. This was an extremely important part of the political campaign for reform, because Obama wanted to assure the "Harry and Louises" of the country that they would not lose the benefits they already had. Many workers who currently don't have job-based benefits will receive coverage starting in 2014, when a limited "employer mandate" kicks in. This requirement that employers provide health benefits applies only to firms with 50 or more workers. The penalty for not complying is a fine that might cost less than group health coverage, so it is unclear how useful this limited mandate will be in covering more people. Therefore, these reforms will still result in rationing by job status and size of business. Workers whose employers are not subject to or who do not comply with the employer mandate will be required to purchase individual coverage in the exchanges. Also, employees who can't afford their employers' insurance will still be eligible for subsidies to purchase coverage in the exchanges. The law does not come close to creating a full employer mandate, which would require that *all* employers provide insurance for *all* their workers.[4]

The 45 million people on Medicare will see substantial benefits from the Affordable Care Act. Coverage of prescription drugs will eventually expand to 75 percent of all seniors' medication costs. The Act increases Medicare payments to family and internal medicine physicians and offers them a temporary bonus, which should increase the availability of primary care for seniors. In a major departure from the traditional Medicare program, the Act will require Medicare—and all health plans—to cover a wide variety of preventive services. As for Medicaid, the Act aims to raise income eligibility to 133 percent of the poverty level, which will bring an estimated 16 million additional people into the program. Medicaid will account for almost half of the increase in coverage expected under the reform.[5]

Even with subsidies and the Medicaid expansion, the law is still expected to leave 15 million to 20 million people without health insurance. Bill Clinton had threatened to veto any legislation that would not result in universal coverage, but Barack Obama never made the same pledge. Instead, he told Congress that he would refuse to back any law that would "add one dime to our deficits," an example of the shift from universalism to cost control. Even though the Affordable Care Act's cost is projected to be $1 trillion, its supporters insist (and the nonpartisan Congressional Budget Office agrees) that it will end up cutting health costs in the long run.

The PPACA has dozens of cost-cutting provisions that, like other aspects of the law, send mixed messages about rights and rationing. In an attempt to reduce premium costs, private insurers will be required to reduce their administration and profit margins, and bring the amount they pay for actual medical care up to 80 or 85 percent of their revenues. Their administration costs will still be far higher than the administrative costs of Medicare or the rejected "public option" (and far higher than administrative costs in any country with universal coverage). Insurers' right to some profit is protected. In addition, the law will tax health plans and drug companies (and tanning salons!) in order to fund subsidies for expanded benefits.

The Act also intends to raise revenues and reduce costs by taxing high-end health insurance, known as "Cadillac plans," that have very generous benefit levels. Some analysts believe that the tax is intended to "prod individuals and businesses to replace Cadillac plans with new plans that force patients to put some skin in the game by requiring them to pay higher deductibles."[6] Replacement of full-benefit plans with high-deductible plans would represent short-term cost savings at the expense of coverage and of economic security for individuals and families, and would mean higher costs for people with the most health problems.

Provisions in the law for more coverage for preventive care and for expansion of community-based clinics are intended to save the system money in the long run. In another cost-control measure, the Act establishes numerous mechanisms to promote electronic medical records, "comparative effectiveness research," evidence-based medicine, and quality incentives. Supporters hope that providing better information about which tests and procedures work, and rewarding physicians for actual improvements in health, will lead physicians and insurance plans to make better and more cost-efficient decisions. They also argue that paying physicians on the basis of effectiveness will remove the "perverse incentive" of fee-for-service payment, which has rewarded quantity over quality. Obama, who was strongly influenced by the health policy experts who have been pushing for these strategies, enthusiastically supports this aspect of reform. Virulent opponents zeroed in on these provisions of the bill, claiming that empowering panels of experts to proclaim the cost-effectiveness of medical procedures will lead to British-style rationing and the imagined "death panels."[7] Much of the success of the new law will hinge on whether these changes will be effective in both curbing costs and distributing medical services more fairly.

"The United States health system has rationed health care in spades for many years, on the economist's definition of rationing," wrote economist Uwe Reinhardt during the health reform campaign, and "President Obama and Congress are now desperately seeking to reduce or eliminate that form of rationing."[8] How far does the Affordable Care Act go in reducing or eliminating US-style rationing by price and other factors? Without universal coverage, and by attempting to preserve the major elements of the current system, the Act still rations coverage by numerous categories. The healthreform.gov website is telling on this score. It has separate sections users can select if they are an "individual," "family with children," "senior," "disabled," or "young adult." Users must also select their individual state to see coverage and pricing options for health plans (national rather than state-based insurance exchanges were negotiated out of the bill, although some multistate plans will be offered). Available options differ on the basis of your age, your health condition, your gender, and your employment status. After users select among these choices, the website presents many different possible types of coverage: employer group insurance, individual insurance via exchanges, Medicaid, Medicare, high-risk pools (which will vanish in 2014 when the new regulations require insurers to take all comers), and community clinics. The new system may cover more people, but it is no less segmented and confusing.

The Affordable Care Act retains and updates many aspects of US-style rationing, including separating people into different groups for different kinds of coverage, means testing (in the case of Medicaid and new government subsidies to buy private insurance), rationing of coverage by age (children may remain on their parents' insurance until age 26), rationing of coverage by location (state exchanges), fragmentation, and complexity.

For health reform to have truly disrupted the American way of rationing and made health coverage a right would have required two features that were absent from the final plan: universal coverage, and the "public option." Although the individual mandate is intended to bring the nation closer to universal coverage than ever before, Obama never promised that the plan would cover everyone; as noted earlier, he saw cost control as far more important (although many argue, and other nations have demonstrated, that universal coverage is one guaranteed way to bring down overall costs). To bring about this cost control, Obama initially supported the public option, a government insurance plan akin to Medicare that would have competed with private insurers in the exchange. This was originally a centerpiece of the president's vision and was strongly supported by liberals in Congress. Senator John D. Rockefeller IV (D-WV) argued that "the inclusion of a strong public plan option in health reform legislation . . . is the only proven way to guarantee that all consumers have affordable, meaningful and accountable options available in the health insurance marketplace."[9] But the administration backed down from the public option and finally dropped it to ensure the support of conservative Democrats in

Congress and counter opposition by business groups. Therefore, unless they are eligible for Medicare or Medicaid, everyone will be required to have (via employment) or buy private health insurance, most of which will be offered by profit-making companies.

To expand health coverage, Obama and his supporters could have built on the existing workplace-based health system by insisting on a broader employer mandate that would have required employers (with subsidies if necessary) to provide health insurance for all their workers. The employer mandate was a major part of both Nixon's and Clinton's reform proposals, and Obama indicated a commitment to the same strategy during the presidential campaign. In fact, he criticized candidate Hillary Clinton for backing the mandate requiring individuals rather than employers to purchase insurance. "If a mandate was the solution," Obama said pointedly in February 2008, "we can try that to solve homelessness by mandating everybody to buy a house."[10] But the employer mandate died when it was removed from the Senate version of the bill. Although the individual mandate replacing it had initially been popular with conservatives—it formed the basis of the 2006 Massachusetts health reform led by Republican Governor Mitt Romney— as the PPACA bill came closer to passage, Republicans and conservative activists increasingly denounced the mandate.

Anger about the individual mandate drives much of the opposition to the Affordable Care Act. Critics charge that a requirement to buy health insurance is a violation of individual rights—the government should not tell Americans what products to buy or not buy. Opponents of compulsory insurance had argued for a century that the choice whether to have health insurance should be up to the individual. State court rulings in Virginia and Florida in 2010–11 declared the Act unconstitutional because the individual mandate, the judges argued, exceeds the powers allowed by the Commerce Clause of the US Constitution. The Commerce Clause allows Congress to regulate economic activity, but the state judges found it unconstitutional for Congress to penalize economic *inactivity* (not buying health insurance). Defenders of the law argue that health insurance falls squarely within the realm of interstate commerce.

Whether further challenges to the PPACA are successful or not, the focus on the constitutionality of the individual mandate misses other issues that are crucial from the perspective of Americans' right to health care. The Affordable Care Act is yet another chapter in the history of how the United States has expanded access to health coverage via subsidies to private entities. The two previous major national reforms, Hill-Burton and Medicare, both channeled significant federal funds to private hospitals and providers. Now that the insurance industry has become the major private player in health care, in the 2010 law it succeeded in winning a massive government subsidy to its business. This was, again, a product of political compromise. Insurance companies would agree to "guaranteed issue" (open enrollment) and the end of preexisting conditions exclusions only in exchange for the individual mandate. By creating the mandate, Congress created a right for private insurance companies to obtain millions of additional customers with taxpayer subsidies. On the other hand for those customers an obligation to purchase insurance is not the same thing as a right to access health care.

Here again, the law sends a mixed message about the desirability of public subsidies to private entities. One of the Act's cost control measures is a major cut to Medicare Advantage programs, the private insurance programs in Medicare that have been heavily subsidized by the government. This ends a taxpayer subsidy that has clearly given these private plans an unfair advantage. Yet the law now extends subsidies to ALL private insurance companies that will participate in the insurance exchanges, without price controls (except for the percentage cap on administrative costs). As Hill-Burton and Medicare showed, government funding to private businesses without planning, budgeting, or price restraints leads to cost inflation. Despite the Affordable Care Act's many cost-saving provisions, both supporters and detractors worry about whether competition in the exchanges will be sufficient to keep the price of private insurance within reach of most Americans.

In the cases of Hill-Burton and Medicare, hospitals and providers succeeded in winning rights to government support while continuing to resist clear rights to access for patients. Private hospitals, providers, and insurance companies also have not hesitated to use their revenues (including government funds) for advertising and lobbying to increase their political clout. Is it possible for the new law to avoid the undesirable outcome of heavily subsidized private interests resisting cost controls and pushing back against any expansion of health care rights? The Obama administration and congressional negotiators, as discussed above, did insist on some basic obligations on the part of insurers to participate in exchanges and to accept anybody, and to reduce their administrative costs. But it is difficult to tell how tensions between the rights of taxpayer-subsidized private insurers and the rights of citizens will be resolved.

Judging from the perspective of rights, the Affordable Care Act falls far short of guaranteeing a right to access and other health rights. There is still a lack of real choice when selecting an insurance plan. Without a public option, most uninsured citizens will be required to buy insurance from a private, and likely for-profit, insurance company. While some of the health exchanges may offer literally hundreds of "choices," there is no guarantee that there will even be a nonprofit option to choose from, although some states will likely choose to do so (again, rationing of choice by region / residence). Without a public or nonprofit option, the only ways for the currently uninsured to escape the obligation to buy insurance from a private, for-profit company would be to be poor enough to qualify for Medicaid, or old or disabled enough to qualify for Medicare, or to opt out of the system altogether by paying a fine. As already noted, by making high-deductible health plans the most likely option, the law does not guarantee economic security for individuals and families who will have trouble affording all of the premiums and out-of-pocket costs, even with a government subsidy. The law still preserves private managed care, allowing access only to participating providers, so truly free choice of doctor will still be denied to most Americans. Medicaid will be expanded (although this too is under challenge), but there is still no requirement that doctors accept Medicare or Medicaid (though there are new financial incentives for them to do so).

It is not surprising that the 2010 health reform sends so many mixed messages about rights and rationing. It was the product of extraordinarily intricate compromises and negotiations that were driven by the complex US political process and many competing interests. There is no doubt the PPACA, if allow to stand, will bring about historic change. The Act may have closed the door on certain possibilities for expanded rights and more just rationing, but it has also opened new ones. Now that public funds are "in the game" of subsidizing private insurers, there is a chance for greater public oversight of insurance company practices and pricing, similar to how Medicare forced hospitals to end racial segregation and, later, to control some costs. The Affordable Care Act's framers ensured that it retained plenty of openings for experimentation at the state level, even including public option plans and single-payer systems. Perhaps most important of all, by requiring every citizen to at least think about whether to participate, the Affordable Care Act will lead to a continuing national debate—ideally an open and democratic one—about how Americans want to organize their health care system, and what kinds of rights and rationing that system should include.

"It has been the imaginative hope and great desire of many thousands of Americans," said physician and civil rights leader Leonidas M. Berry in 1966, that "somehow our vaunted technical know-how will be translated into a great renaissance for human rights and individual human dignity in American Medical Practice."[11] Over the past century, countless health care providers, consumer and labor activists, patient advocates, political leaders, and ordinary Americans have, despite great obstacles, insisted that human rights and dignity must be part of our national discussion of health care, and eventually must be embodied in our health system. If we are to get still closer to that goal, it will be necessary to heed the words of C. Everett Koop, Surgeon General under President Ronald Reagan: "Politics should serve health, not the other way around."[12]

ACKNOWLEDGMENTS

I could never have carried out my ambitions for this book without the extraordinary support offered by a Robert Wood Johnson Foundation Investigator Award in Health Policy Research. I thank the program's director David Mechanic, former deputy director Lynn Rogut, and administrator Cynthia Church for their leadership, encouragement, and vision, and especially for welcoming humanities scholars into the health policy world. I must be sure to add that the views expressed in this book are not necessarily those of the Investigator Awards Program or the Robert Wood Johnson Foundation. This project also received essential support from the National Endowment for the Humanities/ Agency for Healthcare Research and Quality, the American Council of Learned Societies, the Graduate School of Northern Illinois University, the NIU College of Liberal Arts and Sciences Dean's Office, the NIU Department of History, NIU's Social Science Research Institute, and a one-semester NIU faculty sabbatical.

Archivists and librarians at all the institutions listed in the bibliography made this work possible. I especially thank Sara Beazley and Jeannette Harlow of the American Hospital Association Resource Center, Arlene Shaner of the New York Academy of Medicine, and Tim Pennycuff of the University of Alabama-Birmingham Archives. Archivists at the Carl Albert Center, University of Oklahoma, offered generous search assistance. I am humbly grateful to the late, incomparable Walter Lear, a founder of the Medical Committee for Human Rights who devoted much of his life to documenting the history of health care social justice activism in the United States. I was fortunate to be able to work in the unique research collection that, before its donation to the University of Pennsylvania, was housed in Dr. Lear's home in Philadelphia. He is greatly missed.

David Trout and Nathan Hess were brilliant research assistants, advised me on updating my music library so that it extends past 1992, and made me laugh all the time. I also received valuable research assistance from Alyson Roy, John Ray at the University of Alabama, and

Holly Reid, whose work with me was supported by an Undergraduate Research and Artistry Award from NIU. Leane Vandecreek of the NIU Libraries saved the day more than once. I am grateful for the administrative and moral support offered by NIU Department of History staff members Lorraine Scurti, Judy Hendrickson, and the late Sue Manlove.

My work has benefited from the generous readings, comments, and suggestions of Rosemary Stevens, Charles Rosenberg, Gerald Grob, Deborah Stone, David Rosner, Gerald Markowitz, John Murray, Mayer Zald, Ted Brown, Anne-Emmanuelle Birn, Alan Derickson, Eileen Boris, Alex Mold, Robyn Muncy, Nancy Tomes, Rachel Grob, Mark Schlesinger, Elizabeth A. Armstrong, Clark Henderson, Jennifer Nelson, Jim Schmidt, and members of my 2010 Graduate Reading Seminar in the History of Medicine at NIU. Vanessa Gamble offered encouragement early on and led me to invaluable materials at Tuskegee University Archives. Alondra Nelson generously shared her manuscript on the Black Panthers' health activism. Chris Warren, Kirsten Gardner, Allan Kulikoff, Naomi Rogers, and Esyllt Jones kindly extended invitations to present portions of my research to various audiences. Taylor Atkins, Colleen Grogan, David Mechanic, Clint Cargile, Dana Yarak, and two anonymous reviewers generously read and offered crucial suggestions on the manuscript. Clint also tried valiantly (if not always successfully) to eliminate the passive voice from my writing. Karen Darling of the University of Chicago Press has been an extraordinarily supportive and insightful editor, and Mary Corrado provided expert copyediting. Any remaining errors are entirely my own.

Dana Yarak is not just a great writer and editor but also a graphic artist and technician extraordinaire. He organized all of the images and worked hard to salvage some of the lower-resolution photos I wanted to use in this book. He also took the photograph of the New Orleans clinic in chapter 9, translated some Spanish-language newspaper articles, and offered invaluable assistance with the glossary.

Thank you to the Yaraks, Hoffmans, Rasts, Hoefers, and Littletons; I am grateful to be part of your families. Ann Brierly and Carol Brierly Golin, to whom this book is dedicated, still sustain and inspire me every day. My greatest thanks are to Dana and Casey for their love, support, and patience.

NOTES

Introduction

1. Sarah Palin, "Obama and the Bureaucratization of Health Care," *Wall Street Journal*, September 8, 2009, http://online.wsj.com/article/SB10001424052970203 440104574400581157986024.html; Susan Heavey, "Study Links 45,000 Deaths to Lack of Health Insurance," Reuters, September 17, 2009, http://www.reuters. com/article/2009/09/17/us-usa-healthcare-deaths-idUSTRE58G6W520090917. The study was sponsored by Physicians for a National Health Program, an organization that supports single-payer health insurance.

2. Scott Horsley, "Doctors Say Health Care Rationing Already Exists," *All Things Considered*, July 1, 2009, http://www.npr.org/templates/story/story. php?storyId=106168331.

3. Uwe E. Reinhardt, July 3, 2009, "'Rationing' Health Care: What Does It Mean?" *Economix* blog, http://www.NYTimes.com. See also Mechanic, *Truth about Health Care*, chap. 8; Daniels and Sabin, *Setting Limits Fairly*.

4. On FDR and the right to health, see chap. 2; on Obama, see chap. 9. National polls taken from 1968 through 1985 showed from 71 to 86 percent agreeing with statements describing health care as a right: 73%, Roper Report 85–9, 1985; 71%, Roper Report 82–3, 1982; 79%, Roper Report 78–3, 1978; 76%, Roper Report 75–3, 1975; 55% agreed strongly, and 31% agreed somewhat, with the statement "Every person has a right to receive free medical care if he needs it but cannot afford it," National Opinion Research Center, 1968; all available at Kaiser Health Poll Search, http://www.kff.org/kaiserpolls/index2.cfm.

5. Churchill, *Rationing Health Care in America*, 90.

6. On the role of interest group power in the defeat of national health insurance proposals in the United States, see, for example, Gordon, *Dead on Arrival*; Quadagno, *One Nation, Uninsured*.

7. Some countries with universal coverage (e.g., Germany) allow small numbers of people to opt out, and most do not offer coverage to undocumented immigrants.

8. Health Expenditures Per Capita, Public and Private Expenditures, OECD, 2010, http://www.oecd.org/dataoecd/46/33/38979719.pdf.

9. Ezra Klein, "Administrative Costs in Health Care: A Primer," July 7, 2009, http://voices.washingtonpost.com/ezra-klein/2009/07/administrative_costs_in_ health.html.

Rationing and Rights: History and Definitions

1. Mechanic, *Truth about Health Care*, chap. 8.

2. For example, Bentley, *Eating for Victory*.

3. Samuelson, *Collected Scientific Papers*, 1415.

4. Reid, *Healing of America*.

5. For example, Harry Schwartz, "Waiting Room Only," *New York Times*, September 21, 1976, 37.

6. Beauchamp and Childress, *Principles of Biomedical Ethics*, 253.

7. For example, Michael Janofsky, "Oregon Starts to Extend Health Care," *New York Times*, February 19, 1994, 6; Jacobs et al., "Political Paradox."

8. Casalino et al., "What Does It Cost?"

9. *The Dartmouth Atlas of Health Care*, a project led by researcher John Wennberg, documents regional variations in the distribution of health care resources in the United States; http://www.dartmouthatlas.org/.

10. Klein, Day, and Redmayne, *Managing Scarcity*, 7.

11. Not only Americans see "rationing" as a dirty word; it is just as unpalatable in France, for example. Dutton, *Differential Diagnoses*, 8.

12. Marmor, "Right to Health Care."

13. Churchill, *Rationing Health Care in America*, 12–13.

14. Jerome Pollack, "The Voice of the Consumer: Cost, Quality and Organization of Medical Services" (paper presented at Massachusetts General Hospital, May 8, 1963), Davis Papers, NYAM.

15. For analyses of health as a human and social right, see, for example, Mann et al., *Health and Human Rights*; Oppenheimer, Bayer, and Colgrove, "Public Health and Human Rights"; Sunstein, *Second Bill of Rights*.

16. Marshall, *Citizenship and Social Class*; Hunt, *Reclaiming Social Rights*.

17. Duffus, "How to Pay the Doctor?," 360. See also Derickson, *Health Security for All*.

18. For example, Sade, "Medical Care as a Right."

19. Glendon, "Rights in Twentieth-Century Constitutions," 524.

20. On the origins of rights in revolutionary upheavals, see Hunt and Young, *Human Rights and Revolutions*.

21. Tone, *The Business of Benevolence*; Klein, *For All These Rights*.

22. Milmoe McCarrick, "A Right to Health Care," 3.

23. For example, Epstein, *Mortal Peril*; Kluge, "Drawing the Ethical Line."

24. Glendon, "Rights in Twentieth-Century Constitutions," 533.

25. Glendon, *World Made New*.

26. Mechanic, "Rationing Health Care," 34; Abel-Smith, "Minimum Adequate Levels"; Fried, "Equality and Rights."

27. Churchill, *Rationing Health Care in America*, 8–9.

Prologue

1. Markel, *Quarantine!*; Quadagno, "From Poor Laws to Pensions"; Wickenden, "Social Cost."

2. Katz, *Poorhouse*,13–14; Deutsch, "The Sick Poor in Colonial Times," 562; Quadagno, "From Poor Laws to Pensions," 425.

3. Deutsch, "Sick Poor in Colonial Times"; de la Teja and Wheat, "Bexar," 17–18.

4. Smith, "St. Joseph County Poor Asylum,"180; Bonner, *Medicine in Chicago*, 159.

5. Deutsch, "Sick Poor in Colonial Times," 565; for a vivid description of the Philadelphia almshouse, see Newman, *Embodied History*, chap. 1.

6. Newman, *Embodied History*, chap. 3; Rosenberg, *Care of Strangers*, 18–19.

7. De Kruif, *Health Is Wealth*, 98–99. On health rights arguments using the Declaration of Independence, see Derickson, *Health Security for All*, 98–99.

8. On medical regulation and licensing, see Starr, *Social Transformation*.

9. Chapman and Talmadge, "Evolution of the Right to Health Concept."

10. Jensen, "Before the Surgeon General." Thanks to Client Cargile for the phrasing.

11. For a full history of public health care provision, see Grogan, "America's Hidden Health Care State." The Marine Hospital Service later became the US Public Health Service (1912) and its laboratory became the National Institute of Health (1930).

12. The Babylonian Code of Hammurabi (ca. 1700 BCE) specified payments for surgeons (and punishments should they fail!).

13. Baker and Emanuel, "Efficacy of Professional Ethics."

14. John Bell, "Introduction to the Code of Medical Ethics," *Code of Ethics of the American Medical Association* (1847), 83–84, http://www.ama-assn.org/ama/pub/physician-resources/medical-ethics/code-medical-ethics/history-ama-ethics.shtml.

15. Starr, *Social Transformation*.

16. Rosenberg, *Care of Strangers*, 22–23.

17. Rosenberg, *Care of Strangers*, 111–13; Stevens, *Public-Private Health Care State*, 54–55.

18. O'Connell, Joseph S. "The Admission Policy," *Hospital Progress* (October 1932): 361–64.

19. On the history of public hospitals, see Opdycke, *No One Was Turned Away*.

20. Bonner, *Medicine in Chicago*, 160–62.

21. Vanessa Northington Gamble, "The Negro Hospital Renaissance: The Black Hospital Movement, 1920–1945" in Long and Golden, *American General Hospital*, 104; Gamble, *Making a Place for Ourselves*; Byrd and Clayton, *American Health Dilemma*, 209.

22. Emily K. Abel, "'Only the Best Class of Immigration': Public Health Policy toward Mexicans and Filipinos in Los Angeles, 1910–1940," *American Journal of Public Health* 94, no. 6 (2004): 932–39; Enos J. Francisco to John Collier, January 13,

1944, Box 1, Tucson Committee for Interracial Understanding (MS 904), Arizona Historical Society.

23. Goldmann, *Public Medical Care*, 44. The earliest US dispensaries were the Philadelphia, 1786, and the New York, 1791.

24. Rosner, *A Once Charitable Enterprise*, chap. 6; Duffy, *Sanitarians*, 158–59. Duffy is not correct in saying that dispensaries were "virtually eliminated" by World War I, however, as chap. 1 of this book shows. World War II would be more accurate.

25. Starr, *Social Transformation*, chap. 5; Stevens, *In Sickness and in Wealth*, 138.

26. "Report of the Committee on Medical Economics of the CMS," *Chicago Medical Society Bulletin* 37, no. 17 (October 27, 1934).

27. See, for example, Colgrove, Markowitz, and Rosner, *Contested Boundaries*.

28. Stevens, *Public-Private Health Care State*, 57.

29. Rosner, *A Once Charitable Enterprise*. On the Flexner Report, see Starr, *Social Transformation*, 118–23.

30. CCMC, *Medical Care for the American People*.

31. Beito, *From Mutual Aid to the Welfare State*; Murray, *Origins of American Health Insurance*; Hoffman, *Wages of Sickness*, chap. 1.

32. For a lively comparison of national health insurance systems and their histories, see Reid, *Healing of America*.

33. Hoffman, *Wages of Sickness*; Numbers, *Almost Persuaded*.

34. Meckel, *Save the Babies*; Lindenmeyer, *Right to Childhood*.

35. Starr, *Social Transformation*, 263–64.

36. CCMC, *Medical Care for the American People*, 5, 31.

37. CCMC, *Medical Care for the American People*, 160–61.

Chapter One

1. Robison, "Hull-House," 26.

2. Ibid., 27.

3. Joint Committee on Public Emergency Ambulance Service, "Outline of a Plan for Public Emergency Ambulance Service" (Chicago: Hospital Council, 1938), quoted in Robison, "Hull-House," 30.

4. Duffy, *Sanitarians*, 256.

5. CCMC, *Medical Care for the American People*; Edgar Sydenstricker, "Medical Practice and Public Needs," in AAPSS, *Medical Profession and the Public*, 23.

6. Thomas Parran, "Health Services of Tomorrow," in AAPSS, *Medical Profession and the Public*, 79.

7. Perrott, Collins, and Sydenstricker, "Sickness and the Economic Depression." See also Perrott and Collins, "Sickness and the Depression."

8. Trade Union Committee on Unemployment and the WPA (Works Progress Administration), "Report of the Committee on Social Security," March 17, 1938, Box 6, Folder 4, McCulloch Papers, CHM.

9. Grey, *New Deal Medicine*, 5, 7, 21.

10. Drake and Cayton, *Black Metropolis*, 204.

11. Beardsley, *History of Neglect*, 15–17; Smith, *Health Care Divided*.

12. Starr, *Social Transformation*, 259; CCMC, *Medical Care for the American People*, 13; Committee on Economic Security, "Report to the President of the Committee on Economic Security, Final Report on Risks to Economic Security Arising out of Ill Health," March 7, 1935, http://www.ssa.gov / history / reports / health.html.

13. Robison, "Hull-House," 3, 19, 35–36.

14. "Public Hearing of the Cook County Organization of the Illinois Workers Alliance, on the Relief Situation in Cook County, Held Thursday December 5, 1935, at the Hours, of 8:30 pm." McCulloch Papers, Box 4, Folder 10, 37–38, CHM.

15. Starr, *Social Transformation*, 270; Wilma Walker, "Distress in a Southern Illinois County," *Social Service Review* 5 (December 1931), 576; Editorial, *Chicago Medical Society Bulletin*, no. 31 (January 27, 1934), 429.

16. Reverby, *Ordered to Care*, 177.

17. The Joint Committee Representing the Hospital Associations, "The Role of the Voluntary Hospital in National Relief," February 20, 1934 (pamphlet), Subject Files, AHARC.

18. Stevens, *In Sickness and in Wealth*, 142; Cunningham and Cunningham, *Blues*, 10; Ross, "Crisis in the Hospitals," 364; Jennings, "Social Problems of the Depression," 89.

19. Ross, "Crisis in the Hospitals," 364.

20. ICCHWA, *Proceedings: National Health Conference*, 86. See also Derickson, "Take Health from the List."

21. Deutsch, "Great Depression"; Drake and Cayton, *Black Metropolis*, 83–84.

22. Cole, "Relief Crisis," 16–17.

23. ICCHWA, *Proceedings: National Health Conference*, 85.

24. Robison, "Hull-House," 41.

25. Raffensperger, *Old Lady*, 159.

26. Bonner, *Medicine in Chicago*, 174.

27. The Joint Committee Representing the Hospital Associations, "The Role of the Voluntary Hospital in National Relief"; Bonner, *Medicine in Chicago*, 174.

28. Buelow, "Dispensary"; "Illinois Emergency Relief Commission Clinic Program—Confidential," 1935, Box 48, Folder 2, Welfare Council, CHM .

29. Minutes, Executive Committee, Clinic Section, June 29, 1937, Box 48, Folder 3, Welfare Council, CHM.

30. "Minutes of Conference to Consider the Emergency Needs of Dispensaries," August 14, 1931, Box 48, Folder 1, Welfare Council, CHM.

31. "Committee on Expansion of Clinic Facilities under Public Auspices to Chairman of the Health Division," November 20, 1931, Box 48, Folder 1, Welfare Council, CHM.

32. Clinic Section, "Clinic Care in Chicago," November 1935, Box 48, Folder 2, Welfare Council, CHM. Fifteen years earlier, the figure for total visits had been closer to 500,000; Buelow, "Dispensary," 317.

33. Wordell, "Hospital Participation"; Buelow, "Dispensary," 292.

34. Helen Cody Baker, "If Ill and Poor Be Very Ill," reprint from Chicago *Daily News*, March 18, 1939, Box 48, Folder 4, Welfare Council, CHM.

35. ICCHWA, *Proceedings: National Health Conference*, 84.

36. Meeting of the Clinic Section, February 21, 1935, Box 48, Folder 2, Welfare Council, CHM.

37. In 1933 the Council of Social Agencies advised of that "patients should bring referral authorizations with them" but "should not insist upon the patient presenting such a referral in cases where this would involve hardship to the patient." Meeting of the Clinic Section, October 13, 1933, Box 48, Folder 1, Welfare Council, CHM.

38. "Study of Chicago Relief Administration Referrals for Clinic Care and Their Disposition," May 1940, Box 48, Folder 5, Welfare Council, CHM.

39. *Report of the Health Insurance Commission of the State of Illinois*, 358–59; "The Quality of Care Rendered by the University of Chicago Clinics," prepared for the Julius Rosenwald Fund by Emmet B. Bay, MD (September 1931), and "Chicago, University of, Clinics Study," both in File Drawer F-3, Davis Papers, NYAM; Bartlemez, "Applicants Rejected by Admitting Office," 39–44.

40. Council of Social Agencies of Chicago, *Report on Hospital Facilities in Chicago* (1935), 37.

41. "Minutes of the committee appointed by section on clinics and dispensaries, Health Division," June 1, 1932, Box 48, Folder 1; Minutes, Executive Committee, Clinic Section, June 29, 1937, Box 48, Folder 3; "Analysis by Race of New Individuals Admitted to Clinics During January 1937," June 17, 1937, Box 48, Folder 3, Welfare Council, CHM.

42. Baker, "If Ill and Poor Be Very Ill"; "Clinic Care in Chicago," Box 48, Folder 4, Welfare Council, CHM.

43. Robison, "Hull-House," 42.

44. Minutes of the Cooperative Case Committee, April 14, 1936, Box 112, Folder 7, Welfare Council, CHM.

45. "Economic Status of 4,502 Patients Admitted to Sixteen Chicago Clinics during January, 1939," Box 48, Folder 4, Welfare Council, CHM.

46. "Number of Rejections, by Reason, at Nine Chicago Clinics: June 1945 and June 1948," Box 49, Folder 3, Welfare Council, CHM.

47. Minutes of Clinic Section, October 17, 1935, Box 48, Folder 2, Welfare Council, CHM.

48. Minutes, Clinic Section, June 20, 1938, Box 48, Folder 3, Welfare Council, CHM.

49. Minutes of Admitting Committee, August 6, 1938, Box 48, Folder 3, Welfare Council, CHM.

50. Alexander Ropchan, "Recommended Standards for Clinic Admitting Personnel," May 8, 1935, Box 48, Folder 2, Welfare Council, CHM.

51. ICCHWA, *The Nation's Health: Discussion at the National Health Conference*, 5.

52. "An Urban Famine: Summary of Open Hearings Held by the Chicago Workers' Committee on Unemployment," July 1931–January 1932, Box 24, Chicago Commons Records, CHM.

53. "Some situations from May 16, to May 22," n.d., January–June 1939, Box 27, Chicago Commons Records, CHM.

54. Baker, "If Ill and Poor Be Very Ill."

55. "Clinic Care in Chicago," typescript, n.d., ca. 1935, Box 48, Folder 2, Welfare Council, CHM.

56. Wordell, "Hospital Participation."

57. "Resolution on Care of the Indigent Sick, Adopted by American Hospital Association at its 36th Annual Convention, Philadelphia, PA, September 27, 1934," Folder "American Hospital Association Council on Community Relations, 1935–37," File Drawer F-1, Davis Papers, NYAM. For a superb analysis of the AHA's lobbying activities, see Stevens, *In Sickness and in Wealth*.

58. Maurice Dubin, "We Need Help," *Modern Hospital* 47, no. 2 (August 1936), 47–49.

59. "Scientific Meeting of CMS," *Chicago Medical Society Bulletin* 37, no. 1 (July 7, 1934).

60. Letter to Victor Olander, October 9, 1933, Box 72, Folder 1933 October 7–11, Olander Papers, CHM.

61. American Medical Association, *Care of the Indigent Sick*, 46.

62. Medical Advisory Board, Minutes of Meetings, Part 2: Tuesday Afternoon Session, January 29, 1935. The speaker is Edgar Sydenstricker.

63. Jones, "Catholic Charities," 15–16.

64. According to Lizabeth Cohen, "Between 1933 and 1935, the federal government provided 87.6 percent of the dollars spent on emergency relief in Chicago, in contrast to contributions of 11 percent by the state and 1.4 percent by the city . . . private expenditures for relief in Illinois declined from a high of $8.3 million in 1932 to only $942,500 in 1935." Cohen, *Making a New Deal*, 268–69.

65. Alexander Ropchan to Mr. Samuel A. Goldsmith, October 18, 1934, Box 48, Folder 1, Welfare Council. The remainder of the clinics' total budget of $730,000 came from patient fees ($200,000); endowment income and contributions ($200,000); the Community Fund ($45,000); and contributions from medical schools ($85,000). Scientific Meeting of CMS, June 6, 1934, *Chicago Medical Society Bulletin* 37, no. 1 (July 7, 1934), 4, 7; Cole, "Relief Crisis," 143.

66. AMA, *Care of the Indigent Sick*, 48–49; *Chicago Medical Society Bulletin* 36, no. 31 (January 27, 1934), 429.

67. "Public Hearing on the Relief and WPA Situation."

68. Cole, "Relief Crisis," 268.

69. Minutes of the Clinic Section, July 7, 1936, Box 48, Folder 2, Welfare Council, CHM.

70. "Suffering Great as Relief Is Delayed and Slashed," *Chicago Defender*, July 18, 1936, 24.

71. Secretary of the Health Division, "Memorandum on Clinic Service in Chicago," September 9, 1938, Box 48, Folder 3, Welfare Council, CHM.

72. The Joint Committee Representing the Hospital Associations, "The Role of the Voluntary Hospital in National Relief," February 20, 1934 (pamphlet), Subject Files, AHARC.

73. Fred K. Hoehler, Director, American Public Welfare Association, in ICCHWA, *Proceedings: National Health Conference*; Minutes, Clinic Section, July 12, 1935, Box 48,

Folder 2, Welfare Council, CHM; "$55 a Month Pay to WPA Workers Called Too Low," *Chicago Daily Tribune*, October 12, 1935, 5.

74. Works Progress Administration, *Inventory*, 41–44; Stevens, *In Sickness and in Wealth*, 169; Klein, *For All These Rights*, 133.

75. "Payment of Tax Funds to Voluntary Hospitals — Some Current Issues." Report of Joint Committee of AHA and APWA, October 1939. "American Hospital Assn. Council on Community Relations, 1935–37." Davis Papers, NYAM.

76. Parran, "Health Services of Tomorrow," in AAPSS, *Medical Profession and the Public*, 82.

77. Parran, "Health Services of Tomorrow," 82.

78. Morris Fishbein, "The Doctor and the State," in AAPSS, *Medical Profession and the Public*, 99.

79. Editorial, "Health Insurance," *Rockford Register-Republic*, reprinted in the *Chicago Daily Tribune*, January 6, 1935, 16.

Chapter Two

1. "Chicago Workers' Committee on Unemployment, Its Purpose and Platform," 1932, Lundeen Bill & Unemployed Councils, Box A.2.1, ISM.

2. "March for Adequate Cash Relief," 1936, Lundeen Bill and Unemployed Councils, Box A.2.1, ISM.

3. Brinton, *Townsend National Recovery Plan*, 24. For an excellent analysis of the Townsend movement, see Amenta, *When Movements Matter*.

4. Folsom, *Impatient Armies*, 397.

5. James H. S. Brossard, "A Sociologist Looks at the Doctors," in AAPSS, *Medical Profession and the Public*, 5.

6. Roberts, "Social Trends," 1129. Also quoted in Derickson, *Health Security for All*, 71.

7. Kelly Miller, "Views and Reviews," *Chicago Defender*, August 13, 1938, 16.

8. De Kruif, *Health Is Wealth*, 5, 99, 101.

9. "The Townsend Plan Movement," Social Security Online, http://www.ssa. gov/history/towns5.html.

10. Committee on Economic Security (CES), Medical Advisory Board—Minutes of Meetings, Part 2: Tuesday Afternoon Session, January 29, 1935, http://www.ssa. gov/history/reports/ces/ces7minutes2.html. Hereafter, CES Minutes.

11. Blumenthal and Morone, *Heart of Power*, 35, 40.

12. The members of the CES were Frances Perkins, Secretary of Labor, chairman; Henry Morgenthau Jr., Secretary of the Treasury; Homer Cummings, Attorney General; Henry A. Wallace, Secretary of Agriculture; and Harry L. Hopkins, Federal Emergency Relief Administrator.

13. Blumenthal and Morone, *Heart of Power*, 33–34.

14. "Historical Background and Development of Social Security," http://www. ssa.gov/history/briefhistory3.html; Gordon, *Dead on Arrival*, 17.

15. *Nation's Health*, 13.

16. Derickson, *Health Security for All*, 80.

17. *Nation's Health*, 9.

18. ICCHWA, *Proceedings: National Health Conference*, 57, 59, 83.

19. Ben W. Kilgore, Kentucky Farm Bureau, National Health Conference, July 18, 1938, ICCHWA, *The Nation's Health: Discussion at the National Health Conference*, 71–72.

20. Testimony of Watson B. Miller, T. Arnold Hill, ICCHWA, *Proceedings: National Health Conference*, 138.

21. "Dr. Wright Hits Segregated Medical Program at Confab," *Chicago Defender*, July 30, 1938, 5.

22. Wright quoted in "Colored Leaders Endorse President's Plan for Socialized Medicine," March 19, 1938, Box 302, Folder 1, Barnett Papers, CHM.

23. ICCHWA, *Proceedings: National Health Conference*, 119–20.

24. ICCHWA, *Proceedings: National Health Conference*, 84. See also Derickson, "Take Health from the List."

25. *Nation's Health*, 4.

26. Huthmacher, *Wagner*, 264; Biles, "Wagner."

27. "Proceedings of the Fifth State Convention of the Illinois Workers Alliance," November 1938, 6, McCulloch Papers, Box 4, Folder 7, CHM.

28. "Launch Health Campaign," *Chicago Defender*, July 23, 1938, 3; Lorence, *Organizing the Unemployed*, 215.

29. *To Establish a National Health Program*.

30. "Doctors' Group Opposes Wagner Health Aid Bill," *Chicago Daily Tribune*, May 18, 1939, 18.

31. Funigiello, *Chronic Politics*, 45–49; Stevens, *American Medicine*, 194.

32. De Kruif, *Health Is Wealth*, 31.

33. Engel, *Doctors and Reformers*, 67.

34. CES Minutes.

35. Minutes of the Clinic Section, March 1934, Box 48, Folder 1; "Clinic Care in Chicago," 1935, Box 48, Folder 2, Welfare Council, CHM.

36. AMA, *Care of the Indigent Sick*, 45.

37. Nathan B. Van Etten, "Abuses of Medical Charity and the Free Services of Physicians," in AAPSS, *Medical Profession and the Public*, 14, 17.

38. Williams, "Farm Security Administration Borrowers."

39. Grey, *New Deal Medicine*, 139–42.

40. Starr, *Social Transformation*, 303; Klein, *For All These Rights*, 130, 153–54; Cunningham and Cunningham, *Blues*, 37.

41. Berkowitz and Wolff, *Group Health Association*.

42. Cunningham and Cunningham, *Blues*, 40.

43. B. C. MacLean, "Admission of Patients," *Transactions of the American Hospital Association* (1930): 365–70. Subject files, "Admitting and Discharge—Procedures," AHARC.

44. "Pay or Stay?" *Hospitals* 35 (March 1, 1961): 126. *Hoffman v. Clinic Hospital* (1928) upheld the practice; *Gadsden General Hospital v. Hamilton* (1925) awarded damages because threat of force was used.

45. Hortense M. Dillon, "Discharge Practices in 58 General and Special Hospitals," *Modern Hospital* 51 (July 1938): 49–50.

46. Stevens, *In Sickness and in Wealth*, 146; Cunningham and Cunningham, *Blues*, 11.

47. Michael M. Davis, "Change Comes to the Doctor," in AAPSS, *Medical Profession and the Public*, 68.

48. Klein, *For All These Rights*, 128.

49. Rufus Rorem at ICCHWA, *Proceedings: National Health Conference*, 100–101; Klein, *For All These Rights*, 129.

50. Committee on Economic Security, "Report to the President of the Committee on Economic Security, Final Report on Risks to Economic Security Arising out of Ill Health," March 7, 1935, www.ssa.gov/history/reports/health.html.

51. Cunningham and Cunningham, *Blues*, 44–45.

52. Borgwardt, *New Deal*, 136.

53. Sunnstein, *Second Bill of Rights*, 13. For an analysis of economic rights, particularly the right to a job, as the basis for freedom, see MacLean, *Freedom Is Not Enough*.

Chapter Three

1. Dieuaide, *Civilian Health in Wartime*, 19.

2. Dieuaide, *Civilian Health in Wartime*, 19–20; "Our Health and Our Hospitals," *Collier's* 117 (May 11, 1946): 90.

3. Missouri Association for Social Welfare, "Case Illustrations of Existing Health Needs in Missouri," April 10, 1941, 89, Box 148, Central Files 1941–44, Records of the Children's Bureau, National Archives.

4. Missouri Association for Social Welfare, "Case Illustrations of Existing Health Needs in Missouri," April 10, 1941, 85, Box 148, Central Files 1941–44, Records of the Children's Bureau, National Archives. On the history of insulin treatment, see Feudtner, *Bittersweet*.

5. Byrd and Clayton, *American Health Dilemma*, 153–54.

6. Cowdrey, *Fighting for Life*.

7. "US Health Dangers Pictured," *New York Times*, July 12, 1944, 1.

8. "Ask Why 5 Million Unfit for War," *New York Times*, July 8, 1944, 20.

9. "US Health Dangers Pictured."

10. Leonard G. Rowntree, "Fit to Fight," in Fishbein, *Doctors at War*, 45–46.

11. Cowdrey, *Fighting for Life*, 22.

12. Dieuaide, *Civilian Health in Wartime*, 21, 22.

13. "Miracle of 7th Avenue: A History of Phoenix Memorial Hospital," 1981, Arizona Ephemera Collection, Hayden Library, ASU.

14. "City's Hospital and Housing Need Held Acute," *Los Angeles Times*, April 29, 1943, 1; "Hospital Bed Shortage in City More Critical," *Los Angeles Times*, May 13, 1943, A10.

15. Beka Doherty and Arthur Hepner, "The Doctor Shortage," *New Republic*, May 10, 1943, 629–31.

16. "Declare War on Disease," *New Republic*, June 23, 1941, 842.

17. Charles M. McGill to C. L. Williams, March 16, 1942, Box 766, General

Classified Records, Group X–National Defense, Records of the PHS, National Archives.

18. "Doctor Dilemma Caused by the Army's Call Vexes Public Health Meeting and Congress," *Newsweek*, November 9, 1942, 62.

19. Doherty and Hepner, "Doctor Shortage," 629.

20. "Doctor Dilemma."

21. Venice T. Spraggs, "Few Negro Medical Officers to Be Commissioned Due to Set Quota," *Chicago Defender*, January 6, 1945, 6.

22. "More Hospitals: Mississippi's Answer," *Ladies Home Journal*, October 23, 1947.

23. "Hospital Loads Mount; Staff Short of Needs," *Chicago Daily Tribune*, June 4, 1943, 3.

24. Doherty and Hepner, "Doctor Shortage."

25. "You Can Help the War Effort by Conserving Medical and Nursing Care," *American Home*, January 31, 1943, 31.

26. Kate Massee, "Women in War Work," *Chicago Daily Tribune*, August 25, 1943, 23.

27. "Does the Medical Shortage Affect Public Health?" *American Journal of Public Health* 33 (May 1943): 632.

28. "Demand End of Jim Crow in Veteran's Agency," *Chicago Defender*, February 3, 1945, 4.

29. Spraggs, "Few Negro Medical Officers"; "Rural Doctors Won't Be" February 27, 1943, 6.

30. Don Raymond Leveridge, "Doctors in the Draft," *Chicago Daily Tribune*, February 24, 1941, 10.

31. Thomas Parran, "The Public Health Service in the War," in Fishbein, *Doctors at War*, 249, 251, 258–59.

32. Starr, *Social Transformation*, 340–41.

33. Larry DeWitt, "The Civilian War Benefits Program: SSA's First Disability Program." *Social Security Bulletin* (Summer 1997), http://www.ssa.gov/history/civil war.html.

34. Grey, *New Deal Medicine*, 131–36.

35. DeWitt, "The Civilian War Benefits Program."

36. Parran, "Public Health Service in the War," 253–54; Stevens, *In Sickness and in Wealth*, 209–10.

37. Stevens, *In Sickness and in Wealth*, 209.

38. Amy Porter, "Babies for Free," *Collier's* 116 (August 4, 1945): 18–19. For a discussion of EMIC in the context of the history of the US Children's Bureau, see Lindenmeyer, *Right to Childhood*, chap. 8.

39. Porter, "Babies for Free," 28.

40. Sinai and Anderson, EMIC, 19, 21.

41. Lindenmeyer, *Right to Childhood*.

42. Grey, *New Deal Medicine*, 143.

43. Adler, "Dependents of Men in Military Service," 646.

44. Sinai and Anderson, EMIC, 113–14.

45. Eliot, "Wives and Infants of Enlisted Men," 36.

46. "First Lady Points to Maternity Care," New York Times, May 16, 1944, 17.

47. "Baby Aid Given 40,000 Service Wives a Month," Chicago Daily Tribune, May 16, 1944, 15.

48. Auerhan and Loring, "Forty Mothers," 1.

49. Porter, "Babies for Free," 19.

50. Beatrice Oppenheim, "Uncle Sam Looks After Babies: Maternity Care Now Available to Wives of Service Men," New York Times, October 3, 1943, X12.

51. Porter, "Babies for Free," 19.

52. "Babies a Problem to Service Wives," New York Times, December 5, 1943, 63.

53. "Friend of the Yanks," Chicago Daily Tribune, February 15, 1945, 10.

54. Auerhan and Loring, "Forty Mothers," 24.

55. "Jersey Doctors Vote Aid to Service Men," New York Times, April 28, 1944, 10.

56. Elinor Siegel, "Pediatricians Quit Children's Bureau," New York Times, August 3, 1944, 22.

57. "Letter Criticizes Pediatrics Academy Board on Withdrawing Children's Bureau Support," New York Times, October 3, 1944, 20.

58. Siegel, "Pediatricians Quit Children's Bureau."

59. "A Children's Bureau Program," New York Times, October 21, 1944, 16.

60. Porter, "Babies for Free," 28.

61. "Wartime Baby Care Coming to an End," New York Times, July 23, 1947, 26; Porter, "Babies for Free," 19. Today the US military contracts with managed care organizations to provide health coverage to active duty personnel and their dependents.

62. Klein, For All These Rights, 169–71.

63. For example, Sunnstein, Second Bill of Rights; Kessler-Harris, In Pursuit of Equity; MacLean, Freedom Is Not Enough.

64. Somers and Somers, Doctors, Patients, and Health Insurance, 136.

65. John H. Gibbon, "The Army Doctor Comes Home," Harper's, February 1946, 175–80.

66. "Close of the EMIC Program," American Journal of Public Health 39 (December 1949): 1579–81.

67. Arthur J. Lesser to Columlie D. Shiflette, February 15, 1946, Folder 4–18–4–1, Box 148, Central File 1941–44, Records of the Children's Bureau, RG 102, National Archives. Emphasis added.

68. Auerhan and Loring, "Forty Mothers," 31.

69. Gibbon, "Army Doctor Comes Home."

70. "Group Practice Favored by Young Doctors Now in the Armed Services," Science News Letter 46 (December 30, 1944): 426.

71. De Kruif, Health Is Wealth, 237; "Penicillin to Be Free for Needy of City," New York Times, June 24, 1944, 13.

72. Blumenthal and Morone, *Heart of Power*, 75.

73. Grey, *New Deal Medicine*, 144; Charley Cherokee, "National Grapevine," *Chicago Defender*, January 11, 1947, 11.

74. Gambone, *Greatest Generation Comes Home*, 56–61.

75. Quoted in National Council of Jewish Women, "Health Care for All," January 1946, Box 136, Central File 1945–48, Children's Bureau Records, National Archives.

76. Jacobs, *Health of Nations*, 69.

77. "State Insurance and Medicine Advocated for Post-War Britain," *New York Times*, November 27, 1942, 1.

78. "The Universal Declaration of Human Rights," http://www.un.org/en/documents/udhr/index.shtml.

79. http://www.un.org/en/documents/udhr/; Glendon, *World Made New*, 43.

80. Glendon, *World Made New*, 43, 186.

81. Blumenthal and Morone, *Heart of Power*, 81.

82. Quadagno, *One Nation, Uninsured*, 26; Derickson, "Health Security for All?," 1341.

83. Blumenthal and Morone, *Heart of Power*, 65–67.

84. Harry S. Truman, Special Message to the Congress Presenting a 21-Point Program for the Reconversion Period, September 6, 1945; Special Message to the Congress Recommending a Comprehensive Health Program, November 19, 1945. American Presidency Project, http://www.presidency.ucsb.edu/index.php.

85. Quadagno, *One Nation, Uninsured*, 38.

86. "Truman Asks Congress O.K. of Health Plan," *Chicago Daily Tribune*, April 23, 1949, 4. Emphasis added.

87. Derickson, "Health Security for All?"

88. Koojiman, . . . *And the Pursuit of National Health*, 109; Quadagno, *One Nation, Uninsured*, 35–36.

89. Poen, *Truman vs. the Medical Lobby*, 88; Blumenthal and Morone, *Heart of Power*, 78.

90. "National Physicians Renew Opposition to Truman Health Plan," *Chicago Daily Tribune*, January 15, 1948, 3. On McCarthyite tactics in health politics during the Cold War, see Derickson, "House of Falk."

91. Physicians' incomes rose 300 percent between 1939 and 1946. Grey, *New Deal Medicine*, 141.

92. "Warns Truman Medicine Plan Will Hit Unions," *Chicago Daily Tribune*, November 17, 1949, A6.

93. "Laborer," "Budget for Health Care," *Chicago Daily Tribune*, December 10, 1948, 20.

94. Quadagno, *One Nation, Uninsured*, 38.

95. B. Hensel, "Harry Truman's Reluctance in Going Public for National Health Insurance" (paper presented at the annual meeting of the International Communication Association, New Orleans, May 27, 2004), http://www.allacademic.com/meta/p113371_index.html.

96. Quadagno, *One Nation, Uninsured*, 42–43.

Chapter Four

1. Hammond, *Childhood's Deadly Scourge*.

2. Transcript, *Crews v. Birmingham Baptist Hospital*, Tenth Judicial Circuit, Jefferson County, Alabama, April 6, 1933, Alabama State Archives.

3. *Birmingham Baptist Hospital v. Crews*, 6 Div. 468. Supreme Court of Alabama 229 Ala. 398; 157 So. 224; 1934 Ala. LEXIS 365, October 11, 1934.

The incident was not as uncommon as the nurse would have it; newspaper reports of children with diphtheria being turned away from hospitals and dying in their parents' arms can be found in previous decades, for example, "General News from New York: Little Boy Dies on Being Refused Admission to a Hospital," *Chicago Daily Tribune* February 8, 1896, 3; "Baby, Always the Baby . . . Sad Experience of Father Who Could Find No Refuge for His Diphtheria Stricken Girl . . . ," *Chicago Daily Tribune*, December 2, 1902, 3.

Birmingham v. Crews built on a much earlier Supreme Court decision, *McDonald v. Massachusetts General Hospital* (1876), that declared private hospitals to be private corporations, as discussed in the Prologue. What was new about the *Birmingham* decision is that it specifically included emergency care within the hospitals' ability to refuse.

4. Jacobs, *Health of Nations*, 185; Maioni, *Parting at the Crossroads*; Boychuk, *National Health Insurance in the United States and Canada*.

5. National expenditures for medical research increased from $18 million in 1941 to $181 million in 1951; Starr, *Social Transformation*, 343.

6. Stevens, *In Sickness and in Wealth*, 204.

7. *Trained Nurse and Hospital Review* 123 (September 1949): 122.

8. "Hospital Survey and Construction Bill. October 30, 1945."

9. "More Hospitals: Mississippi's Answer."

10. "So Your Community Wants a Hospital," *Ladies Home Journal*, May 1947, 5.

11. "More Hospitals: Mississippi's Answer."

12. "Our Health and Our Hospitals."

13. Starr, *Social Transformation*, 349.

14. "Hospital Survey and Construction Plan in Illinois," 84.

15. D. D. Stephens, MD, Slocomb, Alabama, to Lister Hill, March 6, 1945, Lister Hill Papers, University of Alabama, Tuscaloosa.

16. Claude W. Munger, "A Program for Hospital Development," in *US Senate Hears about Hospitals and Hospital Service*, ed. AHA, 9.

17. Stevens, *In Sickness and in Wealth*, 213; Weeks and Berman, *Shapers of American Health Care Policy*, 29–30. Stevens calls the Commission's membership "a melting pot for middle-of-the-road consensus"; *In Sickness and in Wealth*, 398n37.

18. George Bugbee interview, Weeks and Berman, *Shapers of Health Care Policy*.

19. Stevens, *In Sickness and in Wealth*, 212–16.

20. Starr, *Social Transformation*, 350.

21. "Hospital Survey and Construction Bill. October 30, 1945."

22. Starr, *Social Transformation*, 350.

23. "Hospital Survey and Construction Bill. October 30, 1945," 5–6.

24. Orchard, "Need for Governmental Assistance to Hospitals," 17.

25. "Hospital Construction Bill: Statement by Dr. R. L. Sensenich."

26. George Bugbee quoted in Weeks and Berman, *Shapers of American Health Care Policy*, 38.

27. Abbott, "Hospitals Are Not a Health Program."

28. Means, "Government in Medicine."

29. Stebbins, "Preventive Care." The dangers of hospital infections had been recognized for centuries; see Rosenberg, *Care of Strangers*, chap. 5; Risse, *Mending Bodies, Saving Souls*.

30. "Hill-Burton Hospital Construction Bill."

31. Hoppe, "Hospitals for the People?"

32. In 1954 Hill-Burton would be amended to include some long-term care facilities.

33. Stebbins, "Preventive Care."

34. Teigh, "One Answer." See also Buhler Wilkerson, *No Place like Home*.

35. "Hospital Survey and Construction Bill. October 30, 1945," 19, 21.

36. Quoted in Stevens, *In Sickness and in Wealth*, 218.

37. Means, "Government in Medicine," 48.

38. Matthew Woll to A. C. Bachmeyer, July 12, 1946, MSS 3 Box 58, Ray Lyman Wilbur Collection, Lane Medical Library.

39. Boychuk, *Hospital Policy in the United States and Canada*, 26; Mountin and Perrott, "Health Insurance Programs and Plans of Western Europe."

40. Blumstein, "Court Action, Agency Reaction," 1227n22.

41. Kenneth Williamson interview in Weeks and Berman, *Shapers of American Health Care Policy*, 45.

42. Dowell, "Unfulfilled Promise," 156.

43. Hoppe, "Hospitals for the People?"

44. Bierman, "Health Needs of Low-Income Families," 105; "Wesley Head Tells Private Hospitals' Free Care Problem," *Chicago Daily Tribune*, October 27, 1948, 9; *Presbyterian Hospital Annual Report, 1953–54*, Rush Archives.

45. Roy Gibbons, "Hospital Care Up 116 Percent, Survey Shows," *Chicago Daily Tribune*, November 21, 1948, B23.

46. For example, while around 7 percent of total hospital expenditures in Chicago went to charity care in 1948, individual hospitals might provide significantly less (as little as one-tenth of 1 percent) or significantly more (56 percent at Children's Memorial in 1957). Gibbons, "Hospital Care up 116 Percent"; McCausland, *Element of Love*, 147.

47. Dowell, "Unfulfilled Promise"; Blumstein, "Court Action, Agency Reaction."

48. "Summary of Discussion of Members and Guests at a Meeting of the Commission on Hospital Care, Chicago, Jan 31 and Feb 1," no year, ca. 1946, Ray Lyman Wilbur Collection, Box 58. On Dent, see Richardson, "Albert W. Dent."

49. Thomas, "Expanding Hospital Care for Black Southerners," 831–32.

50. Commission on Hospital Care, *Hospital Care in the United States*. Dent pub-

licly approved of the Commission's recommendation, making him one of the African American "pragmatists" described by Thomas, "Expanding Hospital Care for Black Southerners." Dent, "Available to Negroes," 328.

51. "Statement by U. S. Senator Lister Hill of Alabama before the Committee on Education and Labor of the Senate in Support of the Hospital Construction Bill, February 26, 1945," Folder 1.11, Series 17.1.1, Dean's Administrative Files, UAB Archives.

52. Thomas, "Expanding Hospital Care for Black Southerners."

53. Cobb, "Statement in Support of National Health Bill, S. 1606"; Atlanta Urban League, *Hospital Care of the Negro Population of Atlanta*, 6; Garvin, "Post-War Planning for 'Negro' Hospitals."

54. Thomas, "Expanding Hospital Care for Black Southerners."

55. Thomas, "Expanding Hospital Care for Black Southerners"; Maryland hospital, Southern Conference Educational Fund, "A Survey of Racial Practices and Attitudes in the Hospitals of Southern and Border States," n.d., ca. 1952, Box 143, Health Project, SCHW. The survey data do not indicate whether the responding hospitals were recipients of Hill-Burton funds.

56. "Survey of Racial Practices and Attitudes in the Hospitals of Southern and Border States."

57. National Medical Association, "Statement to the Honorable John F. Kennedy," August 1, 1963, Box 9, Berry Papers, CHM.

58. Truman, "Annual Message to Congress on the State of the Union," January 6, 1947.

59. Starr, *Social Transformation*, 350; Dowell, "Unfulfilled Promise," 154; Stevens, *In Sickness and in Wealth*, 257.

60. West and Raup, "Hospital Use in Hagerstown," 862.

61. "Hospital Care Does Cost Money, BUT," 1953, File 6, Box 1, NHW Collection, AHARC.

62. Ibid.

63. Lucy Freeman, "It's Your Hospital and Your Life!" *Public Affairs* pamphlet No. 187, 1952, File 6, 1953, Box 1, NHW, AHARC.

64. Shortliffe, Hamilton, and Noroian, "Changing Pattern of Medical Care"; 22. Sixty-three percent of the hospitals in this study had expanded their emergency facilities since 1940. For a general history of emergency medicine in the United States, see Zink, *Anyone, Anything, Anytime*.

65. Horgan, "Emergency Room Crisis"; Shortliffe, Hamilton, and Noroian, "Changing Pattern of Medical Care," 22; Duncan, "How to Evaluate Emergency Room Care"; Fahey, "Six Ways."

66. Blalock, "Emergency Care," 51. The rate of increase for ER use exceeded population growth; one author noted that the US population increased at an annual rate of 2 percent from 1955 to 1965, while ER visits increased at 6 percent per year. Seifert and Johnstone, "Meeting the Emergency Department Crisis," 55.

67. Weinerman and Edwards, "'Triage' System Shows Promise," 56.

68. Shortliffe, Hamilton, and Noroian, "Changing Pattern of Medical Care," 23.

69. "Suggestions and Promotional Material for National Hospital Day," 1949, File 2; "Sample Editorial," 1959, File 12, both in Box 1, NHW, AHARC.

70. Fahey, "Six Ways," 66.

71. Duncan, "How to Evaluate Emergency Room Care," 168; "Is the 'Accident Room' Evolving into the Community Medical Center?"

72. Michigan Blue Cross, "Hospital Emergency Room Utilization Study: A Report on Emergency Room Visits in 22 Michigan Hospitals" (hereafter Michigan Blue Cross Study), 1965, 1, File Drawer F-1, Hospital Emergency Units, Michael M. Davis Papers, NYAM.

73. 42 percent, McCarroll and Skudder, "Conflicting Concepts of Function," 37; 70 percent at Good Samaritan Hospital, Phoenix, AZ, and Grace-New Haven Community Hospital, New Haven, CT, Fahey, "Six Ways," 66; 84.5 percent, Duncan, "How to Evaluate Emergency Room Care," 168. Some studies distinguished between "non-emergency" conditions (which might be serious but not requiring immediate care) and "non-urgent" conditions (not requiring care within a few hours, or at all), but others did not.

74. Josephine Robertson, "Emergency Room Crisis," pamphlet, n.d., ca. 1966, Mannix Papers, Box 104, File 4, AHARC.

75. Hoffman, "The Reluctant Safety Net," in Stevens, Rosenberg, and Burns, *History and Health Policy*. Excerpted with permission of Rutgers University Press.

76. Freidson and Feldman, *Public Attitudes toward Health Insurance*, 7–8.

77. Lochridge, "Our Shocking Accident Wards, Part Two."

78. *Afro American* clipping, February 16, 1952, Hospital Discussion folder, Box 131, SCHW.

79. The pamphlet included the example of Maltheus Avery, a World War II veteran who was in an automobile accident in 1949 and died after being turned away from Duke University Hospital because the Jim Crow ward was full. The story of Avery's death was later conflated with that of renowned blood researcher Dr. Charles R. Drew, and created the legend that Drew died after being denied care. Actually, Drew was treated at a white hospital emergency room but could not be saved. Like the legend of Bessie Smith, Drew's story reflected the brutal reality of racial discrimination while not being literally true. Love, *One Blood*.

80. Alfred Maund, *The Untouchables*, Southern Conference Educational Fund Inc., n.d., ca. 1952, File Drawer C-4, "Negro Health," Michael M. Davis Papers, NYAM.

81. Box 122, Hospitals: Misc. cases, 1951–, SCHW; Eleanor Roosevelt, "My Day," October 17, 1952, reprinted in Emblidge, *My Day*.

82. Anonymous reply. "Survey of Racial Practices and Attitudes in the Hospitals of Southern and Border States."

83. Box 122, Hospitals: Misc. cases, 1951–, SCHW.

84. A. M. Mercer to Dr. Marshall, December 5, 1951, Box 122, Hospital Committee, SCHW.

85. Karen Kruse Thomas argues that racial dumping eased after 1952, at least in North Carolina where there was the most hospital capacity for blacks cased

(Thomas, "Hill-Burton Act," 846). However, there is evidence of racial dumping in North Carolina into the early 1960s, when Charlotte Memorial Hospital continued to transfer black patients. Hughie David died of an apparent brain aneurysm at all-black Good Samaritan Hospital, which had no neurosurgeon or angiogram, after being refused help at Charlotte Memorial. Case cited in Quadagno, "Promoting Civil Rights through the Welfare State," 78. See also the North Carolina incidents on p. 83.

86. Scribner, "Quiet Revolution,"131–32n70.

87. Matthew F. McNulty to Berson, January 28, 1961, Folder 11.15, Series 17.1.4, Dean's Administrative Files, UAB Archives; Charles Grainger, "Baby Born in Hospital Yard like Animal Cites Need for Indigent Patient Funds," *Birmingham News*, December 14, 1958, clipping in University Hospital Public Relations Scrapbook, UAB Archives. Thanks to UAB Archivist Tim Pennycuff for alerting me to this incident.

88. Health rights attorney Marilyn Rose, quoted in Smith, *Health Care Divided*, 169.

89. Dr. Quentin Young, interview by the author, June 12, 2003. For a vivid description of this campaign, see also Smith, *Health Care Divided*, 50–53.

90. Box 122, "Hospital Committee," SCEF Records.

91. Anne Braden, "Civil Rights," in Kleber, *Encyclopedia of Louisville*, 191.

92. Wini Young to James Dombrowski, March 19, 1952, Box 122, "Hospital Committee," SCEF Records.

93. Smith, *Health Care Divided*, 49. See also *Hospitals* issue of June 1951 on segregation.

94. Smith, *Health Care Divided*, 54–56.

95. Quadagno, "Promoting Civil Rights Through the Welfare State," 79; Seham, "Discrimination against Negroes in Hospitals"; Smith, *Health Care Divided*, 54–56.

96. Reynolds, "Hospital and Civil Rights, 1945–1963"; "Working Rules for Assuring Non-Discrimination in Hospital Admissions."

97. Albee, *Death of Bessie Smith*; Albertson, *Bessie*, 256–267. Thanks to Taylor Atkins for sharing research materials on this.

98. And only lawsuits that reached at least the state appellate level are readily accessible to the historian. A full accounting of lawsuits brought by patients or families that did not reach the appellate level would require years of painstaking research in county courthouses and local newspapers, and even then local records preservation varies hugely, and many records have not survived. Such a paper trail was successfully followed for this book only for two important emergency care cases, *Birmingham Baptist Hospital v. Crews* and *Guerrero v. Copper Queen*, and even then only limited records were obtained. I could not obtain local court records or transcripts for the other seminal case, *Wilmington General Hospital v. Manlove*.

Hospital records are opaque sources for determining the extent of emergency refusals. Many refusals were likely not recorded at all. Transfers to other hospitals were more likely to be recorded, but reasons for transfers are harder to determine.

In the late 1940s, for example, Wesley Memorial Hospital in Chicago, a private voluntary hospital, regularly and frequently transferred patients from its emergency room to Cook County Hospital, but the reasons for the transfer either are not recorded or are recorded in code. Emergency Room Register 1948–50, Wesley Memorial Hospital, Northwestern University Hospital Archives. Transfers of stable patients for medical reasons do not constitute "dumping," so the reason for the transfer and the patient's condition are crucial in determining whether dumping occurred.

99. In the late 1960s, the *Chicago Defender* newspaper began documenting emergency refusal, and reported that "hundreds" of such cases occurred every year in Chicago; see chap. 7. When emergency room dumping became a national scandal in the 1980s, many more cases began to be documented. One widely accepted study put the number at 250,000 per year; see chap. 8.

100. "Mr. Truman's Memories: On Health and Taxes," *New York Times*, January 23, 1956, 1.

101. After Jones died in surgery, her family brought suit and won in 1954, with the New York Supreme Court ruling that the intern had been negligent. *Jones v. City of New York*. This was a landmark case not because it curbed patient dumping, but because it found the hospital liable for the actions of its intern (generally doctors were treated as free agents by law, not as hospital employees). The few court cases on emergency refusal in the 1940s and '50s had little bearing on the right to access, since they were primarily about malpractice liability. Courts did not raise the issue of public access to emergency rooms until *Wilmington General Hospital v. Manlove* in 1961.

102. AHA, *Emergency Services in the Hospital*. The AHA criticized this practice.

103. *Bourgeois v. Dade County*. See also *Methodist Hospital v. Ball*; John W. Stevens, "Funds Are Asked to Aid Alcoholics," *New York Times*, July 7, 1959, 35. This article reported that all but one of the hospitals in Westchester County refused emergency care to alcoholics except in cases of bodily injury.

104. "Court's Patient Banned; Judge Flays Hospital," *Chicago Daily Tribune*, March 28, 1953, B7.

105. *O'Neill v. Montefiore Hospital*.

106. *Wilmington General Hospital v. Manlove*. This case was a turning point in hospital admissions law because the judges argued that the hospital had an obligation to provide emergency care to the public simply by virtue of having an emergency ward. Although *Wilmington General Hospital v. Manlove* was cited in subsequent decisions affirming a duty to provide emergency care (most significantly, *Guerrero v. Copper Queen*), other courts ignored it and continued to affirm *Birmingham v. Crews* well into the 1970s; for example, *Harper v. Baptist Medical Center–Princeton*.

107. "Engineer Dies, Lake County's 6th Polio Victim," *Chicago Daily Tribune*, September 1, 1952, D11.

108. On the durational residency requirement in health care, see Beatrix Hoffman, "Sympathy and Exclusion: Health Care for Undocumented Immigrants in the United States" in Wailoo, Livingston, and Guarnaccia, *A Death Retold*.

109. Opdycke, *No One Was Turned Away*, 71.

110. Gibbons, "Hospital Care Up 116 Percent."

111. *Rivera v. Misericordia Hospital*. Although the Riveras were clearly Hispanic, no racial discrimination was alleged in the court case.

112. *Stanturf v. Sipes*.

113. "Medicine: The Baby & the Rules," *Time*, February 15, 1954. See also "Hospital Inquiries Set; Death of Baby Turned Away in Chicago Brings Action," *New York Times*, January 28, 1954, 14.

114. Hoffman, "Reluctant Safety Net," 263. Woodlawn Hospital was also notorious for racial exclusion; the Chicago Committee to End Discrimination was founded in response to additional dumping cases by Woodlawn. The Lingo family's ethnicity is not indicated in the sources but this was apparently a case of financial rather than racial refusal.

115. "Backed in Baby's Death; Hospital Absolved by Chicago Medical Society Inquiry," *New York Times*, February 15, 1954, 24.

116. "Doctors Probe, Back Hospital in Baby Death," *Chicago Daily Tribune*, February 15, 1954, 4; "Hospital Taxes," *Chicago Daily Tribune*, March 16, 1954, 20.

117. Leland H. Taylor, "To the Editor," *Southern Patriot* 9, no. 10 (December 1951).

118. "Survey of Racial Practices and Attitudes in the Hospitals of Southern and Border States."

Chapter Five

1. "State Finds Gaps in Health Plans," *New York Times*, May 10, 1959, 39.

2. Reinhardt, "Predictable Managed Care Kvetch." Reinhardt clearly means rationing at the point of service here, while elsewhere he has argued for a more expansive definition of rationing; see Reinhardt, "'Rationing' Health Care: What Does It Mean?"

3. Starr, *Social Transformation*, 327.

4. "State Finds Gaps in Health Plans," *New York Times*, May 10, 1959, 39; CNHI, "Facts of Life, Health, and Health Insurance," 1969; CNHI, "The Failure of Third Party Insurors [*sic*]," fact sheet, ca. 1976, Box 22, Folder 27, CNHI Collection, Reuther Library.

5. US Department of Health, Education, and Welfare, *The Benefit Structure of Private Health Insurance*.

6. Individual policies made up 20–25 percent of all coverage in the 1950s; Somers and Somers, *Doctors, Patients, and Health Insurance*, 366.

7. Starr, *Social Transformation*, 327–28; 7 percent were in independent plans.

8. Klein, *For All These Rights*, chap. 6.

9. Blumenthal and Morone, *Heart of Power*, chap. 3.

10. Blumenthal and Morone, *Heart of Power*, 110–12; Gordon, *Dead on Arrival*, 232–33.

11. Arizona Blue Cross Blue Shield, "Some Important Moves in 1959," Arizona Ephemera Collection, Hayden Library, ASU.

12. *Proceedings: National Congress on Prepaid Health Insurance*, 15.

13. "How Are the Bills Paid?" *Time*, February 8, 1954, http://www.time.com/time/magazine/article/0,9171,860391,00.html.

14. "Memorandum to the Executive Committee from W. H. P. Blandy," May 15, 1950, Box 5, Papers of George Bugbee, AHARC. Later in the century, HIF moved away from its PR activities to focus on academic research, becoming the Center for Health Administration Studies at the University of Chicago.

15. Health Information Foundation, press release, February 13, 1956, Folder 4–18–3–10, Central File, 1953–57, Box 639, Records of the Children's Bureau, National Archives.

16. Health Information Foundation, "Six Letters to Business Leaders: 'Our Stake in Voluntary Health Insurance.' A Project in the Public Interest Sponsored by: HIF," n.d., ca. 1952, Box 10, Bugbee Papers, AHARC.

17. Executive Committee Minutes, March 25, 1955, Box 6, Bugbee Papers, AHARC.

18. Health Information Foundation, no title, n.d., Box 10, Bugbee Papers, AHARC.

19. Enthoven and Fuchs, "Employment-Based Health Insurance," 1540.

20. Social Research, *Attitudes toward Health Insurance*, 26.

21. Health Insurance Institute, *Profile of the Health Insurance Public*, 15.

22. Ibid., 17.

23. Social Research, *Attitudes toward Health Insurance*, 26, 29.

24. Health Insurance Institute, *Profile of the Health Insurance Public*, 20, 28.

25. Frank McLean to Lister Hill, November 19, 1954, Lister Hill Papers, University of Alabama.

26. "Second Meeting of a Series Sponsored by the Health Information Foundation. November 5–6, New York," Box 6, Bugbee Papers, AHARC (hereafter HIF Proceedings 2).

27. Follmann, *Voluntary Health Insurance and Medical Care*, 57.

28. Irv Osthoff, East St. Louis, IL, to Rep. Melvin Price, n.d., ca. 1967, Folder 4–18–3–10, Central File, 1967–68, Box 1156, Records of the Children's Bureau, National Archives. Osthoff could not get coverage for his mentally disabled child. See also DeJong, Batavia, and Griss, "America's Neglected Health Minority," 330–33.

29. Health Insurance Council, "The Health Insurance Story," self-published, 1955, AHARC, 45.

30. In the 2000s, insurance companies went to great lengths to assert that a condition developing years after a policy was sold, including cancer, high blood pressure, and even minor conditions, was actually "pre-existing." See Lisa Girion, "Blue Cross Praised Employees Who Dropped Sick Policyholders, Lawmaker Says," *Los Angeles Times*, June 17, 2009, LAtimes.com. This type of rescission became a target of the Obama health reform law in 2010, as did the practice of exclusion based on preexisting conditions. See epilogue.

31. Not just Blue Cross and indemnity insurance, but most major medical plans excluded "normal maternity" (as opposed to maternity complications). Follmann, *Voluntary Health Insurance and Medical Care*, 57. In the 1970s, two-fifths of plans still did not include maternity care; Hayden, "Gender Discrimination within the Reproductive Health Care System."

32. Klein, *For All These Rights*, 230; Robison, "Insurance Plans of the American Cast Iron Pipe Company," 12; Kessler-Harris, *In Pursuit of Equity*, 247.

33. HIF Proceedings 2, 92.

34. "Proceedings: First Meeting in a Series Sponsored by the Health Information Foundation, September 17 and 18, 1953, Princeton, N.J.," 100, Box 6, Bugbee Papers, AHARC (hereafter HIF Proceedings 1).

35. *Proceedings: National Congress on Prepaid Health Insurance*, 118.

36. Thomasson, "Racial Differences in Health Insurance Coverage and Medical Expenditures," 533; Gordon, *Dead on Arrival*, 192. On the history of racial discrimination by US insurance companies, see Hoffman, "Scientific Racism, Insurance, and Opposition to the Welfare State"; Haller, "Race, Mortality, and Life Insurance."

37. Stone, "Struggle for the Soul of Health Insurance."

38. Health Insurance Council, "Health Insurance Story."

39. Starr, *Social Transformation*, 323; "Prepaid Health Care Cuts Hospital Time, Expert Says," press release, April 29, 1964, Group Health Assn.

40. HIF Proceedings 1, 109–11.

41. Al Hayes, Machinists Union, *Proceedings: National Congress on Prepaid Health Insurance*, 112.

42. Address by Robert E. Van Goor, "Medical Rights Conference, 20 February 1954," File Drawer B-1, "Cooperatives," Michael M. Davis Papers, NYAM. The magazine was *Today's Woman*.

43. *Family Medical Care*, 54.

44. Freidson and Feldman, *Public Attitudes toward Health Insurance*, 12.

45. Kenneth Williamson, "Proceedings—Insurance Meeting, Health Information Foundation," Hampshire House, New York, February 12, 1954, 132, Bugbee Papers, AHARC. Hereafter HIF Proceedings 3.

46. HIF Proceedings 1, 116–17, 232–33. Although speakers are identified by surname in the transcripts, there is no separate list of participants or their affiliations. I have been able to identify the full name and affiliation of some but not all of the participants.

47. HIF Proceedings 1, 96–97, 105.

48. Blandy, HIF Proceedings 1, 233.

49. Follmann, HIF Proceedings 1, 102.

50. Starr, *Social Transformation*, 330.

51. Welch, Normal A., *Proceedings: National Congress on Prepaid Health Insurance*.

52. *Proceedings: National Congress on Prepaid Health Insurance*, 114.

53. Ibid., 97.

54. Klein, *For All These Rights*, 242.

55. Hall, "Deductibles in Health Insurance."

56. HIF Proceedings 3, 105; HIF Proceedings 1, 234.

57. *Family Medical Care*, 68.

58. E. J. Faulkner, *Proceedings: Third National Congress on Voluntary Health Insurance and Prepayment*, 20.

59. Cunningham and Cunningham, *Blues*, 95; Somers and Somers, *Doctors, Patients, and Health Insurance*, 284. For a more detailed discussion of the history of coinsurance, see Hoffman, "Restraining the Health Care Consumer" (excerpted with permission of Duke University Press).

60. Klein, *For All These Rights*, 241–43.

61. Reed and Carr, *Benefit Structure of Private Health Insurance*, 75–76; United States Senate, *Blue Cross and Private Health Insurance Coverage of Older Americans*.

62. Follman, *Voluntary Health Insurance and Medical Care*, 57.

63. Social Research, *Attitudes Toward Health Insurance*, 53–55.

64. Ibid., 52, 56–57.

65. Ibid., 55–56.

66. Ibid., 9, 55–56.

67. *Family Medical Care*, 85–88.

68. Margolius, *Consumer's Guide to Health Insurance Plans*, 23.

69. Anderson, *Voluntary Health Insurance in Two Cities*, 43.

70. Margolius, *Consumer's Guide to Health Insurance Plans*, 23.

71. *Family Medical Care*, 124–25.

72. Margolius, *Consumer's Guide to Health Insurance Plans*, 23; Brecher and Brecher, *How to Get the Most out of Medical and Hospital Benefit Plans*, 16–18.

73. James Brindle, "Medical Rights Conference, 20 February 1954," File Drawer B-1, "Cooperatives," Michael M. Davis Papers, NYAM.

74. "Unions Hit Blue Cross Rate Boost," *A. F. of L. Milwaukee Labor Press*, January 27, 1955; Jerome Pollack, "Major Medical Expense Insurance: An Evaluation," presented to APHA, November 15, 1956, Folder "Major Medical Insurance (Catastrophic)," Davis Papers, NYAM.

75. Raymond Munts, "Catastrophic Illness Insurance: A Barrier . . . on the Road to Health," AFL-CIO Publication, no. 51, May 1957, Folder "Major Medical Insurance (Catastrophic)," Davis Papers, NYAM.

76. Margolius, *Consumer's Guide to Health Insurance Plans*, 11.

77. HIF Proceedings 3, 31.

78. "Proceedings—Voluntary Health Insurance Discussion," October 21–22, 1954, New York City, 141, Box 6, Bugbee Papers, AHARC. This meeting was fourth and last in the series.

79. Cunningham and Cunningham, *Blues*: 103–5.

80. AHA statistic, quoted in Kenneth G. Slocum, "Why You'll Pay More for Health Insurance," *Virgin Islands Daily News*, November 24, 1958, 2.

81. "Unions Hit Blue Cross Rate Boost."

82. Freeman, *Working-Class New York*, 134. See also Markowitz and Rosner, "Seeking Common Ground."

83. Klein, *For All These Rights*, 243.

84. HIF Proceedings 3, 12.

85. Stone, "Struggle for the Soul of Health Insurance."

86. HIF Proceedings 3, 156. On Oseroff, see Weeks and Berman, *Shapers of American Health Care Policy*, 173.

Chapter Six

1. "Annals of Legislation: Medicare."

2. Ball, "Perspectives on Medicare."

3. Quadagno, *One Nation, Uninsured*, 55–58; Oberlander, *Political Life of Medicare*, 28.

4. "40 Elderly Persons Ask Higher Benefits," *New York Times*, October 15, 1959, 26; Claude Sittons, "More Federal Aid for Aging Sought," *New York Times*, December 1, 1959, 22.

5. Blumenthal and Morone, *Heart of Power*, 144.

6. Oberlander, *Political Life of Medicare*, 28.

7. Goldmann, "Problem: The Role of the Federal Government," 162.

8. Somers and Somers, *Doctors, Patients, and Health Insurance*, 439.

9. United States Senate, *Subcommittee on Health of the Elderly to the Special Committee on Aging*, 3.

10. Mrs. Jessie O'Rourke, Indianola, OK to Carl Albert, April 26, 1962, Carl Albert Collection, Box 54, Folder 85; Josephine S. Woods, Tulsa, to Carl Albert, May 29, 1962, Carl Albert Collection, Box 55, Folder 17, both in Albert Center; Mrs. I. (J?) Ehrlich, Montgomery, to Lister Hill, February 23, 1965, Lister Hill Papers, University of Alabama.

11. Mrs. Joseph Tomisek, "Medicare Issue," *Chicago Daily Tribune*, April 29, 1962, 20.

12. Quadagno, *One Nation, Uninsured*, 63–70.

13. Kennedy, "Address at New York Rally in Support of the President's Program of Medical Care for the Aged," 151.

14. Laurence Burd, "Kennedy: Back Medic Bill," *Chicago Daily Tribune*, May 21, 1962, 1; "Mass Senior Citizens' Rally to Support Kennedy's Bill," *Chicago Defender*, May 5, 1962, 5.

15. Marmor, *Politics of Medicare*, 38.

16. Reagan's speech contained the timeless statement that was quoted out of context by vice presidential candidate Sarah Palin in 2008: "If you don't do this and if I don't do it, one of these days you and I are going to spend our sunset years telling our children and our children's children, what it once was like in America when men were free." *Ronald Reagan Speaks Out Against Socialized Medicine*; "Dear Auxiliary Member," April 15, 1961, in possession of the author. I am grateful to Gretchen Galbraith for her gift of the original LP record, transcript, letter, and instructions.

17. "Medical Care Plan Leaders, AMA Clash," *Chicago Tribune*, August 3, 1961, w6.

18. R. J. Rose to Page Belcher, July 2, 1962, Box 70, Folder 36, Page H. Belcher

Collection; Loyde D. McCamry to Tom Steed, May 21, 1962, Tom Steed Collection, Box 26, Folder 11, Albert Center.

19. "Medical Care for the Aged," *Daily Defender*, August 25, 1960, 12.

20. "Reuther Gives His Support to Medicare," *Chicago Daily Tribune*, May 26, 1962, 14.

21. Quoted in Marmor, *Politics of Medicare*, 31.

22. Quadagno, *One Nation, Uninsured*, 72.

23. Quadagno, *One Nation, Uninsured*, 67.

24. Natalie Jaffe, "Hundreds Attend Hearing for Aged," *New York Times*, January 19, 1964, 63.

25. "Transcript of President's News Conference on Foreign and Domestic Matters," *New York Times*, April 26, 1964, 64; Robyn Muncy, "Coal-Fired Reforms: Social Citizenship, Dissident Miners, and the Great Society," *Journal of American History* 96, no. 1 (2009): 72–98.

26. Beschloss, *Reaching for Glory*, 160.

27. Jackie Robinson, "Jackie Robinson Says," *Chicago Defender*, June 30, 1962, 8.

28. "NMA Revolts; Backs Medicare," *Chicago Defender*, August 18, 1962, 1.

29. "Doctors Urged to Provide Leadership in Fight on Medical Discrimination," *Chicago Defender*, November 17, 1962, 3.

30. Martin Luther King Jr., "Civil Right No. 1: The Right to Vote," *New York Times*, March 14, 1965, SM26.

31. For vivid descriptions of the negotiations, see Blumenthal and Morone, *Heart of Power*, chap. 5, and Berkowitz, *Mr. Social Security*, chap. 10.

32. Quadagno, *One Nation, Uninsured*, 75.

33. "Statement of the President Following the Passage of the Medicare Bill by the Senate," July 9, 1965, CMS Speeches, 16.

34. Poen, *Truman vs. the Medical Lobby*, 1.

35. "Signing of Medicare Bill Hailed by NMA Head," *Chicago Defender*, August 7, 1965, 31; "Lauds NMA Doctors on Medicare Stand," *Daily Defender*, August 19, 1965, 10; Hoffman, "Challenge of Universal Health Care."

36. Quadagno, *One Nation, Uninsured*, 92.

37. Smith, *Health Care Divided*, 154–59.

38. J. T. Blasingame Jr., MD, "A Message from the President of the Atlanta Medical Assn.," July 5, 1966, Box 8, Berry Papers, CHM.

39. Smith, *Health Care Divided*, 153–54.

40. Dr. Otis W. Smith and Dr. A. M. Davis comments, untitled typescript (transcript of meeting on Title XI compliance), July 6, 1966, Box 8, Berry Papers, CHM.

41. L. E. Reynolds, Sheffield, Alabama, to Lister Hill, November 10, 1960, Hill Papers.

42. Quadagno, *One Nation, Uninsured*, 98; Oberlander, *Political Life of Medicare*, 109–10.

43. Louis Cassels, "LBJ Warns Hospitals on Bias in Medicare," *Daily Defender*, June 16, 1966, 7.

44. Quadagno, *One Nation, Uninsured*, 98–102; Martin Tolchin, "Doctors' Fees Up as Much as 300% under Medicare," *New York Times*, August 19, 1966, 1.

45. "Medicare Means $7,200 More for Me," *Medical Economics*, September 4, 1967, 156; "Doctors' Fees Up as Much as 300%."

46. Statement of Dr. William A. Nolen, "Costs and Delivery of Health Services to Older Americans," 37, 41.

47. Johnson, "Remarks Before the Annual Convention of the National Medical Association," 52; Starr, *Social Transformation*, 384; Catherine Rampell, "How Much Do Doctors in Other Countries Make?" *Economix* blog, newyorktimes.com, July 15, 2009, http://economix.blogs.nytimes.com/2009/07/15/how-much-do-doctors-in-other-countries-make/; Stevens, *In Sickness and in Wealth*, 286–87.

48. "Television Tape for Medicare," March 15, 1966, Folder 1s1 Accident-Hospital-Medical-Health-11/22/63–3/23/66, EX 1s Box 1, LBJ Library.

49. Thomas J. Lane, Governor's Councillor, State House, Boston, to The President, August 5, 1966; Ivan Allen, Mr., Mayor, City of Atlanta to the President, July 18, 1966, 1s 1 7/15/66 – 8/19/66, GEN 1s 1 12/9/65 Box 3, LBJ Library.

50. Mr. and Mrs. Joseph Sharp, Citrus Heights, CA, to LBJ, October 6, 1966, 1s 1 8/20/66 – 12/31/66; Mrs. Florence Franklin, Glendale, CA, to LBJ, June 10, 1967, 1s1 1/16/67 – 3/31/67, GEN 1s 1 12/9/65 Box 3, LBJ Library.

51. Oberlander, *Political Life of Medicare*, 37–40; "Medicare: A Timeline of Key Developments," Kaiser Family Foundation, http://www.kff.org/medicare/timeline/pf_entire.htm.

52. "The Effect of Deductibles, Coinsurance and Copayment on Utilization of Health Care Services—Opinions and Impressions from Blue Cross and Blue Shield Plans," 1971, Box 8, Folder 20, CNH1 Collection, Reuther Library.

53. Margaret Rackley to George Wallace, October 25, 1978, Folder 4, Box SG4493, Alabama Governor's Files, Alabama State Archives.

54. "New Douglas Bill Would Include Drugs in Medicare," *Daily Defender*, July 6, 1966, 8.

55. Oberlander, *Political Life of Medicare*, 40.

56. "'Medicare Booster' Plan Bows," *Daily Defender*, March 15, 1966, 10.

57. "Statement of the Health Insurance Association of America on the Marketing of Medicare Supplementary Policies," n.d. (1970s), Folder 9–25, CNH1 Collection, Reuther Library.

58. Jack and Susan Smith, Fresno, CA, to National Council for Senior Citizens, February 15, 1977, Folder 11–56; James F. Jessee, Lakewood, CO, to Mr. Woodcock, n.d.; Folder 11–56, "Conference Witnesses—Originals," ca. 1977, Folder 22–15, all in CNH1 Collection, Reuther Library.

59. Jessee to Woodcock; Lloyd Smith, Cave Junction, OR, to CNH1, January 23, 1975, Folder 48–5, CNH1 Collection, Reuther Library. I have standardized unusual spellings in these letters.

60. Leslie Shaver to National Council of Senior Citizens, January 25, 1976, Folder 11–56, CNH1 Collection, Reuther Library.

61. Mrs. E. S. Webster, San Antonio, February 17, 1967, to LBJ, 1s1 1/16/67 – 3/31/67, GEN 1s 1 12/9/65 Box 3, LBJ Library.

62. R. Hirsch to Nelson Cruikshank, March 10, 1977, Folder 11–56, CNHI Collection, Reuther Library.

63. Carl Rhoades, Sullivan, MO, "Dear Sir," n.d., Folder 11–56, CNHI Collection, Reuther Library.

64. MCHR press release, "Heads of Three National Medical Organizations Hit AMA Stand on Health Questions," June 25, 1967, MCHR, Year 67, Box 33, ISM.

65. Moore and Smith, "Legislating Medicaid."

66. Quoted in Poen, *Truman vs. the Medical Lobby*, 97n16.

67. Committee for the Nation's Health, "The Negro, the Government, and Medical Care," n.d., ca. 1946, File Drawer C-4, "Negro Health," Davis Papers, NYAM.

68. "Tax Supported Medical Care for the Needy," 1312.

69. "Hubert and the Means Test."

70. *Medical Assistance for the Aged*, 4.

71. R. J. Rose, Ponca City, OK, to Page Belcher, July 2, 1962, Box 70, Folder 36, Page H. Belcher Collection, Albert Center.

72. Stevens and Stevens, *Welfare Medicine in America*, 45.

73. Stevens and Stevens, *Welfare Medicine in America*, 35; *Medical Assistance for the Aged*, 8.

74. Rosemary and Robert Stevens put it well: "Medicaid's structure embraced the evident flaws of Kerr-Mills as the price of its political acceptability." Stevens and Stevens, *Welfare Medicine in America*, 349.

75. "Title 19," *Chicago Tribune*, July 24, 1966.

76. Grogan and Patashnik, "Between Welfare Medicine and Mainstream Entitlement," 825–26.

77. Engel, *Poor People's Medicine*; Reuters, "Medicaid Improves Health and Budgets of Poor."

78. Testimony of Mrs. Bessie Goodwin, "US Dept. of Health, Education and Welfare, Public Medicaid Hearings, New York City, December 27, 1968," 484–85, Box 1, Papers of Wilbur J. Cohen, LBJ Library (hereafter Cohen Papers); Hoffman, "Don't Scream Alone," excerpted with permission of Rutgers University Press.

79. Testimony of Ethel Mae Matthews, Pin Ria Stinton, and Rev. Austin Ford, all of Atlanta, "Public Hearing on Medicaid, Atlanta, Georgia, December 20, 1968," 16–28, Box 1, Cohen Papers.

80. Testimony of Mrs. Lucy Priggs, "Hearings on Medicaid, Washington, DC, December 30, 1968," 181, Box 2, Cohen Papers.

81. Testimony of Mrs. Odell Young, "HEW Hearings on Medicaid, Columbus, Ohio, December 30, 1968," 167–68, 171, Box 3, Cohen Papers.

82. Ibid., 167–68.

83. "Hearings on Medicaid, Washington, DC, December 30, 1968," 181–88, Box 2, Cohen Papers.

84. "Hearings on Medicaid, San Francisco, December 27, 1968," 108–10, Box 3, Cohen Papers.

85. Testimony of Mrs. Flanagan, "Hearings on Medicaid, Washington, DC, December 30, 1968," Box 2, Cohen Papers.

86. Mrs. Espanola Jackson, "Hearings on Medicaid, San Francisco, December 27, 1968," Cohen Papers.

87. "Hearings on Medicaid, Washington, DC," 189–90, Cohen Papers.

88. "Conference Witnesses—Originals," ca. 1976, Folder 22–15, CNHI Collection, Reuther Library.

89. News clipping, *Huntsville Times*, n.d., in Box SG 4493, Folder 3, Alabama Governor Correspondence, Alabama State Archives.

90. Medical Services Administration, "Medicaid Impact," December 11, 1978, Folder 5, Box SG 4493, Alabama Governor Correspondence, Alabama State Archives.

91. Richard L. Peck, "Can They Make You See Medicaid Patients?" *Medical Economics*, July 11, 1977, 218–24; Hans G. Engel, MD, "Sorry, No More Medicaid Patients for Me," *Medical Economics*, November 11, 1974, 194–95, 201; Wheeler A. Gunnels, MD, to W. H. Kerns, October 25, 1979, Folder 5, Box SG 4493, Alabama Governor Correspondence, Alabama State Archives.

Chapter Seven

1. Leonidas Berry, "The Days of Our Year," NMA Report, August 9, 1966, Box 9, Berry Papers, CHM.

2. Clarence Mitchell and Marilyn G. Rose, "The Failure of the US Department of Health, Education and Welfare to Enforce Title VI of the Civil Rights Act of 1964 with Respect to Health Facilities." Statement of the Health Care Task Force, Leadership Conference on Civil Rights, n.d., ca. 1972, Box 129, Records of the Leadership Conference on Civil Rights I, Library of Congress (hereafter LCCR).

3. "'Direct Action' Planned against Hospital Bias Here, King Says," *Chicago Sun-Times*, March 26, 1966, 12.

4. Leonidas H. Berry, "Human Rights and Regional Medical Programs"; Howard B. Woods, "Weaver Joins Dr. King, Raps SNCC Chiefs," *Daily Defender*, August 9, 1967, 1.

5. Betty Washington, "Hospital Bias in Chicago Blamed for Girl's Death," *Chicago Defender*, November 11, 1967, 1.

6. "Altgeld-Murray Homes, Chicago Housing Authority," Box 66, Folder 10, Welfare Council, CHM.

7. Thomas Picou, "Baby's Death May Eliminate Hospital Bias," *Daily Defender*, February 8, 1968, 4. On Tuskegee, see, for example, Washington, *Medical Apartheid*; Reverby, *Examining Tuskegee*.

8. Mitchell and Rose, "Failure of the US Department of Health, Education and Welfare to Enforce Title VI of the Civil Rights Act of 1964."

9. Office of Don Edwards, press release, September 13, 1973, Box 1: 129, LCCR.

10. On the role of legal services attorneys in the War on Poverty, see Davis, *Brutal Need*.

11. Law, "A Right to Health Care That Cannot Be Taken Away."

12. "Court Cases Filed to Test Right to Health Services."

13. *Cook v. Ochsner Foundation Hospital.*

14. "Poor Protest HEW Changes in Free Care Guidelines."

15. Dowell, "Unfulfilled Promise," 154.

16. Law, "Right to Health Care That Cannot Be Taken Away."

17. Kornbluh, *Battle for Welfare Rights*, 2; Toney, "Revisiting the National Welfare Rights Organization." NWRO occasionally claimed up to 75,000 members, but this included participants who were not dues paying.

18. "Conference Committee on Health Rights, Recommendations to NWRO National Executive Board, ca. 1970," NWRO Papers.

19. "The National Welfare Rights Organization Demands," 1970, Medical Committee for Human Rights, Box 39, NWRO Papers.

20. Hoffman, "'Don't Scream Alone.'"

21. *Modern Hospital* (October 1970): 30–32.

22. Ibid.

23. Ibid.

24. Annas, *Rights of Hospital Patients*, 25–27.

25. Joan Beck, "Civil Rights Overdue for Hospital Patients," *Chicago Tribune*, December 13, 1974, A2.

26. "Acceptance Held Lagging on Patients' Bill of Rights," *Hospital Practice* 9 (February 1974): 56.

27. John F. Horty, "Hospitals Must Adopt Patient Bill of Rights," *Modern Hospital* (June 1973): 33–34.

28. Lee Dembart, "Follow-Up on the News," *New York Times*, June 16, 1974, 29.

29. Kornbluh, *Battle for Welfare Rights*, chap. 7; Silver interview.

Patients' bills of rights did become ubiquitous, but bore little resemblance to the NWRO's demands and excluded a right to access. In 2003 the American Hospital Association actually discontinued its Patients' Bill of Rights, replacing it with a list entitled "The Patient Care Partnership: Understanding Expectations, Rights and Responsibilities." The only "rights" specified in this document are a patient's right to know the identity of practitioners; the right to consent to or refuse treatment; and the right to decide to participate in a research study. The original Point Seven, about the right to care, has completely vanished, replaced by a requirement that the patient must provide information about insurance coverage.

30. Orleck, *Storming Caesar's Palace*, 211–20.

31. "Hospital Group Here Blasts HEW Official," *Daily Defender*, February 3, 1972, 1; Michael L. Culbert, "Dr. Thomas: Blacks Should Run Hospital," *Daily Defender*, January 27, 1972; "US Could Stem Hospital Crisis," *Daily Defender*, February 1, 1972, 2; "St. George Moves to End Discrimination," *Daily Defender*, April 17, 1973, 4.

32. Roger Wilkins, "The Problem of Hospitals' Flight to Suburbs," *New York Times*, February 24, 1978, A14; Clarence Mitchell to Joseph Califano, December 5, 1977, Box II, 41, LCCR; Smith, *Health Care Divided*, 178–79.

33. Smith, *Health Care Divided*, 183; Rose, "Can Hospital Relocations and Closures be Stopped through the Legal System?"

34. See, for example, Sardell, *US Experiment in Social Medicine*, 38–46.

35. For full-length discussions of the program, see Sardell, *US Experiment in Social Medicine*; Lefkowitz, *Community Health Centers*.

36. Nelson, "'Hold Your Head Up and Stick Out Your Chin'"; Dittmer, *Good Doctors*, 229–35.

37. Nelson, *Body and Soul*, 11, 77; Dittmer, *Good Doctors*.

38. Vincent K. Pollard, Chicago Health Research Group, September 2, 1971, "What If Daley Tries to Close Free Clinics Again?" MCHR, Year '70, Box 40, ISM.

39. "Move to Halt Clinic's Closing," *Daily Defender*, February 11, 1970, 2.

40. Dittmer, *Good Doctors*, 227.

41. Donald Janson, "Is Health Care a Right?" *New York Times*, July 2, 1967, 94.

42. Mitchell and Rose, "Failure of the US Department of Health, Education and Welfare to Enforce Title VI of the Civil Rights Act"; transcript of interview with Herbert K. Abrams, MD, February 3, 1993, Medicine and Health Care Delivery in Southern Arizona Oral History Project, 8, Arizona Historical Society.

43. On Latino activist movements, see, for example, MacLean, *Freedom Is Not Enough*, 163–84; Ramos, *American G.I. Forum*; Vargas, *Labor Rights Are Civil Rights*.

44. Abel, "'Only the Best Class of Immigration'"; Cervances, "Failure of Comprehensive Health Services to Serve the Urban Chicano."

45. Aranda, "The Mexican American Syndrome."

46. Ibid.

47. "United Farmworkers' Union Delano Clinic," *El Chicano*, December 7, 1972, 4, Readex Hispanic American Newspapers.

48. "Health Is a Human Right," *El Grito del Norte* (Las Vegas, New Mexico), May 1, 1973, 4, Readex Hispanic American Newspapers.

49. "Lords Give Free X-Rays," July 5, 1970, *El Grito del Norte*, 10, Readex Hispanic American Newspapers.

50. "Lords Give Free X-Rays"; "New Barrio Group Is Born," *El Grito del Norte*, June 1, 1973, 6, Readex Hispanic American Newspapers.

51. "NCHO Seeks Better Chicano Health," *El Chicano*, April 5, 1973, 4, Readex Hispanic American Newspapers.

52. Philip Vargas to Fernando Del Rio, May 12, 1970, Papers of Ernesto Galarza M224, Box 57, Stanford Special Collections.

53. Hogan and Hartson to Hon. Joseph A. Califano, June 15, 1978, Box 41, Folder 10, LCCR II, Library of Congress.

54. Quoted in Warner and Tighe, *Major Problems*, 502.

55. Morgen, *Into Our Own Hands*, 71–73.

56. Ibid., 128–29.

57. See Linda Gordon, *The Moral Property of Women; A History of Birth Control Politics in America*, (Champaign: University of Illinois Press, 2002).

58. Nelson, *Women of Color*; Nelson, "'Hold Your Head Up and Stick Out Your Chin,'" 99.

59. Roth, *Building Bridges*, 24.

60. Olga M. Madar, "Discrimination against Women in Current Health Insurance Programs," Women's Leadership Rally, March 1976, Folder 31–1, Box 31, CNHI.

61. On the MCHR, see Dittmer, *The Good Doctors*; Mullan, *White Coat, Clenched Fist*.

62. Fein, "The Medical Care Section 1994–2005," 838; Ehrenreich and Ehrenreich, *American Health Empire*, vii.

63. For example, Rothman, *Strangers at the Bedside*.

64. Rogers, "Caution," 25.

65. Nancy Tomes, "Patients or Health-Care Consumers? Why the History of Contested Terms Matters," in Stevens, Rosenberg, and Burns, *History and Health Policy*; Cohen, *Consumers' Republic*.

66. "Consumer Directory of Doctors Is Issued by Nader in Maryland," *New York Times*, January 18, 1974, 8; Hoffman, "Challenge of Universal Health Care" (excerpted with permission of Oxford University Press).

67. Freese, *Managing Your Doctor*; Levin, *Talk Back to Your Doctor*; Wolfe, *Pills That Don't Work*.

68. Gregg, *Health Insurance Racket*; Hoyt, *Your Health Insurance*; Law, *Blue Cross: What Went Wrong?*

69. Schorr, *Don't Get Sick in America*, 92. National Broadcasting Corporation, "What Price Health? NBC Reports," broadcast December 19, 1972, 15–17, transcript in Folder 11–41, CNHI Collection.

70. *Miller v. Davis*; Morris, *AARP*.

71. Kennedy, *In Critical Condition*, 146.

72. Jesse W. Baldwin to Edward M. Kennedy, June 18, 1972, Box 48, Folder 7, CNHI Collection; Mrs. R. W. Ferdman, to Nelson Cruikshank, February 10, Folder 11–56, CNHI Collection.

73. Madar, "Discrimination against Women"; Document 41: "Plank 14: Insurance," from National Commission on the Observance of International Women's Year, *The Spirit of Houston: The First National Women's Conference* (Washington, DC: US Government Printing Office, 1978), 60–62; http://womhist.alexanderstreet.com/dp59/doc41.htm.

74. Cunningham and Cunningham, *Blues*, 176–77.

75. "The Horrible Herb Show," *Time*, September 13, 1976; "They Are All Afraid of Herb the Horrible," *Time*, July 10, 1972; www.time.com.

76. Richard D. Lyons, "Americans Now Favor a National Health Plan," *New York Times*, August 9, 1971, 1.

77. Blumenthal and Morone, *The Heart of Power*, 222.

78. Ibid., 116–17.

79. Quadagno, *One Nation, Uninsured*, 116.

80. "What Price Health?"

81. Tom Lawrence, "AFL-CIO Council Dismisses Nixon Health Care Program," *Daily Defender*, May 13, 1971, 4.

82. "What Price Health?"

83. Richard D. Lyons, "Nixon Is Criticized by Auto Union Head over Health Care," *New York Times*, February 24, 1971, 64; Richard D. Lyons, "AMA Presents Its Plan for Health Insurance," *New York Times*, February 26, 1971, 18.

84. Quadagno, *One Nation, Uninsured*, 120–22.

85. "Medicine: Health Care: Supply, Demand and Politics," *Time*, June 7, 1971; Blumenthal and Morone, *Heart of Power*, chap. 7; Richard D. Lyons, "Carter Proposes Law for Tough Controls on Hospital Charges," *New York Times*, April 26, 1977, 81.

86. Quadagno, *One Nation, Uninsured*, 125–28.

87. Quoted in Blumenthal and Morone, *Heart of Power*, 273.

88. Richard D. Lyons, "Rx for Health Care: The Cost Is Staggering," *New York Times*, December 17, 1978, E4.

89. Tom Wicker, "The Health Insurance Minefield," *New York Times*, December 20, 1977, 35.

90. Committee on Technology and Health Care, *Medical Technology and the Health Care System*; Schwartz, "Societal Responsibility for Malpractice"; Cunningham and Cunningham, *Blues*, 175; Wilson, Feldman, and Kovar, "Continuing Trends in Health and Health Care"; Foley, "Editorial: Cost Containment Begins at Home."

91. Fein, *Medical Care, Medical Costs*, 151.

Chapter Eight

1. Fern Schumer and R. C. Longworth, "County Hospital at the Brink," *Chicago Tribune*, May 2, 1982, 33, 40.

2. Schiff et al., "Transfers to a Public Hospital."

3. Judith Feder and Jack Hadley, "Cutbacks, Recession, and Hospitals' Care for the Urban Poor," in Peterson and Lewis, *Reagan and the Cities*, 38.

4. "Ronald Reagan Speaks Out against Socialized Medicine."

5. Heritage Foundation, *Mandate for Leadership: The Project Report on the Department of Health and Human Services*, quoted in Geri Dallek, "Health 'Hit List' Sent to Reagan," *Health Advocate* 117 (February 1981): 1–2.

6. Bernard Weinraub, "Health Chief Gives Plans to Cut Costs," *New York Times*, June 12, 1981, B6; Sandra Blakeslee, "Coast Parley on Medicare and Medicaid Opens amid Protests," *New York Times*, June 20, 1985, B11.

7. Emily Friedman, "The 'Dumping' Dilemma: The Poor Are Always with Some of Us," *Hospitals* (September 1, 1982): 51–56.

8. Betty Washington, "Andelman, Kozoll Attack a Major Health Problem," *Chicago Daily Defender*, January 29, 1968, 5.

9. Friedman, "'Dumping' Dilemma."

10. Ibid., 51–56; Ronald Sullivan, "Care of Poor Is Cut by Private Hospitals," *New York Times*, May 30, 1982, 1.

11. "Hospital Finances Now Sound, but Fund for Poor Is Assailed," *Courier-Journal* (Louisville, KY), undated clipping, (ca. 1985), File 4, Box 170, Mannix Papers, AHARC.

12. Schumer and Longworth, "County Hospital at the Brink."

13. "Dumping the Poor," *American Bar Association Journal* 71 (March 1985): 25; Margaret Engel, "Hospitals Refusing to Admit Poor; Patients Transferred to DC General," *Washington Post*, October 15, 1984, B1.

14. Ansell and Schiff, "Patient Dumping"; Himmelstein et al, "Patient Transfers"; Friedman, "'Dumping' Dilemma."

15. Bard Lineman, "Some Hospitals Turn Away Uninsured Sick People," *Miami Herald*, April 22, 1985, D2; Daniel C. Carson, "Lawmakers Seen near Legislation on 'Patient Dumping,'" *San Diego Union-Tribune*, July 27, 1987, A-3.

16. Kenan Heise, "'Dumping' the Poor at County Hospital Angers Staff," *Chicago Tribune*, September 3, 1982, B3.

17. Larry A. Bedard, Charlotte S. Yeh, and Robert A. Bitterman, "The History of EMTALA," in Bitterman, *Providing Emergency Care under Federal Law*, 7–9.

18. "Equal Access to Health Care," 7.

19. 42 USC 1395dd; COBRA Section 9121; Section 1867 of the Social Security Act.

20. Bedard, Yeh, and Bitterman, "History of EMTALA," 8; Testimony of Lois Salisbury on behalf of Coalition to Stop Patient Dumping, "Equal Access to Health Care," 257–69.

21. "Hospital Faced Penalties for Alleged Dumping," AHA *News*, April 6, 1987, 3.

22. Lauren A. Dame, "The Emergency Medical Treatment and Active Labor Act," *Health Matrix: Journal of Law-Medicine* 8, no. 3 (Winter, 1998); "Equal Access to Health Care," 4.

23. Jack W. Owen, "'Dumping' Charges Reflect Hospitals' Current Financial Stress," AHA *News*, April 6, 1987, 4.

24. Bradford B. Burnett, "To the Editor," *Journal of the American Medical Association* 258, no. 1 (1987): 42, doi: 10.1001 / jama.1987.

25. "Equal Access to Health Care," 101.

26. "Uncompensated Hospital Care."

27. Weinraub, "Health Chief Gives Plans to Cut Costs"; Blakeslee, "Coast Parley on Medicare and Medicaid."

28. John Greenwald, "Those Sky-High Health Costs," *Time* Magazine, July 12, 1982.

29. Frank E. Samuel Jr., President, Health Industry Manufacturers Assn., "To the Editor," *New York Times*, November 11, 1985, A18.

30. Rosenberg and Browne, "Impact of the Inpatient Prospective Payment System and Diagnosis Related Groups," 88.

31. "Equal Access to Health Care," 9.

32. "Medicaid and Medicare Expenditures," http://www.bcbs.com / blueresources / mcrg / chapter2 / ch2_slide_21.html; Boccuti and Moon, "Comparing Medicare and Private Insurers." On the history of Medicare regulation, see Oberlander, *Political Life of Medicare*, 120–26.

33. The amount of cost shifting varied depending on the type of hospital; hos-

pitals with fewer insured patients were less able to engage in the practice. Wu, "Hospital Cost Shifting Revisited."

34. Oberlander, *Political Life of Medicare*, 53–73; Quadagno, *One Nation, Uninsured*, 149–59.

35. For example, Brandt, *No Magic Bullet*.

36. "Panel Finds No Valid Excuse for Not Treating AIDS Case," *New York Times*, September 22, 1983, 22; Michael T. Isbell, "AIDS and Access to Care: Lessons for Health Care Reformers," *Cornell Journal of Law and Public Policy* 3, no. 1 (1993): 44.

37. Susan Duerksen, "Ethics Crisis: AIDS Patients Denied Care by Some Doctors," *San Diego Union-Tribune*, September 30, 1987, A-1.

38. "Equal Access to Health Care," 3.

39. On the history of Ward 5B, see Risse, *Mending Bodies, Saving Souls*, chap. 12.

40. Isbell, "AIDS and Access to Care," 14–15.

41. Howard H. Hiatt, "Why Did Wilson Roberts Have to Suffer Needlessly?" *New York Times*, August 9, 1988, clipping in ACT UP/NY Records, NYPL.

42. Jonathan Freedman, "Insurers Put Our Health at Risk," *Los Angeles Times*, November 19, 1990, clipping in ACT UP / NY Records.

43. *Kenneth Westhoven v. Lincoln Foodservice Products Inc.*, State of Indiana Civil Rights Commission, December 3, 1990; Beverly Gaucher, "PWA Sues Storehouse over AIDS Cap," *Southern Voice*, November 22, 1992, ACT UP / NY Records.

44. Wayne Kawadler to R. Steve Bell, November 19, 1990, Box 41, Folder 2, ACT UP / NY Records.

45. Great Republic Insurance Company, "Agent Guidelines," n.d., Box 41, Folder 3, ACT UP / NY Records.

46. Bayer, *Private Acts, Social Consequences*, 257.

47. Epstein, *Impure Science*.

48. Orland Outland to John Garamendi, December 3, 1990, and January 18, 1991, Box 41, Folder 2, ACT UP / NY Records.

49. ACT UP / NY Chronology, http://www.actupny.org/documents/cron-90.html; "DC Marchers Fault Insurance Industry's Approach to AIDS," *Washington Post*, May 14, 1991, B2.

50. Henry J. Kaiser Family Foundation, "Ryan White Comprehensive AIDS Resources Emergency Act," November 2008, http://www.kff.org/hivaids/upload/7582.pdf.

51. ACT UP Healthcare Campaign Working Group, Memo #1 (n.d.), Box 42, File 1, ACT UP / NY Records.

52. "Medical Insurance Bill of Rights for People with HIV Disease," ACT UP/NY Records.

53. Isbell, "AIDS and Access to Care," 9–53.

54. Bruce Lambert, "Flaws in Health Care System Emerge as Epidemic Rages," *New York Times*, February 8, 1989, A1.

55. Bayer, *Private Acts, Social Consequences*, 258–60.

56. Lawrence K. Altman, "Deaths from AIDS Decline Sharply in New York City; Access to Care Is Cited," *New York Times*, January 25, 1997, 1.

57. "The Crisis in Health Insurance, Part 1," *Consumer Reports*, August 1990, 533–49.

58. US Department of Labor, "A Look at Employers' Costs of Providing Health Benefits," July 31, 1996, http://www.dol.gov/oasam/programs/history/reich/reports/costs.htm.

59. Statement of Barbara Lyons, Kaiser Commission on the Future of Medicaid, "Health Care Coverage for the Uninsured," Hearing of the US Senate Committee on Finance, February 20, 1994, http://www.archive.org/stream/healthcarecover-a00unit/healthcarecovera00unit_djvu.txt.

60. Quadagno, *One Nation, Uninsured*, 144; Milt Freudenheim, "A Health-Care Taboo is Broken," *New York Times*, May 8, 1989, D1.

61. US Department of Labor, "A Look at Employers' Costs of Providing Health Benefits," July 31, 1996, http://www.dol.gov/oasam/programs/history/reich/reports/costs.htm.

62. Daschle, *Critical*, 77.

63. Transcript of Speech by Clinton Accepting Democratic Nomination, *New York Times*, July 17, 1992, A14.

64. Robin Toner, "Hillary Clinton's Potent Brain Trust on Health Care Reform," *New York Times*, February 28, 1993.

65. Rhoda H. Karpatkin, "To the Editor," and Andres F. Costas, MD, "To the Editor," both *New York Times*, March 14, 1993, F11; Robert Pear, "White House Shuns Bigger AMA Voice in Health Changes," *New York Times*, March 5, 1993, A1.

66. Steffie Woolhandler and David U. Himmelstein, "Universal Care? Not from Clinton," *New York Times*, June 12, 1994, HR7; Blumenthal and Morone, *Heart of Power*, 374.

67. Quadagno, *One Nation, Uninsured*, 192; Robert Pear, "AMA Rebels over Health Plan in Major Challenge to the President," *New York Times*, September 30, 1993.

68. For a detailed discussion of the employer mandate, see Marie Gottschalk, *The Shadow Welfare State: Labor, Business, and the Politics of Health Care in the United States* (Ithaca: Cornell University Press, 2000).

69. Quadagno, *One Nation, Uninsured*, 190.

70. Hacker, *Road to Nowhere*, 87.

71. Hacker, *Road to Nowhere*, 100; Potter, *Deadly Spin*.

72. Skocpol, *Boomerang*, 137–38; "They're Back: Harry and Louise on Health Insurance," *USA Today*, August 18, 2008.

73. Blumenthal and Morone, *Heart of Power*, 375. Skocpol describes a "vacuum of top-level White House leadership" when it came to politics; Hacker writes that Clinton "had a bill but no coalition to defend it." Hacker, *Road to Nowhere*, 151.

Chapter Nine

1. Quadagno, *One Nation, Uninsured*, 196–97.

2. Lucy Ament, "SCHIP Seen Contributing to a Steep Drop in Number of Uninsured Children," *AHA News Now*, August 21, 2006.

3. "The American Uninsured Crisis," *State Legislatures* 35, no. 5 (May 2009); Quadagno, *One Nation, Uninsured*, 195.

4. "Number of Nonelderly Uninsured Americans, 1994–2006," Kaiser Fast Facts, http://www.kff.org.

5. "New Carsey Institute Report Finds That Over One-Third of Rural Children Rely on SCHIP and Medicaid," press release, May 10, 2007, http://www.unh.edu/news/cj_nr/2007/may/as10schip.cfm.

6. Sered and Fernandopulle, *Uninsured in America*.

7. Angel, Lein, and Henrici, *Poor Families in America's Health Care Crisis*, 89.

8. Elise Gould, "The Chronic Problem of Declining Coverage," EPI *Issue Brief* 202, Economic Policy Institute, September 16, 2004, http://www.epi.org/publications/entry/issuebrief202/.

9. Steven Findlay, "To Reform Health Care, Bust Myths," *USA Today*, May 13, 2003.

10. Institute of Medicine, *Care without Coverage*.

11. Skocpol, *Boomerang*, 168–71.

12. Anders, *Health against Wealth*, 244.

13. Bradford H. Gray, "The Rise and Decline of the HMO: A Chapter in US Health-Policy History," in Stevens, Rosenberg, and Burns, *History and Health Policy*, 315–28, quote on 323; Cohn, *Sick*, 66.

14. "Managed Care Museum Timeline," http://www.managedcaremuseum.com/timeline.htm. This number does not include enrollment in Preferred Provider Organizations, another, less restrictive, form of managed care.

15. Anders, *Health against Wealth*, 78–79; Spencer Rich, "Managed Care, Once an Elixir, Goes under the Legislative Knife," *Washington Post*, September 25, 1996.

16. Kavaler and Spiegel, *Risk Management in Health Care Institutions*, 387.

17. Potter, *Deadly Spin*, 24–25; Caroline Roche, Steven M. Shapiro, and Michael J. Painter, "Drive-By Deliveries Increase the Risk of Neonatal Brain Damage," *Neurology Today* 4, no. 3 (March 2004): 4.

18. Lillian Polak, "To the Editor," *New York Times*, November 20, 1998.

19. Public Citizen, "Hospital Emergency Rooms and Patient Dumping," press release, n.d., ca. 1998, http://www.citizen.org/publications/release.cfm?ID=4891.

20. George J. Church, Sam Allis, John F. Dickerson, et al., "Backlash against HMOs," *Time*, April 14, 1997; Illinois State Medical Society press release, November 25, 1996, http://www.managedcaremuseum.com/archives/Artc1102.htm.

21. Quadagno, *One Nation, Uninsured*, 162.

22. Ibid., 163; Church et al., "Backlash against HMOs."

23. Church et al, "Backlash against HMOs."

24. Peter D. Jacobsen, *Strangers in the Night: Law and Medicine in the Managed Care Era* (New York: Oxford University Press, 2002).

25. Church et al., "Backlash against HMOs."

26. Marc A. Rodwin, "Patient Appeals as Policy Disputes: Individual and Collective Action in Managed Care" in Hoffman et al., *Patients as Policy Actors*; Gray, "Rise and Decline of the HMO," 309.

27. Elizabeth Armstrong and Eugene DeClercq, "Is It Time to Push Yet?" in Hoffman et al., *Patients as Policy Actors*.

28. Church et al., "Backlash against HMOs;" Reinhardt, "The Predictable Managed Care Kvetch."

29. Mechanic, "Managed Care Backlash," 37.

30. Cohn, *Sick*, 84.

31. Henry J. Kaiser Family Foundation, *Health Care Costs: A Primer*, August 2007, 9, http://www.kff.org/insurance/upload/7670.pdf.

32. St. Louis presidential debate, October 17, 2000.

33. Second debate transcript, October 11, 2000, http://abcnews.go.com/Politics/story?id=122736&page=1.

34. Herzlinger, *Market-Driven Health Care*. For critiques of consumer-driven health care, see Mark Schlesinger, "The Dangers of the Market Panacea," in James A. Morone and Lawrence R. Jacobs, eds., *Healthy, Wealthy, and Fair: Health Care and the Good Society* (New York: Oxford University Press, 2007); Jost, *Health Care at Risk*: 93, 101.

35. For example, Robert Kuttner, "Bush's Troubling Medicare Plan," *American Prospect*, September 10, 2000, http://prospect.org/cs/articles?article=bushs_troubling_medicare_plan.

36. Blumenthal and Morone, *Heart of Power*, 393.

37. Robin Toner, "Rival Visions Led to Rocky Start for Drug Benefit," *New York Times*, February 6, 2006, http://www.NYTimes.com.

38. Bush, George W. Transcript of third Bush-Kerry Presidential Debate, October 13, 2004, Arizona State University, Tempe. http://www.debates.org/pages/trans2004d.html.

39. Ron Lieber, "Hefty Tax Break Spared in Health Care Bill," *New York Times*, March 26, 2010, http://www.NYTimes.com.

40. "The Many Hidden Costs of High-Deductible Health Insurance," *New York Times*, May 29, 2009, http://www.NYTimes.com; Hoffman, "Restraining the Health Care Consumer."

41. Eric Dash, "Health Savings Accounts Attract Wall Street," *New York Times*, January 27, 2006.

42. For a more detailed discussion, see Hoffman, "Blown Away: Health Care, Health Coverage, and American Public Health after 9/11 and Katrina," in Colgrove et al., *Contested Boundaries* (excerpted with permission of Rutgers University Press).

43. Stephanie Armour, "Bad Times Make Choice to Help Victims Tough," *USA Today*, October 7, 2001, 3B.

44. Armour, "Bad Times."

45. www.windowsofhope2001.org.

46. Disaster Relief Medicaid: Testimony of James R. Tallon Jr., President, United Hospital Fund, before the New York State Assembly Standing Committee on Health, December 3, 2001, http://www.uhfnyc.org/homepage3219/homepage_show.htm?doc_id=192218.

47. Testimony of James R. Tallon Jr.

48. Albor Ruiz, "Disaster Medicaid Plan Set to Expire," *New York Daily News*, January 24, 2002, 1.

49. Katherine E. Finkelstein, "Disaster Gives the Uninsured Wider Access to Medicaid." *New York Times*, November 23, 2001, D1.

50. Michael Perry, "New York's Disaster Relief Medicaid: Insights and Implications for Covering Low-Income People," a study sponsored by the Kaiser Commission on Medicaid and the Uninsured and the United Hospital Fund, Washington, DC, August 2002, iii-iv, 5, 9.

51. Perry, "New York's Disaster Relief Medicaid," 16–17.

52. Joyce Purnick, "The Doctor Will See You, for Now," *New York Times*, March 7, 2002, B1.

53. Dale Russakoff, "Out of Tragedy, N. Y. Finds Way to Treat Medicaid Need," *Washington Post*, November 26, 2001, A2.

54. Purnick, "Doctor Will See You, for Now"; Eugene LeCoutuer, "New York's Disaster Relief Medicaid: What Happened When It Ended?" Commonwealth Fund Report 737 (July 9, 2004), http://www.commonwealthfund.org.

55. Raymond Hernandez, "Senate Passes 9 / 11 Health Bill as Republicans Back Down," *New York Times*, December 22, 2010.

56. "Deal Reached on Package for 9 / 11 Aid Responders," *Crain's New York Business*, December 22, 2010.

57. *Characteristics of the Uninsured: A View from the States*, prepared by the State Health Access Data Assistance Center at the University of Minnesota on behalf of the Robert Wood Johnson Foundation, May 2005, http://www.rwjf.org/files/research/Full_SHADAC.pdf.

58. January W. Payne, "At Risk before the Storm Struck: Prior Health Disparities Due to Race, Poverty Multiply Death, Disease," *Washington Post*, September 13, 2005, HE01.

59. Richard Morin and Lisa Rein, "Some of the Uprooted Won't Go Home Again." *Washington Post*, September 16, 2005, A1.

60. Leigh Hopper, "Houston's 'Katrina Clinic': A Safety Net That Held Strong, Breaking the Fall of 15,000." *Houston Chronicle*, September 19, 2005, A1.

61. Nicholas D. Kristof, "A Health Care Disaster," *New York Times*, September 25, 2005, A11.

62. Judith Graham, "Storm Sweeps Away Health Insurance," *Chicago Tribune*, December 29, 2005; BlueCross BlueShield of Louisiana, Memorandum to Providers, November 9, 2005, available at www.lsms.org.

63. Seattle Times News Service, "Many Evacuees Rejected for Medicaid," *Seattle Times*, October 6, 2006, A14.

64. Ricardo Alonso-Zaldivar, "A Long Road to Recovery," *Los Angeles Times*, October 9, 2005, A1.

65. Judith Graham, "Hurricane-Battered Louisiana Mulls Deep Medicaid Cuts," *Chicago Tribune*, October 21, 2005.

66. Kaiser Commission on Medicaid and the Uninsured, "Health Coverage for Individuals Affected by Hurricane Katrina: A Comparison of Different Approaches to Extend Medicaid Coverage," October 10, 2005, http://www.kff.org.

67. Kevin Freking, "Senators, Administration Battle over Care for Katrina Victims," *Associated Press*, September 28, 2005.

68. Mary Curtius, "Senators Fume at White House Disdain for Katrina Healthcare Plan," *Los Angeles Times*, September 29, 2005, A13.

69. Curtius, "Senators Fume."

70. Freking, "Senators, Administration Battle."

71. Kaiser Commission on Medicaid and the Uninsured, "Health Coverage for Individuals Affected by Hurricane Katrina"; Tom Baxter, "Evacuees Intensify Medicaid Burdens," *Cox News Service*, October 17, 2005.

72. Editorial, "The High Cost of Health Care," *New York Times*, November 25, 2007.

73. Potter, *Deadly Spin* Kindle edition; statistic from "National Health Expenditures Historicals, 1960–2007," Centers for Medicare and Medicaid Services.

74. Peter R. Orszag to Jeb Hensarling, March 8, 2007, http://www.cbo.gov. For a conservative rejoinder, see Andrew Biggs, "The Entitlement Crisis is More Than a Health Care Crisis," February 24, 2009, FrumForum, http://www.frumforum.com/the-entitlement-crisis-is-more-than-a-health-care-crisis.

75. Mahar, *Money-Driven Medicine*; Bill Moyers, "Money-Driven Medicine" transcript, August 28, 2009, http://www.pbs.org/moyers/journal/08282009/watch.html; Angell, *Truth about the Drug Companies*.

76. Kathy A. Gambrell, "Bush Seeks Medical Malpractice Reform," *Consumer Watchdog*, January 16, 2003, http://www.consumerwatchdog.org/story/bush-seeks-medical-malpractice-reform; Baker, *Medical Malpractice Myth*; Kohn, Corrigan, and Donaldson, *To Err Is Human*.

77. National Priorities Partnership, "Reducing Emergency Department Overuse," November 2010, http://www.qualityforum.org/NPP/docs/Reducing_ED_Overuse_CAB.aspx; James Arvantes, "Emergency Room Visits Climb amid Primary Care Shortages," *American Academy of Family Physicians News Now*, August 27, 2008.

78. Hoffman, "Sympathy and Exclusion"; American College of Emergency Physicians, "Illegal Immigrant Care in the Emergency Department," http://www.acep.org/content.aspx?id=25206; Epstein, *Mortal Peril*. For arguments that EMTALA has not been a major driver of ER use, see, for example, Hermer, "Scapegoat"; Hoffman, "Reluctant Safety Net."

79. Brownlee, *Overtreated*, 8. On medical mistakes, see Kohn, Corrigan, and Donaldson, *To Err Is Human*.

80. Potter, *Deadly Spin*.

81. Connecticut Center for a New Economy, "Yale, Don't Lien on Me," 2003, www.ctneweconomy.org. Sara Austin, "Think You're Covered? Think Again," *Self*, October 2004, 247–49, 255.

82. John Carreyrou and Barbara Martinez, "Nonprofit Hospitals, Once for the Poor, Strike It Rich," *Wall Street Journal*, April 4, 2008, A1.

83. "AMA Study Shows Competition Disappearing," *AMA News*, February 23, 2010.

84. "Send Me Your Health Care Horror Stories: An Appeal from Michael Moore,"

February 3, 2006, http://www.michaelmoore.com/words/mikes-letter/send-me-your-health-care-horror-stories-an-appeal-from-michael-moore.

85. Box Office Mojo, http://boxofficemojo.com/movies/?id=sicko.htm.

86. For example, Michael D. Tanner, "Michael Moore Goes Sicko on Health Care Reform," June 18, 2007, http://www.cato.org/pub_display.php?pub_id=8336; Paul Guppy, "Moore's Sicko Offers No Cure for US Health Care," October 2007, http://www.washingtonpolicy.org/publications/opinion/moores-sicko-offers-no-cure-us-health-care.

87. Transcript of second McCain, Obama debate, articles.cnn.com.

Epilogue

1. Obama offers health care details in speech to Congress, September 9, 2009, articles.can.com.

2. "Patient Protection and Affordable Care Act," Part II–Other Provisions, Sec. 1251, https://www.annualmedicalreport.com/text-of-health-care-bill-patient-protection-and-affordable-care-act-hr-3590-text-of-bill/.

3. Rebecca Veseley, "Spending Caps Will Benefit Public: Families USA," *Modern Healthcare*, March 17, 2011, http://www.modernhealthcare.com/article/20110317/NEWS/303179968#.

4. "Employers That Don't Offer Minimum Essential Health Coverage May Face Penalties," *ReformAlert* (Blue Cross / Blue Shield), March 25, 2011, http://www.bcbsm.com/healthreform/reform-alerts/ra_03_25_2011.shtml.

5. Robert Pear, "Cuts Leave Patients with Medicaid Cards, but No Specialist to See," *New York Times*, April 3, 2011, http://www.NYTimes.com.

6. Jacobs and Skocpol, *Health Care Reform and American Politics*, 141; http://www.NYTimes.com.

7. Pipes, *Truth About Obamacare*, 131.

8. Reinhardt, "'Rationing' Health Care: What Does It Mean?"

9. Sheryl Gay Stolberg, "'Public Option' in Health Plan May Be Dropped," *New York Times*, August 17, 2009, http://www.NYTimes.com.

10. American Morning transcript, CNN, February 5, 2008, http://transcripts.cnn.com/TRANSCRIPTS/0802/05/ltm.02.html.

11. Leonidas Berry, "Statement of President National Medical Association at Final Briefing Conference before Briefing of Medicare" [*sic*], June 1966, Box 9, Berry Papers, CHM.

12. Koop, "Health and Health Care for the 21st Century," 2092.

GLOSSARY

ACT UP AIDS Coalition to Unleash Power, an activist organization of people with AIDS and supporters formed in New York in 1987.

Acute (vs. chronic) When referring to a disease or condition, acute means of short duration (and typically severe), while chronic implies a long-term or recurring condition without reference to severity.

Adverse selection In health insurance, the presumed likelihood of those at greater medical risk to buy insurance, knowing that they will need to use it.

American Federation of Labor Founded in 1886 by skilled craft workers. Led by Samuel Gompers, the AFL grew rapidly through the early part of the 20th century and became the primary voice of organized labor, although it initially excluded unskilled, minority, and women workers. These policies and other issues gave rise to the rival CIO (see **Congress of Industrial Organizations** below) in the 1930s. The two merged to become the AFL-CIO in 1955.

American Medical Association Founded in 1847 by US physicians to elevate standards for medical education and eliminate competition by "irregular" practitioners. Eventually became a political and trade force on behalf of physicians. The AMA describes its mission as promoting "the art and science of medicine and the betterment of public health."

Black Panther Party Radical civil rights / black power organization founded in Oakland, California, in 1966 by Bobby Seale and Huey Newton.

Blue Cross / Blue Shield Blue Cross started in 1929 as a nonprofit plan developed by Justin Ford Kimball of Baylor University to cover teachers' hospital expenses out of monthly fees paid by the users. This method of prepaid hospital insurance was endorsed and publicized by the American Hospital Association, which adopted the Blue Cross symbol for plans meeting its approval. Starting in 1939, doctors' groups created Blue Shield plans to cover some physicians' fees. Blue Cross and Blue Shield merged in 1982 and announced its move into for-profit insurance in 1994.

Capitation Payment for medical services made at a fixed rate per patient, regardless of what services are actually provided during the covered period.

Catastrophic health insurance Plans usually including high deductibles and designed to cover serious medical emergencies instead of more routine medical care.

Cherry picking Insurance company practice of selecting younger and healthier participants and excluding older and unhealthier ones in order to minimize insurance payouts.

Chronic (vs. acute) See **acute** above.

Clinic A facility where patients receive outpatient or ambulatory care, as distinct from a hospital, which offers inpatient care.

COBRA The Consolidated Omnibus Budget Reconciliation Act (COBRA) requires employers with 20 or more employees to offer continued health coverage to terminated employees and dependents for a specified period (18 or 36 months), with the insured paying the full cost of the group premium.

Community Rating Used by insurance companies to set premium costs on the basis of the demographic characteristics and claims history of a group or locality, as opposed to the specific health conditions of the covered population. Everyone in the population pays the same rates. See **Experience Rating** below.

Comprehensive health insurance Insurance designed to cover a wide range of medical expenses.

Congress of Industrial Organizations Debate within the American Federation of Labor (see AFL above) about whether unions should organize entire workplaces instead of only along craft lines led to the formation of the Committee of Industrial Organizations within the AFL in 1935. The CIO organized widely in the rubber, steel, mining, automotive, and other industries and remained a rival of the AFL until their merger in 1955.

Cooperative health association A health insurance plan, group medical practice, and/or hospital that is owned and run by subscribers.

Copayment A fixed fee that patients covered by health insurance must pay themselves for a given medical service, usually at the time the service is given. Also known as Coinsurance and Cost sharing. See also **Out-of-Pocket** below.

Cost sharing The mechanism whereby medical expenses are distributed between insurer and insured, through such methods as premiums, copayments, deductibles, and the like.

Deductible A specified amount that a covered patient must pay before insurance coverage kicks in. Higher deductibles sometimes imply lower premiums, and vice versa.

Dispensary A facility to dispense medicines, either freestanding or connected to a hospital. In the late nineteenth and early twentieth centuries, dispensaries also offered a wide variety of medical care, usually free to the public but sometimes on a sliding scale or fee basis.

Emergency Room The part of a hospital specializing in the treatment of unscheduled patients with acute medical problems.

Employer Mandate A requirement that employers provide health coverage for their workers.

ERISA The Employment Retirement Income Security Act of 1974 is a federal law that sets guidelines for employer-provided benefit plans. One of its provisions made employer-provided managed care plans immune from civil lawsuits.

Experience Rating Medical underwriting of an insurance plan (cost projection and setting of premium costs) varies according to the particular health conditions and experience of the individual or group. See also **Cherry Picking** and **Community Rating**.

Fee for service Payment of medical providers based on the services provided rather than salary or some other form of compensation.

Group practice The provision of medical services by a group of physicians sharing a common facility and resources.

Health Maintenance Organization A type of managed care organization that contracts with doctors and hospitals to provide health services to members. Members are required to use participating providers or be subject to additional costs.

Health savings accounts / medical savings accounts Tax-advantaged savings account available to US taxpayers with high-deductible health plans.

Hill-Burton Act The Hospital Survey and Construction Act, passed by the federal government during the Truman administration in 1946 and designed to improve the physical plant and expand the number of hospitals nationwide by providing federal grants and guaranteed loans to states and municipalities.

HIPAA The Health Insurance Portability and Accountability Act of 1996. Included privacy rules to protect individually identifiable health care information and placed limits on insurers' ability to impose preexisting conditions exclusions in group health plans.

Indemnity insurance Insurance that requires the insured to pay for services out of pocket, and then be reimbursed for eligible expenses by the insurance company after filing a claim.

Indigent Impoverished and / or requiring economic assistance to obtain needed medical care.

Individual mandate A requirement that individuals buy or otherwise obtain health insurance.

Kaiser Permanente The largest non-profit **managed care** (see below) organization in the United States, founded by industrialist Henry J. Kaiser in 1945.

Long-term care The provision of health care and other services to address chronic illness, disability, or old age.

Major medical insurance See **Catastrophic insurance** above.

Malpractice In medicine, negligence or misconduct by a physician, or failure of a physician to meet a proper standard of care.

Managed Care A method of providing health care while controlling costs, via organizations such as HMOs.

Medicare The federal program signed into law by President Lyndon Johnson in 1965, designed to cover many medical expenses incurred by Americans aged 65 and older.

Medicaid Part of the Social Security Amendments passed in 1965, along with **Medicare** (see above). Medicaid is a federal / state system providing medical assistance to the poor.

National Association for the Advancement of Colored People (NAACP) Prominent US civil rights organization founded in 1909. The NAACP's Legal Defense and Education Fund initiated the legal case that became *Brown v. Board of Education* (1954), which outlawed segregation in public schools.

National Medical Association (NMA) Founded in 1895, the largest national organization representing African American physicians.

Office of Economic Opportunity The federal agency responsible for implementing many of the programs comprising the **War on Poverty** (see below).

Out of pocket Refers to expenses paid by a patient for services rendered, as opposed to being covered by an insurance plan.

Overutilization Excessive, unnecessary use of medical services, laboratory tests, etc., by physicians and/or patients.

Patient dumping The transfer or premature discharge of a patient from a hospital for other than medical reasons.

Patient Protection and Affordable Care Act National health reform law signed by President Barack Obama on March 23, 2010. Major provisions include requiring insurance companies to accept all applicants and requiring uninsured individuals to purchase health insurance from state exchanges.

Primary care Refers to health care services most commonly needed by patients, or to the initial point of contact for patients within a health care system. In the United States, the primary care provider has commonly been the family physician or a general practitioner, as contrasted to a specialist.

Public health As distinct from health care, public health focuses on prevention of illness rather than cure, and on the health of populations rather than individuals. Public health activities may be carried out by governments or private organizations.

Public hospital A hospital owned by a local, state, or federal government.

Rationing Restriction or control of the consumption of a commodity or service.

Rights Something to which an individual is entitled. Rights also "represent articulations—public or private, formal or informal—of claims that people use to persuade others (and themselves) about how they should be treated and about what they should be granted," as stated by Martha Minow in her article "Interpreting Rights" (page 1867).

Single payer An insurance system in which a single agency, usually public, collects and administers all health care funding. Hospitals and health care providers remain private. Medicare and the Canadian health care system are single payer systems.

Sliding scale A payment rate based on ability to pay.

Social insurance The provision of support for the unemployed, aged, disabled, etc., by general tax revenue and/or contributions by employers and employees.

Social rights As distinct from political or civil rights, rights to social provision such as unemployment insurance, old age assistance, and medical care, and/or rights to economic security.

Social Security Act Programs including contributory old age pensions, unemployment insurance, and aid to dependent children passed by the US Congress at the height of the Great Depression in 1935.

Social movement A sustained campaign of people who come together to achieve a common goal. Social movement tactics vary and may include organizing, protesting, publicity campaigns, political campaigns, and/or civil disobedience.

Socialized medicine A health system in which the government runs both the financing of health care and its delivery. Examples: Cuba, British National Health Service, and US Veterans' Administration Health System.

State Children's Health Insurance Program Created in 1997, allows states to expand health coverage to families with children whose incomes are too high to qualify for standard Medicaid.

Voluntary health insurance Health insurance provided by private nonprofit or for-profit groups, organizations, or companies. The term was most commonly used from the 1920s through the 1950s to distinguish from the compulsory health insurance advocated by some reformers.

War on Poverty The unofficial name given to measures taken during the administration of President Lyndon B. Johnson to reduce poverty rates in the United States. Major legislation included the Economic Opportunity Act of 1964, which created programs such as Head Start and VISTA, the Community Health Centers program, and amendments to the Social Security Act (see **Medicare** and **Medicaid** and **Office of Economic Opportunity** above).

BIBLIOGRAPHY

Archival and Manuscript Collections

Alabama State Archives, Montgomery, AL
Alabama Circuit Court Records
Alabama Governor Correspondence

Albert Center, University of Oklahoma, Norman, OK
Carl Albert Collection
Page H. Belcher Collection
Tom Steed Collection

Arizona Historical Society, Tucson, AZ
Medicine and Health Care in Southern Arizona Oral History Project

Arizona State Library, Phoenix, AZ
Governor's Files

Center for Hospital and Health Administration History, American Hospital
Association Resource Center (AHARC), Chicago, IL
Subject Files
George Bugbee Papers
Malcolm MacEachern Papers
John Robert Mannix Papers
National Hospital Week (NHW) Collection

Chicago History Museum (CHM), Chicago, IL
Claude Barnett Papers
Leonidas M. Berry Papers
Chicago Commons Records
Raymond Hilliard Papers
Frank McCulloch Papers
Victor Olander Papers
Seymour Simon Papers
Welfare Council of Metropolitan Chicago Records (Welfare Council)

Hayden Library, Arizona State University (ASU), Phoenix, AZ
Arizona Ephemera Collection
Chicanos por la Causa
Human Rights of Arizona Collection

Institute for Social Medicine (ISM), Philadelphia, PA
    Individuals' Files
    Medical Committee for Human Rights (MCHR)
    Organizations' Files

Joint Commission for the Accreditation of Health Care Organizations, Oak
Brook, IL (JCAHO)
    Annual Reports

Lane Medical Library Special Collections, Stanford University, Palo Alto, CA
    Ray Lyman Wilbur Collection

Library of Congress, Washington, DC
    Leadership Council on Civil Rights (I and II) (LCCR)

Louisiana State Archives, Baton Rouge
    Files of David L. Ramsey
    Human Rights Bureau Files

Lyndon B. Johnson Presidential Library, Austin, TX
    Papers of Wilbur J. Cohen
    White House Central Files, Subject Files

Moorland Spingarn Research Collection, Howard University, Washington, DC
    Records of the National Welfare Rights Organization (NWRO)

New Orleans Health Department, New Orleans, LA
    Correspondence//Subject Files, 1949–95
    Victor Hugo Schiro Collection

New York Academy of Medicine, New York, NY (NYAM)
    Michael M. Davis Papers

New York Public Library, New York, NY (NYPL)
    ACT UP/NY Records

National Archives, Washington, DC
    Records of the Children's Bureau
    Records of the Public Health Service (PHS)

National Library of Medicine, Washington, DC (NLM)
    Leonidas M. Berry Papers

Northwestern University Hospital Archives, Chicago, IL
    Wesley Memorial Hospital Records

Rush-Presbyterian-St. Luke's Hospital Archives, Chicago, IL (Rush Archives)
    Annual Reports

Special Collections and Archives, Stanford University, Palo Alto, CA
    Mexican American Legal Defense and Education Fund Records

National Council of La Raza Records
Papers of Ernesto Galarza
Papers of Phillip Shapiro

Walter Reuther Collection, Wayne State University, Detroit, MI
Committee on National Health Insurance Collection (CNHI)

Tuskegee University Archives, Tuskegee, AL
Southern Conference for Human Welfare Records (SCHW)

University of Alabama at Birmingham (UAB), University Archives
Dean's Administrative Files

University of Alabama, Tuscaloosa
Lister Hill Papers

Audio Recording

Ronald Reagan Speaks Out against Socialized Medicine (1960)

Legal Decisions

Birmingham Baptist Hospital v. Crews, 229 Ala. 398 (1934).
Bourgeois v. Dade County, 99 So. 2d 575 (1957).
Cook v. Ochsner Foundation Hospital, 319 F. Supp. 603 (1970).
Gadsden General Hospital v. Hamilton, 212 Ala. 531. 103 So. 553 (1925).
Guerrero v. Copper Queen, 112 Ariz. 104, 1975.
Harper v. Baptist Medical Center–Princeton, 341 So. 2d 133 (1976).
Hoffman v. Clinic Hospital, 213 N.C. 669 (1928).
Jones v. City of New York, 134 N.Y.S. 2d 779 (1954).
McDonald v. Massachusetts General Hospital, 120 Mass. 432 (1876).
Methodist Hospital v. Ball, 50 Tenn. App. 460 (1961).
Miller v. Davis, 464 F. Supp. 458 (1978).
O'Neill v. Montefiore Hospital, 11 A.D. 2d 132 (1960).
Rivera v. Misericordia Hospital, 15 Wis. 2d 351 (1962).
Simkins v. Cone, 376 U.S. 938 (1964).
Stanturf v. Sipes, 447 S.W. 2d 558 (1969).
Wilmington General Hospital v. Manlove, 54 Del. 15 (1961).

Periodicals

American Home
American Hospital Association (AHA) News
American Journal of Public Health
Bulletin of the American College of Surgeons
Chicago Defender / Chicago Daily Defender
Chicago Medical Society Bulletin

Chicago Sun-Times
Chicago Tribune / Chicago Daily Tribune
Collier's
Consumer Reports
El Chicano
El Grito del Norte
Harper's
Health Advocate
Hospital Practice
Hospitals
Houston Chronicle
Illinois Medical Journal
Journal of the American Medical Association (JAMA)
Journal of the National Medical Association (JNMA)
Ladies' Home Journal
Los Angeles Times
Medical Economics
Miami Herald
Modern Hospital
Nation
New England Journal of Medicine
New Republic
Newsweek
New York Daily News
New Yorker
New York Times
San Diego Union-Tribune
Science News Letter
Seattle Times
Social Service Review
State Legislatures
Time
Trained Nurse and Hospital Review
Transactions of the American Hospital Association
USA Today
Wall Street Journal
Washington Post
Woman's Home Companion

Government Documents, Speeches, and International Agreements

"Costs and Delivery of Health Services to Older Americans." Hearings before the Subcommittee on Health of the Elderly of the Special Committee on Aging, United States Senate, June 22 and 23, 1967. Washington, DC: US Government Printing Office, 1967.

"Equal Access to Health Care: Patient Dumping." Hearing before a Subcommittee of the Committee on Government Operations, House of Representatives, July 22, 1987. Washington, DC: US Government Printing Office, 1987.

"Hospital Survey and Construction Bill. October 30, 1945." Serial Set Vol. No. 10927, Session Vol. No. 3, 79th Congress, 1st Session, S. Rpt. 674, 3. Readex US Congressional Series Set.

Kennedy, John F. "Address at New York Rally in Support of the President's Program of Medical Care for the Aged," May 2, 1962. https://www.presidency.ucsb.edu/ws/?pid=8669. Accessed May 15, 2011.

Johnson, Lyndon B. "Remarks before the Annual Convention of the National Medical Association, Houston, Texas," August 14, 1968, CMS Speeches, https://www.cms.gov/History/.

———. "Statement of the President Following the Passage of the Medicare Bill by the Senate," July 9, 1965, CMS Speeches, https://www.cms.gov/History/.

Organization of American States, American Declaration of the Rights and Duties of Man, adopted by the Ninth International Conference of American States (1948).

Truman, Harry S. "Annual Message to Congress on the State of the Union." January 6, 1947. *Public Papers of the Presidents of the United States*, http://www.presidency.ucsb.edu/ws/index.php.

"Uncompensated Hospital Care." Hearing before the Subcommittee on Health of the Committee on Ways and Means, House of Representatives, March 12, 1987. Washington, DC: US Government Printing Office, 1987.

United Nations, Universal Declaration of Human Rights. http://www.un.org/en/documents/udhr/.

United States Senate, Subcommittee on Health 1964. *Blue Cross and Private Health Insurance Coverage of Older Americans: A Report to the Special Committee on Aging*. Washington, DC: US Government Printing Office, 1964.

Books, Articles, Proceedings, and Theses

Abbott, Edith. "Hospitals Are Not a Health Program." *Social Service Review* 14 (March 1940): 138–39.

Abel, Emily K. "'Only the Best Class of Immigration': Public Health Policy Toward Mexicans and Filipinos in Los Angeles, 1910–1940." *American Journal of Public Health* 94, no. 61 (June 2004): 932–39.

Abel-Smith, Brian. "Minimum Adequate Levels of Personal Health Care: History and Justification." *Milbank Memorial Fund Quarterly* 56, no. 1 (Winter 1978): 7–21.

Adler, Stuart W. "Medical Care for Dependents of Men in Military Service." *American Journal of Public Health* 33 (June 1943): 645–50.

Albee, Edward. *The Death of Bessie Smith*. New York: Samuel French Ltd., 1995.

Albertson, Chris. *Bessie*. New Haven, CT: Yale University Press, 2003.

Amenta, Edwin. *When Movements Matter: The Townsend Plan and the Rise of Social Security*. Princeton, NJ: Princeton University Press, 2006.

American Academy of Political and Social Science (AAPSS). *The Medical Profession and the Public: Current and Counter-Currents*. Philadelphia: American Academy of Political and Social Science, 1934.

American Hospital Association (AHA). *Emergency Services in the Hospital: A Guide to Organization and Management*. Chicago: American Hospital Association, 1962.

———. *The US Senate Hears about Hospitals and Hospital Service*. Chicago: American Hospital Association, 1944.

American Medical Association (AMA). *Care of the Indigent Sick*. Chicago: American Medical Association, 1945.

Anders, George. *Health against Wealth: HMOs and the Breakdown of Medical Trust*. New York: Houghton Mifflin, 1996.

Anderson, Odin, and the staff of the National Opinion Research Center. *Voluntary Health Insurance in Two Cities: A Survey of Subscriber-Households*. Cambridge, MA: Harvard University Press, 1957.

Angel, Ronald, Laura Lein, and Jane Henrici. *Poor Families in America's Health Care Crisis*. New York: Cambridge University Press, 2006.

Angell, Marcia. *The Truth about the Drug Companies: How They Deceive Us and What to Do about It*. New York: Random House, 2004.

"Annals of Legislation: Medicare." *New Yorker*, July 2, 1966: 35.

Annas, George J. *The Rights of Hospital Patients*. New York: Avon Books, 1975.

Ansell, David A., and Robert L. Schiff. "Patient Dumping: Status, Implications, and Policy Recommendations." *JAMA* 257, no. 11 (March 20, 1987): 1500–1502.

Aranda, Robert G. "The Mexican American Syndrome." *American Journal of Public Health* 61, no. 1 (January 1971): 104–9.

Atlanta Urban League. *A Report on Hospital Care of the Negro Population of Atlanta, Georgia, 1947*. Atlanta: Atlanta Urban League, 1947.

Auerhan, Gloria, and Jeanette Loring. "A Study of Forty Mothers Who Received Maternity Care under the Emergency Maternity and Infant Care Plan at Sloane Hospital for Women." Master's thesis, New York School of Social Work, Columbia University, May 1945.

Baker, Robert, and Linda Emanuel. "The Efficacy of Professional Ethics: The AMA Code of Ethics in Historical and Current Perspective." *Hastings Center Report* 30, no. 4 (July–August 2000): S13-S17.

Baker, Tom. *The Medical Malpractice Myth*. Chicago: University of Chicago Press, 2005.

Ball, Robert M. "Perspectives on Medicare: What Medicare's Architects Had in Mind." *Health Affairs* 14, no. 4 (1995): 62–72.

Bartlemez, Carol Jane. "Applicants Rejected by Admitting Office at Children's Memorial Hospital (Part One)." Master's thesis, University of Chicago School of Social Service Administration, 1937.

Bayer, Ronald. *Private Acts, Social Consequences: AIDS and the Politics of Public Health*. New Brunswick, NJ: Rutgers University Press, 1991.

Beardsley, Edward H. *A History of Neglect: Health Care for Blacks and Mill Work-*

ers in the Twentieth-Century South. Knoxville: University of Tennessee Press, 1987.

Beauchamp, Tom L., and James F. Childress. *Principles of Biomedical Ethics.* New York: Oxford, 2001.

Beito, David. *From Mutual Aid to the Welfare State: Fraternal Societies and Social Services, 1890–1967.* Chapel Hill: University of North Carolina Press, 2000.

Bentley, Amy. *Eating for Victory: Food Rationing and the Politics of Domesticity.* Urbana: University of Illinois Press, 1998.

Berkowitz, Edward. *Mr. Social Security: The Life of Wilbur J. Cohen.* Lawrence: University Press of Kansas, 1995.

Berkowitz, Edward, and Wendy Wolff. *Group Health Association: A Portrait of a Health Maintenance Organization.* Philadelphia: Temple University Press, 1988.

Berry, Leonidas H. "Human Rights and Regional Medical Programs." *Journal of the National Medical Association* 58, no. 5 (September 1966): 387–88.

Beschloss, Michael. *Reaching for Glory: Lyndon Johnson's Secret White House Tapes.* New York: Simon & Schuster, 2002.

Bierman, Pearl. "Meeting the Health Needs of Low-Income Families." *Annals of the American Academy of Political and Social Science* 337 (September 1961): 103–13.

Biles, Roger. "Robert F. Wagner, Franklin D. Roosevelt, and Social Welfare Legislation in the New Deal." *Presidential Studies Quarterly* 28, no. 1 (Winter 1998): 139–52.

Bitterman, Robert A., ed. *Providing Emergency Care under Federal Law:* EMTALA. Dallas: American College of Emergency Physicians, 2000.

Black, Kathryn. *In the Shadow of Polio: A Personal and Social History.* Reading, MA: Addison-Wesley, 1996.

Blalock, William R. "Emergency Care." *Hospitals* 40 (April 1, 1966): 51–54.

Blumenthal, David, and James A. Morone. *The Heart of Power: Health and Politics in the Oval Office.* Berkeley: University of California Press, 2009.

Blumstein, James F. "Court Action, Agency Reaction: The Hill-Burton Act as a Case Study." *Iowa Law Review* 69 (July 1984):1227.

Boccuti, Christina, and Marilyn Moon. "Comparing Medicare and Private Insurers: Growth Rates in Spending over Three Decades." *Health Affairs* 22, no. 2 (2003): 230–37.

Bole, Thomas J., and W. B. Bondeson, eds. *Right to Health Care.* New York: Springer, 1991.

Bonner, Thomas Neville. *Medicine in Chicago, 1850–1950: A Chapter in the Social and Scientific Development of a City.* 2nd ed. Urbana: University of Illinois Press, 1991.

Borgwardt, Elizabeth. *A New Deal for the World: America's Vision for Human Rights.* Cambridge, MA: Harvard University Press, 2005.

Boston Women's Health Book Collective. *Our Bodies, Ourselves: A Book by and for Women.* New York: Simon & Schuster, 1971.

Boychuk, Gerard W. *National Health Insurance in the United States and Canada: Race,*

Territory, and the Roots of Difference. Washington, DC: Georgetown University Press, 2008.

Boychuk, Terry. *The Making and Meaning of Hospital Policy in the United States and Canada*. Ann Arbor: University of Michigan Press, 1999.

Brandt, Allan M. *No Magic Bullet: A Social History of Venereal Disease in the United States since 1880*. New York: Oxford University Press, 1987.

Brecher, Ruth, and Edward Brecher. *How to Get the Most out of Medical and Hospital Benefit Plans: A Program for Labor and Management*. Englewood Cliffs, NJ: Prentice-Hall, 1961.

Brinton, J.W. *The Townsend National Recovery Plan: The Solution of Your Problem*. Chicago: Townsend National Weekly, 1936.

Brownlee, Shannon. *Overtreated: Why Too Much Medicine Is Making Us Sicker and Poorer*. New York: Bloomsbury, 2007.

Buelow, Paul A. "The Dispensary Comes to Chicago: Health Care and the Poor before 1920." PhD diss., University of Illinois at Chicago, 1997.

Buhler Wilkerson, Karen. *No Place like Home: A History of Nursing and Home Care in the United States*. Baltimore: Johns Hopkins University Press, 2001.

Byrd, W. Michael, and Linda A. Clayton. *An American Health Dilemma*. Vol. 2. *Race, Medicine, and Health Care in the United States, 1900–2000*. New York: Routledge, 2002.

Casalino, Lawrence P., Sean Nicholson, David N. Gans, et al. "What Does It Cost Physician Practices to Interact with Health Insurance Plans?" *Health Affairs* 28, no. 4 (July/August 2009): 533–43.

Cervances, Robert A. "The Failure of Comprehensive Health Services to Serve the Urban Chicano." *Health Services Reports* 87, no. 10 (December 1972): 932–40.

Chapman, Carleton B., and John M. Talmadge. "The Evolution of the Right to Health Concept." *Pharos* 34 (1971): 30–51.

Churchill, Larry R. *Rationing Health Care in America: Perceptions and Principles of Justice*. South Bend, IN: University of Notre Dame Press, 1988.

Clark, Dean A., I. S. Falk, Dora Goldstine, et al. "Tax Supported Medical Care for the Needy: A Statement of the Joint Committee on Medical Care of the American Public Health Association and the American Public Welfare Association." *American Journal of Public Health* 42, no. 10 (October 1952): 1310–27.

Cobb, W. Montague. "Statement in Support of National Health Bill, S. 1606, on behalf of the National Association for the Advancement of Colored People." *Journal of the National Medical Association* 38, no. 4 (July 1946): 133–37.

Cohen, Lizabeth. *Making a New Deal: Industrial Workers in Chicago*. New York: Cambridge University Press, 1990.

———. A Consumers' Republic: The Politics of Mass Consumption in Postwar America. New York: Knopf, 2003.

Cohn, Jonathan. *Sick: The Untold Story of America's Health Care Crisis—and the People Who Pay the Price*. New York: HarperCollins, 2007.

Cole, Dwayne Charles. "The Relief Crisis in Illinois during the Depression, 1930–1940." PhD diss., St. Louis University, 1973.

Colgrove, James, Gerald Markowitz, and David Rosner, eds. *The Contested Boundaries of American Public Health*. New Brunswick, NJ: Rutgers University Press, 2008.

Columbia University School of Public Health and Administrative Medicine / National Opinion Research Center. *Family Medical Care under Three Types of Health Insurance*. New York: Foundation of Employee Health, Medical Care, and Welfare, 1962.

Commission on Hospital Care. *Hospital Care in the United States*. New York: Commonwealth Fund, 1947.

Committee for National Health Insurance (CNHI). "Facts of Life, Health, and Health Insurance." Washington, DC: Committee for National Health Insurance, 1969.

Committee on Technology and Health Care, Assembly of Engineering, National Research Council and Institute of Medicine. *Medical Technology and the Health Care System: A Study of the Diffusion of Equipment-Embodied Technology*. Washington, DC: National Academy of Sciences, 1979.

Committee on the Costs of Medical Care (CCMC). *Medical Care for the American People: The Final Report*. Chicago: University of Chicago Press, 1932.

"Court Cases Filed to Test Right to Health Services." *Hospital Practice* 6 (June 1971): 148–52.

Cowdrey, Albert E. *Fighting for Life: American Military Medicine in World War II*. New York: Free Press, 1994.

Cunningham, Robert, III, and Robert Cunningham Jr. *The Blues: A History of the Blue Cross Blue Shield System*. DeKalb: Northern Illinois University Press, 1999.

Curran, William J. "Legal History of Emergency Medicine from Medieval Common Law to the AIDS Epidemic." *American Journal of Emergency Medicine* 18 (November 1997): 658–70.

Daniels, Norman, and James E. Sabin. *Setting Limits Fairly: Learning to Share Resources for Health*. New York: Oxford, 2008.

Daschle, Tom. *Critical: What We Can Do about the Health Care Crisis*. New York: Thomas Dunne Books, 2008.

Davis, Martha F. *Brutal Need: Lawyers and the Welfare Rights Movement, 1960–1973*. New Haven: Yale University Press, 1995.

DeJong, Gerben, Andrew I. Batavia, and Robert Griss. "America's Neglected Health Minority: Working-Age Persons with Disabilities." *Milbank Quarterly* 67 (1989): 311–51.

de Kruif, Paul. *Health Is Wealth*. New York: Harcourt Brace, 1940.

de la Teja, Jesús F., and John Wheat. "Bexar: Profile of a Tejano Community, 1820–1832." *Southwestern Historical Quarterly* 89, no. 1 (July 1985): 7–34.

Dent, Albert W. "Hospital Services and Facilities Available to Negroes in the United States." *Journal of Negro Education* 18, no. 3 (Summer 1949): 326–32.

Derickson, Alan. *Health Security for All: Dreams of Universal Health Care in America*. Baltimore: Johns Hopkins University Press, 2005.

——. "Health Security for All? Social Unionism and Universal Health Insurance, 1935–1958." *Journal of American History* (March 1994): 1333–56.

——. "The House of Falk: The Paranoid Style in American Health Politics." *American Journal of Public Health* 87, no. 11 (November 1997): 1836–43.

——. "Take Health from the List of Luxuries: Labor and the Right to Health Care, 1915–1949." *Labor History* 41 (May 2000): 171–87.

Deutsch, Albert. "The Sick Poor in Colonial Times." *American Historical Review* 46, no. 3 (April 1941): 560–79.

Deutsch, Tracey. "Great Depression." In *Encyclopedia of Chicago*, edited by James R. Grossman, Ann Durkin Keating, and Janice L. Reiff. Chicago: University of Chicago Press, 2004.

Dieuaide, Francis R. *Civilian Health in Wartime*. Cambridge, MA: Harvard University Press, 1942.

Dittmer, John. *The Good Doctors: The Medical Committee for Human Rights and the Struggle for Social Justice in Health Care*. New York: Bloomsbury, 2009.

Dowell, Michael A. "Hill-Burton: The Unfulfilled Promise." *Journal of Health Politics, Policy, and Law* 12, no. 1 (Spring 1987): 153–75.

Drake, St. Clair, and Horace R. Cayton. *Black Metropolis: A Study of Negro Life in a Northern City*. Chicago: University of Chicago Press, 1993, reprint of 1945 edition.

Duffus, R. L. "How to Pay the Doctor?" *North American Review* 232, no. 4 (October 1931): 358–63.

Duffy, John. *The Sanitarians: A History of American Public Health*. Urbana: University of Illinois Press, 1990.

Duncan, Margaret. "How to Evaluate Emergency Room Care." *Modern Hospital* 99 (1961): 168.

Dutton, Paul V. *Differential Diagnoses: A Comparative History of Health Care Problems and Solutions in the United States and France*. Ithaca, NY: Cornell University Press, 2007.

"Effect of Changing Technology on Hospital Costs." *Social Security Bulletin*, May 1972: 28–30.

Ehrenreich, Barbara, and John Ehrenreich. *The American Health Empire: Power, Profits and Politics*. New York: Vintage, 1971.

Eliot, Martha M. "Experience with the Administration of a Medical Care Program for Wives and Infants of Enlisted Men." *American Journal of Public Health* 34 (January 1944): 34–39.

Emblidge, David, ed. *My Day: The Best of Eleanor Roosevelt's Acclaimed Newspaper Columns*. Cambridge, MA: DaCapo Press, 2001.

Engel, Jonathan. *Doctors and Reformers: Discussion and Debate over Health Policy, 1925–1950*. Columbia: University of South Carolina Press, 2002.

——. *Poor People's Medicine: Medicine and American Charity Care since 1965*. Durham, NC: Duke University Press, 2005.

Enthoven, Alain C., and Victor R. Fuchs. "Employment-Based Health Insurance: Past, Present, and Future." *Health Affairs* 25, no. 6 (November/December 2006): 1538–47.

Epstein, Richard. *Mortal Peril: Our Unalienable Right to Health Care?* New York: Basic Books, 1997.

Epstein, Steven. *Impure Science: AIDS, Activism, and the Politics of Knowledge.* Berkeley: University of California, 1996.

Fahey, John M. "Six Ways to Deal with the Emergency Room Crisis." *Medical Economics* 65, no. 103 (November 20, 1964): 69.

Fein, Oliver. "The Medical Care Section 1994–2005: Reflections on Our Past and Future." *Medical Care* 37, no. 8 (August 1999): 837–41.

Fein, Rashi. *Medical Care, Medical Costs: The Search for a Health Insurance Policy.* Cambridge, MA: Harvard University Press, 1999.

Feudtner, Chris. *Bittersweet: Diabetes, Insulin, and the Transformation of Illness.* Chapel Hill: University of North Carolina Press, 2006.

Fishbein, Morris, ed. *Doctors at War.* New York: Dutton, 1945.

Foley, Henry A. "Editorial: Cost Containment Begins at Home." *Public Health Reports* 93, no. 4 (July–August 1978).

Follmann, J. F., Jr. *Voluntary Health Insurance and Medical Care: Five Years of Progress, 1952–1957.* Chicago: Health Insurance Association of America, 1958.

Folsom, Franklin. *Impatient Armies of the Poor: The Story of Collective Action of the Unemployed, 1808–1942.* Boulder: University Press of Colorado, 1991.

Freeman, Joshua B. *Working-Class New York: Life and Labor since World War II.* New York: New Press, 2000.

Freese, Arthur S. *Managing Your Doctor: How to Get the Best Possible Health Care.* New York: Stein and Day, 1974.

Fried, Charles. "Equality and Rights in Medical Care." *Hastings Center Report* 6 (February 1976): 29–34.

Freidson, Eliot, and Jacob J. Feldman. *Public Attitudes toward Health Insurance.* New York: Health Information Foundation Research Series 5, 1958.

Funigiello, Phillip. *Chronic Politics: Health Care Security from FDR to George W. Bush.* Lawrence: University of Kansas Press, 2005.

Gamble, Vanessa Northington. *Making a Place for Ourselves: The Black Hospital Movement, 1920–1945.* Oxford: Oxford University Press, 1995.

Gambone, Michael. *The Greatest Generation Comes Home: The Veteran in American Society.* College Station: Texas A&M Press, 2005.

Garvin, Charles Herbert. "Post-War Planning for 'Negro' Hospitals." *Journal of the National Medical Association* 37 (January 1945): 28–29.

Glendon, Mary Ann. "Rights in Twentieth-Century Constitutions." *University of Chicago Law Review* 59, no. 1 (Winter 1992): 519–38.

———. *A World Made New: Eleanor Roosevelt and the Universal Declaration of Human Rights.* New York: Random House, 2001.

Goldmann, Franz. "The Problem: The Role of the Federal Government." *American Journal of Public Health* 49, no. 2 (February 1959): 161–68.

———. *Public Medical Care: Principles and Problems.* New York: Columbia University Press, 1945.

Goodman, John C., Gerald L. Musgrave, and Devon M. Herrick. *Lives at Risk:*

Single-Payer National Health Insurance around the World. Lanham, MD: Rowman and Littlefield, 2004.

Gordon, Colin. *Dead on Arrival: The Politics of Health Care in Twentieth-Century America.* Princeton, NJ: Princeton University Press, 2004.

Gregg, John E. *The Health Insurance Racket and How to Beat It.* Chicago: Regnery, 1973.

Grey, Michael R. *New Deal Medicine: The Rural Health Programs of the Farm Security Administration.* Baltimore: Johns Hopkins University Press, 1999.

Grogan, Colleen. "America's Hidden Health Care State." Manuscript in progress.

Grogan, Colleen, and Eric Patashnik, "Between Welfare Medicine and Mainstream Entitlement: Medicaid at the Political Crossroads," *Journal of Health Politics, Policy, and Law* 28, no. 5 (October 2003): 821–58.

"Group Practice Favored by Young Doctors Now in the Armed Services." *Science News Letter* 46 (December 30, 1944): 426.

Hacker, Jacob. *The Road to Nowhere: The Genesis of President Clinton's Plan for Health Security.* Princeton, NJ: Princeton University Press, 1996.

Hall, Charles P., Jr. "Deductibles in Health Insurance: An Evaluation," *Journal of Risk and Insurance* 33 (June 1966): 254–63.

Haller, John S. "Race, Mortality, and Life Insurance: Negro Vital Statistics in the Late Nineteenth Century." *Journal of the History of Medicine and Allied Sciences* 25, no. 3 (July 1970): 247–61.

Hammond, Evelyn. *Childhood's Deadly Scourge: The Campaign to Control Diphtheria in New York City, 1880–1930.* Baltimore: Johns Hopkins University Press, 1999.

Hartog, Hendrick. "The Constitution of Aspiration and 'The Rights That Belong to Us All.'" *Journal of American History* 74 (1987): 1013–34.

Hayden, Lisa A. "Gender Discrimination within the Reproductive Health Care System: Viagra v. Birth Control." *Journal of Law and Health* 13 (1998): 96–171.

Health Insurance Institute (HII). *A Profile of the Health Insurance Public: A National Study of the Pattern of Health Insurance, Public Attitudes and Knowledge.* New York: Health Insurance Institute, 1959.

Hermer, Laura D. "The Scapegoat: EMTALA and Emergency Department Overcrowding." *Journal of Law and Policy* 14 (2006): 695–732.

Herzlinger, Regina. *Market-Driven Health Care: Who Wins, Who Loses in the Transformation of America's Largest Service Industry.* New York: Perseus, 1997.

"The Hill–Burton Hospital Construction Bill." *Journal of the American Medical Association* 129 (November 17, 1945): 804.

Himmelstein, D., S. Woolhandler, M. Harnley, et al. "Patient Transfers: Medical Practice as Social Triage." *American Journal of Public Health* 74 (1984): 74–77.

Hoffman, Beatrix. "The Challenge of Universal Health Care: Social Movements, Presidential Leadership, and Private Power." In *Social Movements and the Transformation of American Health Care,* edited by Jane C. Banaszak-Holl, Sandra R. Levitsky, and Mayer N. Zald. New York: Oxford University Press, 2010.

——. "'Don't Scream Alone': The Health Care Activism of Poor Americans in the 1970s." In *Patients as Policy Actors*, edited by Beatrix Hoffman, Nancy Tomes, Rachel Grob, and Mark Schlesinger. New Brunswick, NJ: Rutgers University Press, 2011.

——."Restraining the Health Care Consumer: The History of Deductibles and Copayments in US Health Insurance." *Social Science History* 30, no. 4 (2006): 501–28.

——. "Scientific Racism, Insurance, and Opposition to the Welfare State: Frederick L. Hoffman's Transatlantic Journey." *Journal of the Gilded Age and Progressive Era* 2 (2003): 150–90.

——. *The Wages of Sickness: The Politics of Health Insurance in Progressive America*. Chapel Hill: University of North Carolina Press, 2001.

Hoffman, Beatrix, Nancy Tomes, Rachel Grob, and Mark Schlesinger, eds. *Patients as Policy Actors*. New Brunswick, NJ: Rutgers University Press, 2011.

Hoge, Vane M. "The Hospital as an Instrument in a Public Health Program," *American Journal of Public Health* 37 (December 1947): 1519–24.

Hoppe, A.W. "Hospitals for the People?" *Nation* 175 (September 13, 1952): 200.

Horgan, Patricia D. "The Emergency Room Crisis: How One Hospital Is Handling It." *R.N.* (October 1962): 46–57, 94.

"The Hospital Construction Bill: Statement by Dr. R. L. Sensenich." *Hospital Progress* 26, no. 3 (March 1945): 76.

"Hospital Survey and Construction Plan in Illinois Gets Under Way." *Illinois Medical Journal* 94 (August 1948): 84–88.

Hoyt, Edwin P. *Your Health Insurance: A Story of Failure*. New York: John Day, 1970.

"Hubert and the Means Test." *American Academy of General Practice* 23 (May 1961): 79–80.

Hunt, Lynn, and Marilyn B. Young, eds. *Human Rights and Revolutions*. Lanham, MD: Rowman and Littlefield, 2000.

Hunt, Paul. *Reclaiming Social Rights: International and Comparative Perspectives*. Aldershot, UK: Ashgate, 1996.

Huthmacher, J. Joseph. *Senator Robert F. Wagner and the Rise of Urban Liberalism*. New York: Atheneum, 1968.

Institute of Medicine. *Care without Coverage: Too Little, Too Late*. Washington, DC: National Academies Press, 2002.

Interdepartmental Committee to Coordinate Health and Welfare Activities (ICCHWA). *Proceedings: National Health Conference*. Washington, DC: US Government Printing Office, 1938.

"Is the 'Accident Room' Evolving into the Community Medical Center?" *Bulletin of the American College of Surgeons* (March–April 1961), 43.

Jacobs, Lawrence R., and Theda Skocpol. *Health Care Reform and American Politics: What Everyone Needs to Know*. New York: Oxford University Press, 2010.

——. *The Health of Nations: Public Opinion and the Making of American and British Health Policy*. Ithaca, NY: Cornell University Press, 1993.

Jacobs, Lawrence R., Theda Skocpol, Theodore Marmor, and Jonathan Oberlander. "The Oregon Health Plan and the Political Paradox of Rationing." *Journal of Health Politics, Policy, and Law* 24, no. 1 (1999): 161–80.

Jennings, Babette S. "How Hospitals Are Meeting the Social Problems of the Depression." *Modern Hospital* 42, no. 5 (May 1934): 87–90.

Jensen, John. "Before the Surgeon General: Marine Hospitals in Mid-Nineteenth Century America." *Public Health Reports* 112, no. 6 (November–December 1997): 525–27.

Johnson, Haynes, and David Broder. *The System: The American Way of Politics at the Breaking Point.* Boston: Back Bay Books, 1997.

Jones, Gene D. L. "The Chicago Catholic Charities, the Great Depression, and Public Monies." *Illinois Historical Journal* 83, no. 1 (Spring 1990): 13–30.

Jost, Timothy Stoltzfus. *Health Care at Risk: A Critique of the Consumer-Driven Movement.* Durham, NC: Duke University Press, 2007.

Katz, Michael B. *In the Shadow of the Poorhouse.* New York: Basic Books, 1986.

Katz, Steven J., Karen Cardiff, Marina Pascali, Morris L. Barer, and Robert G. Evans. "Phantoms in the Snow: Canadians' Use of Health Care Services in the United States." *Health Affairs* (May/June 2002).

Kavaler, Florence, and Allen D. Spiegel. *Risk Management in Health Care Institutions: A Strategic Approach.* Sudbury, MA: Jones and Bartlett Learning, 2003.

Kennedy, Edward M. *In Critical Condition: The Crisis in America's Health Care.* New York: Pocket Books, 1973.

Kessler-Harris, Alice. *In Pursuit of Equity: Women, Men, and the Quest for Economic Citizenship in 20th-Century America.* New York: Oxford University Press, 2003.

Kleber, John E., ed. *The Encyclopedia of Louisville.* Louisville: University Press of Kentucky, 2001.

Klein, Jennifer. *For All These Rights: Business, Labor, and the Shaping of America's Public-Private Welfare State.* Princeton, NJ: Princeton University Press, 2006.

Klein, Rudolf, Patricia Day, and Sharon Redmayne. *Managing Scarcity: Priority Setting and Rationing in the National Health Service.* Buckingham: Open University Press, 1996.

Kluge, E. H. "Drawing the Ethical Line between Organ Transplantation and Lifestyle Abuse." *Canadian Medical Association Journal* 150, no. 5 (1994): 745–46.

Kohn, Linda T., Janet M. Corrigan, and Molla S. Donaldson. *To Err Is Human: Building a Safer Health System.* Washington, DC: National Academies Press, 2000.

Kooijman, Jaap. . . . *And the Pursuit of National Health: The Incremental Strategy toward National Health Insurance in the United States of America.* Amsterdam: Rodopi, 1999.

Koop, C. Everett. "Health and Health Care for the 21st Century: For All the People." *American Journal of Public Health* 96, no. 12 (December 2006): 2090–92.

Kornbluh, Felicia. *The Battle for Welfare Rights: Politics and Poverty in Modern America.* Philadelphia: University of Pennsylvania Press, 2007.

Law, Sylvia A. *Blue Cross: What Went Wrong?* New Haven, CT: Yale University Press, 1974.

——. "A Right to Health Care That Cannot Be Taken Away: The Lessons of Twenty-Five Years of Health Advocacy." *Tennessee Law Review* 61 (Spring 1994): 771.

Lefkowitz, Bonnie. *Community Health Centers: A Movement and the People Who Made It Happen.* New Brunswick, NJ: Rutgers University Press, 2007.

Levin, Arthur. *Talk Back to Your Doctor: How to Demand and Recognize High Quality Health Care.* Garden City, NY: Doubleday, 1975.

Lindenmeyer, Kriste. *A Right to Childhood: The US Children's Bureau and Child Welfare, 1912–46.* Urbana: University of Illinois Press, 1997.

Lochridge, Patricia. "Our Shocking Accident Wards, Part One." *Collier's* 123 (March 12, 1949): 21–22.

——. "Our Shocking Accident Wards, Part Two." *Collier's* 123 (March 19, 1949): 22, 51–52.

Long, Diana Elizabeth, and Janet Golden, eds. *The American General Hospital: Communities and Social Contexts.* Ithaca, NY: Cornell University Press, 1989.

Longman, Philip. *Best Care Anywhere: Why VA Health Care Is Better than Yours.* Sausalito, CA: Polipoint, 2010.

Lorence, James J. *Organizing the Unemployed: Community and Union Activists in the Industrial Heartland.* Albany: State University of New York Press, 1996.

Love, Spencie. *One Blood: The Death and Resurrection of Charles R. Drew.* Chapel Hill: University of North Carolina Press, 1996.

MacLean, Nancy. *Freedom Is Not Enough: The Opening of the American Workplace.* Cambridge, MA: Harvard University Press, 2008.

Mahar, Maggie. *Money-Driven Medicine: The Real Reason Health Care Costs So Much.* New York: HarperCollins, 2006.

Maioni, Antonia. *Parting at the Crossroads: The Emergence of Health Insurance in the United States and Canada.* Princeton, NJ: Princeton University Press, 1998.

Mann, Jonathan M., Michael A. Grodin, Sofia Gruskin, and George J. Annas, eds. *Health and Human Rights: A Reader.* New York: Routledge, 1999.

Margolius, Sidney. *A Consumer's Guide to Health Insurance Plans.* Public Affairs Pamphlet no. 325. New York: Public Affairs Committee, 1962.

Markel, Howard. *Quarantine! East European Jewish Immigrants and the New York City Epidemics of 1892.* Baltimore: Johns Hopkins University Press, 1999.

Markowitz, Gerald, and David Rosner. "Seeking Common Ground: A History of Labor and Blue Cross." *Journal of Health Politics, Policy, and Law* 16, no. 4 (1991): 695–718.

Marmor, Theodore. *The Politics of Medicare.* 2nd ed. New York: Aldine de Gruyter, 2000.

——. "The Right to Health Care: Reflections on Its History and Politics." In *Right to Health Care*, edited by Thomas J. Bole and W. B. Bondeson. New York: Springer, 1991.

Marshall, T. H. *Citizenship and Social Class.* Cambridge: Cambridge University Press, 1950.

Mayo, William J. "The Right to Health." *North American Review* 211, no. 771 (February 1920): 194–202.

McCarroll, James R., and Paul A. Skudder. "Conflicting Concepts of Function Shown in National Survey." *Hospitals* 34 (December 1, 1960): 35–38.

McCausland, Clare. *An Element of Love: A History of the Children's Memorial Hospital of Chicago, Illinois.* Chicago: Children's Memorial Hospital, 1981.

Means, James Howard. "Government in Medicine." *Atlantic Monthly* 191 (March 1953): 46–50.

Mechanic, David. "The Managed Care Backlash: Perceptions and Rhetoric in Health Care Policy and the Need for Reform." *Milbank Quarterly* 79, no. 1 (2001): 35–54.

———. "Rationing Health Care: Public Policy and the Medical Marketplace." *Hastings Center Report* 6, no. 1 (February 1976): 34–37.

———. *The Truth about Health Care: Why Reform Is Not Working in America.* New Brunswick, NJ: Rutgers University Press, 2008.

Meckel, Richard. *Save the Babies: American Public Health Reform and the Prevention of Infant Mortality, 1850–1929.* Baltimore: Johns Hopkins University Press, 1990.

Milmoe McCarrick, Pat. "A Right to Health Care." National Reference Center for Bioethics Literature, reprint from *Kennedy Institute of Ethics Journal* (January 1993).

Minow, Martha. "Interpreting Rights: An Essay for Robert Cover." *Yale Law Journal* 96, no. 8 (July 1987): 1860–1915.

Moore, Judith D., and David G. Smith. "Legislating Medicaid: Considering Medicaid and Its Origins." *Health Care Financing Review* 27, no. 2 (Winter 2005–2006): 45–52.

Morgen. Sandra. *Into Our Own Hands: The Women's Health Movement in the United States, 1969–1990.* New Brunswick: Rutgers University Press, 2002.

Morris, Charles R. *The AARP: America's Most Powerful Lobby and the Clash of Generations.* New York: Times Books, 1996.

Mountin, Joseph W., and George S. J. Perrott. "Health Insurance Programs and Plans of Western Europe: A Summary of Observations." *Public Health Reports* 62, no. 11 (March 14, 1947): 369–99.

Mullan, Fitzhugh. *White Coat, Clenched Fist.* New York: Macmillan, 1976.

Murray, John E. *Origins of American Health Insurance: A History of Industrial Sickness Funds.* New Haven, CT: Yale University Press, 2007.

The Nation's Health: Discussion at the National Health Conference. Washington, DC: US Government Printing Office, 1939.

Nelson, Alondra. *Body and Soul: The Black Panther Party and the Fight against Medical Discrimination.* Minneapolis: University of Minnesota Press, 2011.

Nelson, Jennifer. "'Hold Your Head Up and Stick Out Your Chin': Community Health and Women's Health in Mound Bayou, Mississippi." *National Women's Studies Association Journal* 17, no.1 (2005): 99–118.

———. *Women of Color and the Reproductive Rights Movement.* New York: New York University Press, 2003.

Newman, Simon P. *Embodied History: The Lives of the Poor in Early Philadelphia.* Philadelphia: University of Pennsylvania Press, 2003.

Numbers, Ronald. *Almost Persuaded: American Physicians and Compulsory Health Insurance, 1912–1920.* Baltimore: Johns Hopkins University Press, 1978.

Oberlander, Jonathan. *The Political Life of Medicare.* Chicago: University of Chicago Press, 2003.

Oblinger, Walter L. "Medico-Legal Aspects of Treatment in Automobile Accidents." *Illinois Medical Journal* 114 (September 1958): 111.

Opdycke, Sandra. *No One Was Turned Away: The Role of Public Hospitals in New York City since 1900.* New York: Oxford University Press, 1999.

Oppenheimer, Gerald, Ronald Bayer, and James Colgrove. "Public Health and Human Rights: Old Wine in New Bottles?" *Journal of Law, Medicine & Ethics* 30 (2002): 522–32.

Orchard, William J. "The Need for Governmental Assistance to Hospitals and Its Effect upon the Voluntary Hospital System." *Hospitals* (March 1940): 13–17.

Orleck, Annelise. *Storming Caesar's Palace: How Black Mothers Fought Their Own War on Poverty.* Boston: Beacon Press, 2005.

"Our Health and Our Hospitals." *Collier's* 117 (May 11, 1946): 90.

Perrott, George S. J., and Selwyn D. Collins. "Sickness and the Depression: A Preliminary Report upon a Survey of Wage-Earning Families in Ten Cities." *Milbank Memorial Fund Quarterly* 12, no. 2 (April 1934): 218–24.

Perrott, George S. J., Selwyn D. Collins, and Edgar Sydenstricker. "Sickness and the Economic Depression." *Public Health Reports* 48, no. 41 (October 13, 1933): 1251–65.

Peterson, George E., and Carol Weiss Lewis. *Reagan and the Cities.* Washington, DC: Urban Institute, 1986.

Pipes, Sally. *The Truth about Obamacare: What They Don't Want You to Know about Our New Health Care Law.* Washington, DC: Regnery, 2010.

Poen, Monte. *Harry S. Truman vs. the Medical Lobby: The Genesis of Medicare.* Columbia: University of Missouri Press, 1996.

"Poor Protest HEW Changes in Free Care Guidelines." *Hospital Practice* 7 (September 1972): 171.

Potter, Wendell. *Deadly Spin: An Insurance Company Insider Speaks Out on How Corporate PR Is Killing Health Care and Deceiving Americans.* New York: Bloomsbury, 2010.

Proceedings: National Congress on Prepaid Health Insurance. Chicago: American Medical Association, 1960.

Proceedings: Third National Congress on Voluntary Health Insurance and Prepayment. Chicago: American Medical Association, 1963.

Quadagno, Jill. "From Poor Laws to Pensions: The Evolution of Economic Support for the Aged in England and America." *Milbank Memorial Fund Quarterly* 62, no. 3 (Summer 1984): 417–46.

——. *One Nation, Uninsured: Why the US Has No National Health Insurance.* New York: Oxford University Press, 2006.

——. "Promoting Civil Rights through the Welfare State: How Medicare Integrated Southern Hospitals." *Social Problems* 47, no.1 (2000): 68–89.

Raffensperger, John G. *The Old Lady on Harrison Street: Cook County Hospital, 1833–1995*. New York: Peter Lang, 1997.

Ramos, Henry. *The American G.I. Forum: In Pursuit of the Dream, 1948–1983*. Houston, TX: Arte Publico Press, 1998.

Reed, Louis S., and Willine Carr. *The Benefit Structure of Private Health Insurance, 1968*. Social Security Administration Research Report, no. 32. Washington, DC: Social Security Administration, 1970.

Reid, T. R. *The Healing of America: A Global Quest for Better, Fairer, and Cheaper Health Care*. New York: Penguin, 2009.

Reinhardt, Uwe E. "The Predictable Managed Care Kvetch on the Rocky Road from Adolescence to Adulthood." *Journal of Health Politics, Policy, and Law* 24, no. 5 (1999): 897–910.

Report of the Health Insurance Commission of the State of Illinois. Springfield: Illinois State Journal, 1919.

Reuters. "Medicaid Improves Health and Budgets of Poor." Reuters.com. July 7, 2011. http://www.reuters.com/article/2011/07/07/us-medicaid-study-idUSTRE7665UU20110707.

Reverby, Susan M. *Ordered to Care: The Dilemma of American Nursing, 1850–1945*. Cambridge: Cambridge University Press, 1987.

———. *Examining Tuskegee: The Infamous Syphilis Study and Its Legacy*. Chapel Hill: University of North Carolina Press, 2009.

Reynolds, P. Preston. "Hospital and Civil Rights, 1945–1963: The Case of *Simkins v. Moses H. Cone Memorial Hospital*." *Annals of Internal Medicine* 126 (1997): 898–906.

Richardson, Joe M. "Albert W. Dent: A Black New Orleans Hospital and University Administrator." *Louisiana History* 37, no. 3 (Summer 1996): 309–23.

Risse, Guenter B. *Mending Bodies, Saving Souls: A History of Hospitals*. New York: Oxford University Press, 1999.

Roberts, Stewart. "Social Trends Underlying Health and Hospital Insurance." *New England Journal of Medicine* 212 (1935): 1123–29.

Robison, Clara Elliott. "The Medical Care and Insurance Plans of the American Cast Iron Pipe Company, Birmingham, Alabama." Master's thesis, Tulane University, 1945.

Robison, Ruth Louise. "Medical Care in the Neighborhood of Hull-House." Master's thesis, School of Social Service Administration, University of Chicago, 1940.

Rogers, Naomi. "Caution: The AMA May Be Dangerous to Your Health." *Radical History Review* 80 (Spring 2001): 5–34.

Rose, Marilyn G. "Can Hospital Relocations and Closures Be Stopped through the Legal System?" *Health Services Research* 18, no. 4 (Winter 1983): 551–74.

Rosenberg, Charles E. *The Care of Strangers: The Rise of America's Hospital System*. New York: Basic Books, 1987.

Rosenberg, Marjorie A., and Mark J. Browne. "The Impact of the Inpatient Prospective Payment System and Diagnosis Related Groups: A Survey of the Literature." *North American Actuarial Journal* 5, no. 4: 84–94.

Rosner, David. *A Once Charitable Enterprise: Hospitals and Health Care in Brooklyn and New York, 1885–1915*. Cambridge: Cambridge University Press, 1982.

Ross, Mary. "Crisis in the Hospitals." *Survey Graphic* 22 (July 22, 1933): 364–66.

Roth, Silke. *Building Bridges: The Coalition of Labor Union Women*. Westport, CT: Greenwood, 2003.

Rothman, David J. *Strangers at the Bedside: A History of How Law and Bioethics Transformed Medical Decision Making*. New York: Aldine de Gruyter, 2003.

Sade, Robert M. "Medical Care as a Right: A Refutation." *New England Journal of Medicine* 285, no. 23 (December 2, 1971): 1288–92.

Samuelson, Paul A. *The Collected Scientific Papers of Paul A. Samuelson*. Cambridge, MA: MIT Press, 1966.

Sarat, Austin, and Thomas R. Kearns, eds. *Legal Rights: Historical and Philosophical Perspectives*. Ann Arbor: University of Michigan Press, 1997.

Sardell, Alice. *The US Experiment in Social Medicine: The Community Health Center Program, 1965–1986*. Pittsburgh: University of Pittsburgh Press, 1988.

Schiff, Robert L., David A. Ansell, James E. Schlosser, Ahamed H. Idris, Ann Morrison, and Steven Whitman. "Transfers to a Public Hospital: A Prospective Study of 467 Patients." *New England Journal of Medicine* 314 (February 27, 1986): 552–57.

Schorr, Daniel. *Don't Get Sick in America*. Nashville: Aurora Publishers, 1970.

Schwartz, Daniel H. "Societal Responsibility for Malpractice." *Milbank Memorial Fund Quarterly* 54, no. 4 (Autumn 1976): 469–88.

Scribner, Christopher. "The Quiet Revolution: Federal Funding and Change in Birmingham, Alabama, 1933–1965." PhD diss., Vanderbilt University, 1996.

Seham, Max. "Discrimination against Negroes in Hospitals." *New England Journal of Medicine* 271 (October 29, 1964): 940–43.

Seifert, Vernon D., and J. Stanley Johnstone. "Meeting the Emergency Department Crisis." *Hospitals* 40 (November 1, 1966): 55–59.

Sered, Susan Starr, and Rushika Fernandopulle. *Uninsured in America: Life and Death in the Land of Opportunity*. Berkeley: University of California Press, 2006.

Shortliffe, Ernest C., Stewart Hamilton, and Edward H. Noroian. "The Emergency Room and the Changing Pattern of Medical Care." *New England Journal of Medicine* 2 (January 2, 1958): 20–25.

Sinai, Nathan, and Odin W. Anderson. EMIC: *A Study of Administrative Experience*. Ann Arbor: University of Michigan School of Public Health, 1948.

Skocpol, Theda. *Boomerang: Health Care Reform and the Turn against Government*. New York: Norton, 1996.

Smith, Bruce. "Poor Relief at the St. Joseph County Poor Asylum, 1877–1891." *Indiana Magazine of History* 86, no. 2 (June 1990): 178–96.

Smith, David Barton. *Health Care Divided: Race and Healing a Nation*. Ann Arbor: University of Michigan Press, 1999.

Social Research. *Attitudes toward Health Insurance, I: The Extended Benefits Study*. Chicago: Blue Cross and Blue Shield Commission, 1956.

Somers, H. M., and A. R. Somers. *Doctors, Patients, and Health Insurance: The Organization and Financing of Medical Care*. Washington, DC: Brookings Institution, 1961.

Sparer, Edward V. "Gordian Knots: The Situation of Health Care Advocacy for the Poor Today." *Clearinghouse Review* 15, no. 1 (1981).

Starr, Paul. *The Social Transformation of American Medicine*. New York: Basic Books, 1984.

Stebbins, Ernest L. "Preventive Care Calls for Increased Utilization of Hospitals." *Hospitals* 20 (February 1946): 56–59.

Stevens, Robert, and Rosemary Stevens. *Welfare Medicine in America: A Case Study of Medicaid*. New York: Free Press, 1974.

Stevens, Rosemary. *American Medicine and the Public Interest*. New Haven, CT: Yale University Press, 1971.

———. *In Sickness and in Wealth: American Hospitals in the Twentieth Century*. New York: Basic Books, 1989.

———. *The Public-Private Health Care State: Essays on the History of American Health Care Policy*. New Brunswick, NJ: Transaction Publishers, 2007.

Stevens, Rosemary, Charles Rosenberg, and Lawton Burns, eds. *History and Health Policy: Putting the Past Back In*. New Brunswick, NJ: Rutgers University Press, 2006.

Stone, Deborah. "The Struggle for the Soul of Health Insurance." *Journal of Health Politics, Policy, and Law* 18, no. 2 (1993): 287–317.

Sunnstein, Cass. *The Second Bill of Rights: FDR's Unfinished Revolution and Why We Need It More than Ever*. New York: Basic Books, 2004.

Teigh, Murray. "One Answer to Our Hospital Shortage," *Woman's Home Companion* 75 (November 1948): 4, 187.

Thomas, Karen Kruse. "The Hill-Burton Act: Expanding Hospital Care for Black Southerners, 1939–1960." *Journal of Southern History* 72, no. 4 (November 2006): 823–70.

Thomasson, Melissa A. "Racial Differences in Health Insurance Coverage and Medical Expenditures in the United States: A Historical Perspective." *Social Science History* 30, no. 4 (2006): 529–50.

To Establish a National Health Program: Hearings before a Subcommittee of the Committee on Education and Labor, United States Senate, Seventy-Sixth Congress, First Session on S.1620. Part 1. April 27, May 4, 5, 11, and 12, 1939. Washington, DC: US Government Printing Office, 1939.

Tone, Andrea. *The Business of Benevolence: Industrial Paternalism in Progressive America*. Ithaca, NY: Cornell University Press, 1997.

Toney, Mark. "Revisiting the National Welfare Rights Organization." *Color Lines: The National Magazine on Race and Politics* (Fall 2000). http://www.colorlines.com.

Vargas, Zaragosa. *Labor Rights Are Civil Rights: Mexican-American Workers in Twentieth-Century America*. Princeton, NJ: Princeton University Press, 2007.

Wailoo, Keith, Julie Livingston, and Peter Guarnaccia, eds. *A Death Retold: Jesica Santillan, the Bungled Transplant, and Paradoxes of Medical Citizenship*. Chapel Hill: University of North Carolina Press, 2006.

Warner, John Harley, and Janet Tighe. *Major Problems in the History of American Medicine and Public Health*. Boston: Houghton Mifflin, 2001.

Washington, Harriet A. *Medical Apartheid: The Dark History of Medical Experimentation on Black Americans from Colonial Times to the Present*. New York: Harlem Moon, 2006.

Wasserstrom, Jeffrey N., Lynn Hunt, and Marilyn B. Young, eds. *Human Rights and Revolutions*. Lanham, MD: Rowman and Littlefield, 2000.

Weeks, Lewis E., and Howard J. Berman. *Shapers of American Health Care Policy: An Oral History*. Ann Arbor, MI: Health Administration Press, 1985.

Weinerman, E. Richard, and Herbert R. Edwards. "'Triage' System Shows Promise in Management of Emergency Department Load." *Hospitals* 38 (November 16, 1964): 55–62.

West, Margaret D., and Ruth M. Raup. "Hospital Use in Hagerstown." *Public Health Reports* 74, no. 10 (October 1959): 861–69.

Wickenden, Elizabeth. "The Social Cost of Residence Laws." *Social Casework* 37 (June 1956).

Williams, R. C. "The Medical Care Program for Farm Security Administration Borrowers." *Law and Contemporary Problems* 6, no. 4 (Autumn 1939): 583–94.

Wilson, Ronald W., Jacob J. Feldman, and Mary Grace Kovar. "Continuing Trends in Health and Health Care." *Annals of the American Academy of Political and Social Science* 435 (January 1978): 140–56.

Wolfe, Sidney M. *Pills That Don't Work*. Washington, DC: Public Citizen Health Research Group, 1980.

Wordell, Charles A. "Hospital Participation in Funds Raised for Unemployment and Other Relief." *Transactions of the American Hospital Association* (1932): 188–93.

"Working Rules for Assuring Non-discrimination in Hospital Admissions." *Yale Law Journal* 74, no. 1 (November 1964): 151–69.

Works Progress Administration. *Inventory: An Appraisal of Results of the Works Progress Administration*. Washington, DC: Works Progress Administration, 1938.

Wu, Vivian Y. "Hospital Cost Shifting Revisited: New Evidence from the Balanced Budget Act of 1997." *International Journal of Health Care Finance and Economics* 10, no. 1 (August 12, 2009): 61–83. doi: 10.1007/s10754-009-9071-5.

Zink, Brian J. *Anyone, Anything, Anytime: A History of Emergency Medicine*. Philadelphia: Mosby/Elsevier, 2006.

INDEX

government / public responsibility, xx,
xxiv, xxvii, xxviii, 48; for indigent
care, 5, 15, 16–17, 19, 174; for subsidy
of private hospitals, 16
government subsidies / funding: of
clinics, 18, 19; of hospitals, xxviii,
16, 19, 20, 64, 77, 128, 152, 209; of
indigent care, 29, 30; of insurance
companies, xiii, 60, 94, 164, 214,
215, 216, 217, 220; of managed care,
191; of private entities / system,
xiii–xiv, 15, 16, 20, 46, 60, 184, 197,
198, 218–19. *See also* Affordable Care
Act; Hill-Burton (Hospital Survey
and Construction) Act of 1946;
Medicare
Grady Hospital (Atlanta, GA), 138
Grant, Anna, 172
Grant Hospital, 14
Grassley, Charles, 203, 205
grassroots mobilization, 22–23, 60, 120,
122, 150, 153, 166. *See also* activism;
social movements; *and individual
organizations*
Great Britain. *See* Britain
Great Depression, xiv, xxxv, Part 1,
268
Great Society, 170. *See also* Johnson,
Lyndon B. (LBJ); War on Poverty
Gregg, Alan, 56
Gregg, H. Robert, 171
Green, William, 60
Greenberg, Florence, 8, 9, 11, 28, 158
Grey, Michael, 6
grievance mechanisms, 148
Grisham, John, 210
Group Health Association, 33
group practice, 30, 55, 100, 101, 110,
267; in health reform proposals,
xxxv; prepaid, 32–33, 101–2, 163, 199
guaranteed issue, 219
Guerrero v. Copper Queen, 242 n, 98,
243n106
gynecological care, 194

Hacker, Jacob, 185, 259n73
Hamilton, Alice, 27
Hamilton Memorial Hospital, 81
Hansen, Clifford, 164
*Harper v. Baptist Medical Center-
Princeton*, 243n106
"Harry and Louise," 185–86, 192, 214
Harvard Business School, 195
Harvard Law School, 209
Harvard Medical School, ix, 42
Harvard Pilgrim Health Care, 192
Hatch, Orrin, 179
Hayden, Charles, 103, 106, 111,
Health, Education, and Welfare,
Department of (HEW), 137, 151,
139–40, 146, 151–52. *See also*
Health and Human Services,
Department of
health alliances, 183–86
Health and Hospitals Corporation
(New York), 181, 199
Health and Human Services, Depart-
ment of, 170, 205. *See also* Health,
Education, and Welfare, Depart-
ment of (HEW)
Healthcare Campaign (ACT UP), 180
Health Care Finance Administration
(HCFA), 174
health care reform, xiv, 188; and AIDS
activism, 181; during Bush (George
W.) administration, 196–98, 206,
207; during Carter administration,
165–66; during Clinton administration, 169, 183–87, 190, 192; during
Eisenhower administration, 93–94;
incremental, 187; during Kennedy
administration (*see* Medicare);
during Johnson administration (*see*
Medicare); in Massachusetts, 218;
during New Deal, 23, 24–33, 35; during Nixon administration, xvi, 162,
163–64; during Obama administration (*see* Affordable Care Act);
during Progressive Era, xxxiii–xxxiv,